NURSING ACROSS THE
HEALTH CARE
CONTINUUM

Pocket Companion for

MEDICAL-SURGICAL NURSING ACROSS THE HEALTH CARE CONTINUUM

3rd Edition

Donna D. Ignatavicius, MS, RN, Cm

Clinical Nurse Specialist
Calvert Memorial Hospital
Prince Frederick, Maryland
Former Professor
Charles County Community College
La Plata, Maryland

Kathy A. Hausman, PhD, RNc

Director of Patient Care Services
Emergency Department
Franklin Square Hospital
Baltimore, Maryland

W. B. SAUNDERS COMPANY
A Division of Harcourt Brace & Company
Philadelphia   London   Toronto   Montreal   Sydney   Tokyo

W. B. SAUNDERS COMPANY

A Division of Harcourt Brace & Company

The Curtis Center
Independence Square West
Philadelphia, PA 19106

Pocket Companion for
**Medical-Surgical Nursing Across the
Health Care Continuum,** 3/e   ISBN 0–7216–6992–1

Printed in the United States of America
Last digit is the print number: 9   8   7   6   5   4   3   2   1

Preface

The third edition of *Pocket Companion for Medical-Surgical Nursing Across the Health Care Continuum* is a quick reference to the vital information you need for dealing with conditions commonly seen in the clinical setting. It is designed to be used as a stand-alone reference or as a companion to Ignatavicius, Workman, and Mishler's *Medical-Surgical Nursing Across the Health Care Continuum*, Third Edition.

The book is divided into two parts. Part I covers special concerns of the clinical nurse, such as nursing care of the dying client and postoperative nursing care. Part II, by far the larger part of the book, provides need-to-know information about the diseases and disorders that nurses in clinical practice encounter most frequently. Approximately 280 disorders are included. They are organized alphabetically for ease of use in all clinical settings. An A-to-Z thumb tab facilitates finding these disorders.

We also include extensive cross-references. With these cross-references, you can look up any of the common diseases and disorders in a variety of ways, and still find quickly whatever it is that you need to know. For example, you are assigned the care of a client with ALS and you can't quite recall, in the fast pace of the clinical setting, that the acronym *ALS* stands for *amyotrophic lateral sclerosis.* You look up ALS in Part II of the *Pocket Companion,* and you are quickly referred to the coverage of amyotrophic lateral sclerosis.

Again, suppose that you are assessing a client who has Lou Gehrig's disease. Not being familiar with the condition, you step out of the room and look up Lou Gehrig's disease in the *Pocket Companion.* You are referred to the coverage of amyotrophic lateral sclerosis.

Also included are highlighted Transcultural, Elderly, and Women's Health Considerations for these clients with unique needs. A diamond-shaped symbol (◆) follows the unique trade names of drugs in Canada.

The third edition includes four appendices. Appendix 1 is a quick reference guide to head-to-toe physical assessment of the adult. Appendix 2 highlights considerations for ethical decision-making. Appendix 3 summarizes electrocardiographic complexes, segments, and intervals. Finally, Appendix 4, a new appendix, features Internet and other sources of additional information.

Whether you use the *Pocket Companion* as a stand-alone reference or as a companion to *Medical-Surgical Nursing Across the Health Care Continuum,* we hope that it will become a trusted companion to your clinical practice.

DONNA D. IGNATAVICIUS
KATHY A. HAUSMAN

Contents

PART I

SPECIAL NURSING CONCERNS

NURSING CARE OF THE CLIENT EXPERIENCING LOSS

OVERVIEW

- *Loss* is being deprived of or being without something valued that one once had.
- The types of loss include
    1. Material loss—loss of a physical object to which one has important attachment
    2. Relationship loss—ending of opportunities to relate to another human being
    3. Intrapsychic loss—loss of an emotionally important image of self, loss of emotions such as faith, courage
    4. Functional loss—loss of functional ability due to illness, injury, aging, etc.
    5. Role loss—loss of one's accustomed place in the social network (retirement, promotions,change in marital status, etc.)
    6. Systemic loss—loss of contact with certain interactional behaviors within a system; for example, when a child leaves the home
- *Grieving* is the psychologic, social, and physical reaction to the perception of significant loss.
- *Mourning* is the process of doing the grief work.
- Common responses to loss are grief, shock and disbelief, denial, anger, bargaining, depression, acceptance, guilt, identification with the deceased, "grief attacks," and visual or auditory hallucinations.
- There is no fixed timetable by which a person passes through grieving.
- Processes of mourning for healthy accomodation to loss:
    1. Recognizing loss through acknowledgment and understanding
    2. Reacting to the separation by experiencing the pain and some form of expression to all the psychological reactions
    3. Realistic recollections and review of the relationship of the lost object or person

4. Relinquishing old attachments to the lost object or person
5. Readjusting and adapting to the new world
6. Reinvesting in the new world

- Complicated mourning—a state of compromise, distortion, or failure of one of the six processes of mourning

COLLABORATIVE MANAGEMENT

- The nurse records the client's description of
    1. Relationship and age of the deceased
    2. Cause of death and length of illness
    3. Length of preparation for the death
    4. Degree of intimacy or intensity of the relationship
    5. Characteristics of the grieving individual:
        a. Age, education, and employment
        b. Economic status
        c. History of losses
        d. History of depressions
        e. Personality or mental health problems
        f. Substance abuse history
        g. Ethnic background, family structure
        h. Social and spiritual support
        i. Coping strategies
- Grief may cause physiologic distress in addition to emotional pain, which may lead to serious illness; therefore the nurse assesses the client for signs and symptoms of serious disease.
- The nurse
    1. Is physically and psychologically "with" the client, empathizing to provide emotional support
    2. Actively listens to the client and acknowledges the legitimacy of the client's pain
    3. Provides physical support such as gentle touching, holding hands, and hugging
    4. Shows through manner and words that the expression of grief is not only acceptable and expected but healthy
    5. Can say something such as "just let the tears come. Don't hold back"
    6. Avoids stereotypical assurances such as "things will be fine. Don't cry" or "In a year from now . . ."
    7. Avoids explaining the loss in philosophical or religious terms

8. Respects the religious, cultural, and social mores of the client
9. Refers the mourner to bereavement counselors

NURSING CARE OF THE DYING CLIENT

OVERVIEW

- Death is defined as cessation of respiration and heartbeat.
- As death nears, clients may manifest fear, anxiety, and physical symptoms of distress that require treatment and control.
- Hospice care attempts to facilitate quality of life and death with dignity for clients with terminal disease, using a multidisciplinary approach.

COLLABORATIVE MANAGEMENT

- The nurse obtains information on
    1. Client's diagnosis
    2. Past medical history
    3. Recent state of health
- The nurse assesses for
    1. Signs and symptoms of impending death
        a. Pain
        b. Dyspnea
        c. Delirium
        d. Nausea and vomiting
        e. Coolness of extremities
        f. Increased sleeping
        g. Decreased desire for fluid and food
        h. Incontinence
        i. Congestion and gurgling
        j. Breathing pattern change
        k. Disorientation
        l. Restlessness
    2. Vital signs
    3. Breath sounds, cough
    4. Bowel sounds, abdominal distention
    5. Urine output

6. Pain level
   a. Visual or verbal analogue scale is used if possible
   b. Location, character
   c. Level of intensity in the past
   d. Reaction to medications
   e. Effect on activities
   f. Effect on sleep
   g. Frequency and amount of medications needed to treat and control

➤ Transcultural Considerations

1. Dying process for Americans frequently oriented to high-tech hospital setting; family demands for testing and treatment are common even when clients themselves prefer a palliative approach.
2. Hispanic-Americans see dying as a family affair; a primary caretaker (wife or daughter) takes responsibility for care.
3. Southeast Asians feel that discussion of dying brings bad luck, and hospitals and treatments are alien. Some family members may avoid visiting terminally ill client for fear of contracting the disease.
4. A variety of values, religious beliefs, practices of healing, and family structure may impact dying in both positive/challenging and negative ways.

- The nurse provides care for the dying client:
  1. Keeps the client in bed or a recliner if desired
  2. Refrains from providing food and drink to the client with impaired swallowing or no desire to eat
  3. Reinforces to the family that cessation of food and liquids is thought to be a natural process and that hydration can cause more discomfort than good
  4. Provides frequent mouth care
  5. Administers medications for nausea and vomiting
  6. Administers pain medication and bolus dosages as needed
  7. Adminsters medication and other treatments for the client in respiratory distress
     a. Hyoscyamine (Levsin) or a diuretic may be used to decrease secretions.
     b. Morphine is used to treat dyspnea and/or labored respirations; clients already receiving morphine for pain may require a 50% increase for relief of dyspnea.

5

      c. Antianxiety drugs such as lorazepam (Ativan)
      d. Changes client's position, elevates the head slightly
      e. Administers oxygen
   8. Manages anxiety/agitation by:
      a. Assessing and treating pain and urinary retention
      b. Ensuring adequate sedation around the clock to prevent further restlessness and terminal agitation
   9. Provides appropriate skin care
  10. Covers the client with a light blanket

- The nurse encourages the family to
    1. Engage in normal conversation with the dying client
    2. Touch and gently stroke the client
    3. Play the client's favorite music or television shows

- The nurse provides care of the client after death:
    1. Ensures that the death certificate is completed
    2. Prepares the body for viewing by the family according to institutional or home policy
    3. Closes the client's eyes
    4. Places dentures (if available) in the mouth
    5. Places the client flat in bed; removes all pillows except one supporting the head
    6. Places a pad around the perineum to absorb fecal material and fluid
    7. Supports the family to say their last words and perform their farewell gestures freely and naturally around the bed
    8. Notifies the hospital chaplain or religious leader at the family's request
    9. Follows agency procedure for preparing the client for transfer to the morgue or funeral home

PREOPERATIVE NURSING CARE

OVERVIEW

- Preoperative care begins when the client is scheduled for surgery and ends at the time of transfer to the surgical suite.

- The primary role of the nurse is as an educator, an advocate and promoter of health.
- *Inpatient* refers to a client who is admitted to a hospital the day before or the same day of surgery and who requires hospitalization after surgery.
- *Outpatient* refers to a client who goes to the surgical area (surgical center, ambulatory care center) the day of surgery and returns home on the same day.
- Primary reasons for surgery are
  1. Diagnostic
  2. Curative
  3. Restorative
  4. Palliative
  5. Cosmetic
- The urgency of the surgery may be
  1. Elective
  2. Urgent
  3. Emergency
- The extent of surgery can be
  1. Simple
  2. Modified
  3. Radical

Considerations for Elderly Clients

1. Normal aging process decreases immune system functioning and delays wound healing.
2. Decreased ability to withstand the stresses of surgery and anesthesia.
3. Increased risk of a change in mental status.
4. Often have cardiovascular, respiratory, renal, musculoskeletal, and nutritional deficits that increase the risk of surgery.
5. Greater incidence of chronic illness, malnutrition, and allergies.

COLLABORATIVE MANAGEMENT
Assessment

- The nurse records the client's
  1. Age
  2. Allergies to medication and food
  3. Current medications (prescription and over-the-counter)
  4. History of medical and surgical problems

      a. Myocardial infarction within the past 6 months
      b. Congestive heart failure or coronary artery disease
      c. Dysrhythmias
      d. Pneumonia
      e. Pulmonary disease such as chronic obstructive pulmonary disease or asthma

5. Prior surgical procedures and experiences
6. Prior experience with anesthesia
7. Tobacco, alcohol, and illicit substance use
8. Family medical history and problems with anesthetics that may indicate possible intraoperative needs and reactions to anesthesia, such as malignant hyperthermia
9. Blood transfusion status:
      a. Autologous
      b. Directed blood donation
10. Knowledge and understanding about events during the perioperative period
11. Support system availability

- Preoperative assessment is performed to determine baseline data, hidden medical problems, potential complications related to the administration of anesthesia, and potential complications of surgery.
- The nurse assesses the client's
  1. Vital signs
  2. Cardiovascular system:
     a. Palpates peripheral pulses; observes for indications of arteriosclerosis
     b. Auscultates the heart for rate, regularity, and abnormal heart sounds
     c. Records blood pressure to determine presence of hypertension or increased diastolic pressure
     d. Reports symptoms such as chest pain, shortness of breath, or dyspnea to the physician
  3. Respiratory system:
     a. Observes
        (1) Posture and fingers (for clubbing)
        (2) Rate, rhythm, depth of respirations
        (3) Lung expansion
     b. Auscultates the lungs to determine the quality and presence of adventitious sounds and abnormal breath sounds
  4. Renal system:
     a. Observes

      (1) Frequency of urination

      (2) Dysuria

      (3) Nocturia

      (4) Difficulty starting urine flow

      (5) Oliguria

      (6) Appearance and odor of urine

  b. Questions the client about usual fluid intake and continence

  c. Recalls that scopolamine, morphine, meperidine, and barbiturates may cause confusion, disorientation, apprehension, and restlessness when administered to clients with decreased renal function

5. Neurologic system:
  a. Level of consciousness
  b. Orientation
  c. Ability to follow commands and communicate
  d. Motor or sensory changes
  e. Risk of falling

6. Musculoskeletal system (the following may affect positioning):
  a. Arthritis
  b. Joint replacement
  c. Skeletal deformities
  d. Length of neck and shape of thoracic cavity, which may interfere with respiratory and cardiac function

7. Nutritional status:
  a. Recognizes that malnutrition and obesity can cause poor wound healing and increase surgical risk
  b. Assesses for indicators of fluid and electrolyte imbalance and malnutrition:
      (1) Brittle nails
      (2) Wasting muscles
      (3) Dry, flaky skin
      (4) Dull, sparse, dry hair
      (5) Decreased skin turgor
      (6) Postural hypotension
      (7) Decreased serum albumin
      (8) Abnormal electrolytes

8. Psychosocial status:
  a. Anxiety and fear
  b. Coping mechanisms

9. Laboratory findings:
  a. Complete blood count

    b. Electrolytes
    c. Urinalysis
    d. Type and cross-match
    e. Coagulation studies
  10. Other diagnostic studies:
    a. Chest x-ray
    b. Electrocardiogram

Planning and Implementation

✦ NDx: Knowledge Deficit

- Informed consent for the surgical procedure is obtained by the physician; the nurse may witness the client's signature.
- Consent implies that the client has been provided with information necessary to understand the
  1. Nature of and reasons for surgery
  2. Available options and risks associated with each option
  3. Risks of surgical procedure and potential outcomes
  4. Risks associated with the administration of anesthesia
- The nurse
  1. Notifies the physician of any indications that the client did not understand the information given concerning the procedure or is not adequately informed
  2. Clarifies facts presented by the physician
  3. Dispels myths about surgery
  4. Ensures that special permits that may be needed are obtained by the physician
- The client is allowed *nothing by mouth* (NPO) for 6 to 8 hours before surgery; it is customary to place the client on NPO status after midnight.
- The nurse
  1. Emphasizes the consequences of not adhering to NPO restrictions:
     a. Surgery may be cancelled
     b. There is an increased risk of aspiration during surgery
  2. Consults the physician concerning the administration of medications such as corticosteroids and those used for hypertension, diabetes mellitus, cardiac disease, glaucoma, and epilepsy

- *Bowel preparation* is usually done for clients having major abdominal, pelvic, perineal or perianal surgery or diagnostic procedures such as a colonoscopy.
- Repeated enemas can cause
  1. Electrolyte imbalance, especially potassium
  2. Fluid deficit
  3. Postural hypotension
  4. Vagal stimulation
  5. Anorectal discomfort in the client with hemorrhoids
  6. Fatigue
- *Skin preparation* varies depending on the procedure and facility/physician preference.
- Shaving is generally not done until immediately before the start of the surgical procedure or not at all.
- The nurse prepares the client for the possibility of tubes, drains, and intravenous lines postoperatively:
  1. Foley catheter, nasogastric tube
  2. Drains that promote the evacuation of fluid from the surgical wound
  3. Intravenous line, which is usually used for all clients
- The nurse teaches the client and family postoperative *exercises* preoperatively to reduce apprehension and to increase postoperative cooperation and participation:
  1. Ensures client mastery by observing correct performance on return demonstration
  2. Encourages the client to frequently practice
     a. Diaphragmatic breathing
     b. Incentive spirometry
     c. Coughing and deep breathing
     d. Splinting the wound
     e. Turning and leg exercises
     f. Early ambulation
     g. Range-of-motion exercises
- The nurse explains the use and importance of antiembolism stockings and sequential compression devices.
- The nurse informs the family about the client's care and allows them to participate if they desire to do so.

✦ **NDx:** Anxiety

- The nurse
  1. Assesses the client's anxiety level and knowledge base

2. Provides information about the surgical procedure and allows time for questions
3. Provides the client with rest and sleep
4. Uses distraction techniques, such as television, radio, or books as intervention
5. Assesses the readiness and desire of the family to take an active part in the client's care

- The nurse reviews the chart for
  1. Operative permit and other special permits
  2. Results of all laboratory, radiographic, and diagnostic tests
  3. Allergies, and documents any on the front of the chart
  4. Abnormal results that are documented and reported to the physician
  5. Height and weight
  6. Current vital signs
  7. Special needs flagged (e.g., client refusal to allow blood transfusion)

- Client preparation includes
  1. Hospital gown
  2. Antiembolism stockings or Ace bandages, if ordered
  3. Security of all client valuables; if rings cannot be removed, cover with tape and note on preoperative checklist
  4. Identification band, allergy band
  5. Removal of dentures (including partial plates), hairpins and clips of any type, wigs and toupees, prosthetic devices, all jewelry such as earrings and watches
  6. Checking facility policy regarding removal of hearing aids and fingernail polish
  7. Instructing the client to void

- If preoperative medication is given, the client should remain in bed with the side rails up.

- Common preoperative medications:
  1. Sedatives and hypnotics (e.g., pentobarbital sodium, secobarbital sodium, and chloral hydrate [Novochlorhydrate◆])
  2. Tranquilizers (e.g., chlorpromazine hydrochloride, hydroxyzine hydrochloride, diazepam, and promethazine hydrochloride)
  3. Opioids (e.g., meperidine hydrochloride, morphine sulfate, and hydromorphone hydrochloride)

4. Anticholinergics (e.g., atropine sulfate, glyco-pyrrolate, and scopolamine)

INTRAOPERATIVE NURSING CARE

OVERVIEW

- Intraoperative care begins when the client enters the surgical suite.
- A *surgeon* is responsible for the surgical procedure and surgical judgments about the client.
- An *anesthesiologist* is a physician who specializes in the administration of anesthesia.
- A *certified registered nurse anesthetist* is a registered nurse who administers anesthetics under the supervision of an anesthesiologist, a surgeon, a dentist, or a podiatrist.
- A *circulating nurse* is a registered nurse who ensures that the necessary supplies and equipment are available, safe, and functional before surgery; helps to position the client on the operating room table; comforts and reassures the client; ensures that sterile technique and the sterile field are maintained by the surgical team; documents that drains or catheters are in place; and documents the length of surgery and the count of sponges, sharps, and instruments.
- A *surgical assistant,* who might be another surgeon, resident, nurse, physician assistant, or sugical technologist, holds retractors, suctions the wound, cuts tissue, sutures and dresses the wound.
- A *scrub nurse* or *technologist* sets up surgical instruments; hands them to the surgeon and the assistants; and maintains an accurate count of sponges, sharps, and instruments.
- There are multiple types of anesthesia:
    1. *General anesthesia,* which induces depression of the central nervous system, causing analgesia, amnesia, and unconsciousness
    2. *Balanced anesthesia,* which is a combination of agents used to provide hypnosis, amnesia, analgesia, muscle relaxation, and relaxation of reflexes

with minimal disturbance to the client's physiologic function

3. *Local or regional anesthesia,* which temporarily interrupts the transmission of nerve impulses to and from a specific area or region; motor function may or may not be involved, and the client does not lose consciousness

   a. *Topical anesthesia* involves the use of a regional anesthetic applied directly to the surface of the area to be anesthetized, usually in the form of an ointment or spray.

   b. *Local infiltration* is the injection of an anesthetic agent intracutaneously and subcutaneously into the tissue surrounding an incision, wound, or lesion.

   c. *Field block* is produced by a series of injections around the operative field.

   d. A *nerve block* involves the injection of a local anesthetic into or around a nerve or nerve supply.

   e. *Spinal* or *intrathecal anesthesia* is administered by injecting an anesthetic into the subarachnoid space at L2–3 or L3–4.

   f. A *caudal block* is the injection of an anesthetic agent into the epidural space through the sacral hiatus and caudal canal.

   g. An *epidural block* is the injection of an anesthetic agent into the epidural space through the interspace of the vertebrae.

- *Conscious sedation* is given to dull or reduce the intensity of pain or awareness during a procedure without loss of defensive reflexes.
- Complications of general anesthesia may include

  1. Malignant hyperthermia—an acute, life-threatening complication manifested by hyperthermia, tachycardia or other dysrhythmias, muscle rigidity, hypotension, tachypnea, and cola-colored urine

  2. Overdose, if the client's pharmacokinetics are such that they do not respond or react as expected.

  3. Difficult intubation, resulting in broken or injured teeth or caps, swollen lips, or trauma to vocal cords

- Complications of local or regional anesthesia are usually attributed to overdosage, incorrect administration technique, systemic absorption, or client sensitization to the anesthetic (anaphylaxis)

ℰ Considerations for Elderly Clients

1. Allow the client to retain eyeglasses and hearing aids until anesthesia is administered.
2. Use a small pillow under the client's head if it is normally bent slightly forward.
3. Lift the client when transferring to prevent shearing forces on fragile skin.
4. Carefully position the client with arthritic joints; extra padding is needed.
5. Use a cap or stockinette on the extremities to prevent heat loss and to conserve body heat.
6. Warm prepping solution.

COLLABORATIVE MANAGEMENT
Assessment

- The nurse validates
  1. For the correct client by checking the client's identification bracelet and chart using the client's name and hospital-assigned number
  2. All aspects of the preoperative checklist are complete and information is on the chart
     a. Allergies are noted
     b. Previous anesthesia and any reactions are documented
     c. History of blood transfusions and reaction, if any, are noted
     d. Reports on laboratory, radiographic, and diagnostic tests are complete
     e. The client's history and physical examination are reported
     f. Medications routinely taken by the client are noted
  3. Correct attire and removal of items such as jewelry, hearing aids, contact lenses, and dentures
  4. Whether an autologous blood transfusion is being used

Planning and Implementation

✦ **NDx:** Risk for Injury

- The surgical team observes for and treats complications of general anesthesia.

15

- The nurse
  1. Pads the operating bed or table with foam, silicone gel pads, or both
  2. Properly places the grounding pads
- The nurse ensures proper *positioning* by assessing for
  1. Physiologic alignment
  2. Minimal interference with circulation
  3. Protection of skeletal and neuromuscular structures
  4. Optimal exposure of the operative site and intravenous line
  5. Access for the anesthesiologist
  6. Preservation of the client's dignity
  7. Client comfort and safety
- The nurse observes for complications of special positioning, such as wrist or foot drop, loss of sensation, and inflammation.

✦ NDx: Impaired Skin Integrity

- The surgeon applies a plastic drape after the skin has been prepped and is dry.
- Skin closures include
  1. Sutures:
     a. Absorbable
     b. Nonabsorbable
  2. Clamps
  3. Staples
  4. Steri-Strips
- After the wound is sutured, the plastic drape is carefully removed and the surgeon applies a sterile dressing.
- Special attention is paid to elderly clients and clients with fragile skin to prevent skin tearing when the adhesive drape is removed.

POSTOPERATIVE NURSING CARE

OVERVIEW

- Postoperative care begins when the client is admitted to the postanesthesia care unit (PACU, or recovery

room) and extends through discharge from the hospital or ambulatory care facility.
- Time spent in the PACU varies with the client's age and physical health, type of procedure, anesthesia used, and postoperative complications.

COLLABORATIVE MANAGEMENT

Assessment

- The nurse assesses for
  1. Postanesthesia score (PACU nurse)
  2. Respiratory function:
     a. Patent airway
     b. Adequate respiratory exchange
     c. Breath sounds bilaterally
     d. Symmetric movement of the chest wall
     e. Indications of diaphragmatic breathing and sternal retraction
  3. Cardiovascular function:
     a. Vital signs
     b. Peripheral pulses
     c. Presence of Homans' sign
     d. Edema, redness, and pain (indications of thrombophlebitis)
  4. Fluid and electrolyte balance:
     a. Intake and output
     b. Complete blood count
     c. Electrolytes
     d. Complications, which occur more often in the elderly
  5. Neurologic system:
     a. Level of consciousness
     b. Eye opening
     c. Ability to follow commands
     d. Motor movement
     e. Sensation and pain
     f. Orientation
  6. Genitourinary system:
     a. Output and color of urine
     b. Inspection, palpation, and percussion of the client's abdomen for bladder distention
  7. Gastrointestinal system:
     a. Auscultation for bowel sounds
     b. Palpation of the abdomen
     c. Patency of the nasogastric tube or any abdominal tubes and drains
     d. Nausea and vomiting

17

8. Integumentary system, integrity of the wound site
9. Dressings and drains:
   a. Color, amount, and consistency of drainage
   b. Integrity of Penrose drains (a single-lumen, soft latex tube inserted into or close to the surgical site)
   c. Patency and integrity of Hemovac, VacuDrain, or Jackson-Pratt drains to ensure maintenance of suction
   d. Patency of all other drains or tubes
10. Pain
11. Psychosocial:
    a. Anxiety, restlessness, fear

Planning and Implementation

- The nurse
  1. Monitors vital signs every 4 hours or more frequently if clinically indicated (significant changes in blood pressure may indicate myocardial depression, hemorrhage, oversedation, and/or pain)
  2. Performs a complete systems assessment every shift
  3. Measures and records intake and output
  4. Observes for and reports postoperative complications:
     a. Urinary retention
     b. Pulmonary atelectasis, pneumonia, emboli
     c. Infection or alterations in wound healing
     d. Urinary tract infection
     e. Thrombophlebitis

✦ NDx: Impaired Gas Exchange

- The nurse in the PACU
  1. Positions the client on the side or with the head turned to prevent possible aspiration
  2. Keeps the head of the bed flat until the client regains a gag reflex and to prevent hypotension as long as it is not contraindicated
  3. Raises the head of the bed to promote respiratory function, when appropriate
  4. Monitors for stridor or snoring, which are signs of upper airway obstruction from tracheal or laryngeal spasm, mucus in the airway, or occlusion of the airway from relaxation of the tongue
- The nurse (after client transfer from PACU)

1. Completes a respiratory assessment once each shift for at least 48 hours after surgery
2. Administers oxygen, if needed
3. Encourages the client to turn, cough, and deep breathe (splints wound as needed)
4. Provides incentive spirometry and/or chest physiotherapy, as clinically indicated
5. Suctions the client, as needed
6. Monitors for complications, such as atelectasis, pneumonia, pulmonary edema, and emboli

✦ **NDx:** Impaired Skin Integrity

- The nurse
  1. Observes the wound for separation
     a. Checks for *dehiscence,* the partial or complete separation of the upper layers of the wound
        (1) Applies a sterile nonadherent or saline dressing and binder to the wound
        (2) Notifies the surgeon immediately
     b. Checks for *evisceration,* the total separation of the layers and extrusion of internal organs or viscera through an open wound
        (1) Covers the wound with a sterile towel or nonadherent dressing moistened with normal saline
        (2) Notifies the surgeon immediately
        (3) Does not attempt to reinsert the protruding organ or viscera
     c. Monitors vital signs and assesses for signs of shock
     d. Supports and reassures the client
     e. Prepares the client for surgery to repair the wound
  2. Performs dressing changes, as ordered (with the first change usually done by the physician)
     a. Reinforces the dressing if it becomes wet from drainage
     b. Documents the color, type, amount, and odor of drainage and notes time of observation on the client's chart
     c. Notifies the surgeon of excessive drainage; documents the time of the call and the physician's response
     d. Recognizes that wet dressings are a source of infection; obtains an order from the surgeon for dressing changes using aseptic technique

     e. Follows facility procedure for dressing changes and wound care

  3. Observes the wound for infection; may administer antibiotics prophylactically

✦ NDx: Pain

- Opioids and nonopioids, such as meperidine hydrochloride (Demerol), morphine sulfate (Epimorph◆, Statex◆), codeine sulfate, butorphanol tartrate (Stadol), oxycodone hydrochloride with aspirin (Percodan), and oxycodone with acetaminophen (Tylox, Percocet) are routinely given immediately postoperatively.
- The nurse
  1. Assesses the type, location, and intensity of the pain before giving the medication
  2. Assesses and documents the effectiveness of the medication
  3. Monitors patient-controlled analgesia (PCA), as ordered, via an intravenous or internal pump, with the rate or dosage of infusion of an opioid analgesic adjusted by the client on the basis of his or her pain level and physical response to the drug
  4. Tapers pain medication as recovery progresses and administers nonopioid medication such as acetaminophen (Tylenol, Atasol◆) and nonsteroidal anti-inflammatory drugs such as ibuprofen (Motrin, Novoproten◆, Amersol◆, Advil), as ordered
  5. Positions the client based on surgical procedure and medical condition
  6. Turns the client every 2 hours or more often as needed
  7. Provides back rubs, relaxation techniques, and distraction to control pain

Continuing Care

- The nurse
  1. Collaborates with the client and family to identify and correct any safety hazards in the home before discharge
  2. Identifies strategies that can be used to modify the environment to accommodate any client limitations, meal preparation, or dressing changes
  3. Teaches the care of the surgical wound and provides written instruction as needed:
     a. Importance of hand washing

b. Disposal procedure for the soiled dressing
c. Return demonstration of wound care
4. Reinforces diet therapy and obtains a dietary consultation if necessary; advises a high-protein, high-calorie diet to promote wound healing unless client is on a restricted or special diet
5. Provides information on drug therapy, instructing the client to notify the physician if pain is not relieved or suddenly increases
6. Reinforces restrictions in activity and exercise

REHABILITATION

OVERVIEW

- Chronic disease is characterized by
  1. Duration longer than 3 months
  2. The need for special training of the client in rehabilitation
- *Rehabilitation* is the process of learning to live with chronic and disabling conditions. Impairment is an abnormality of a body structure or structures or an alteration in a system function resulting from any cause.
- *Disability* is the consequence of an impairment; a *handicap* is the disadvantage experienced by an individual as a result of impairments and disabilities.
- Settings for rehabilitation include
  1. Freestanding rehabilitation hospitals
  2. Rehabilitation units within acute care hospitals or within skilled nursing or long-term care facilities
  3. Outpatient hospital rehabilitation centers
  4. Transitional living centers, a step between a rehabilitation center and an independent living center (ILC), with the goal of preparing the client to live at home or in the ILC
  5. ILCs, in which the client shares an apartment or home with other disabled clients and has supervision and support available
- Rehabilitation team members typically include the
  1. Nurse
  2. Occupational therapist

3. Orthotist
4. Physicians
5. Physical therapist
6. Psychologist
7. Recreational therapist
8. Respiratory therapist
9. Speech language pathologist
10. Social worker and/or case manager
11. Vocational counselor
12. Cognitive therapist

COLLABORATIVE MANAGEMENT

Assessment

- The nurse records the client's health history with a rehabilitation focus
    1. History of present condition
    2. Occupation
    3. Educational background
    4. Home situation:
        a. Architectural features
        b. Proximity of shopping centers, transportation
        c. Availability of support for help in the home such as cooking and cleaning
    5. Daily schedule and activities of daily living (ADL)
    6. Bowel and bladder routine and habits
    7. Sexuality patterns
    8. Sleep habits, bedtime routine
- The nurse assesses for
    1. Cardiovascular system:
        a. Routine cardiovascular assessment
        b. Alteration in cardiac status such as chest pain and diuresis
        c. Manifestations of activity intolerance and unwillingness to return to *any* activity
    2. Respiratory system:
        a. Routine respiratory assessment
        b. Level of activity the client can perform without becoming short of breath
    3. Gastrointestinal (GI) system:
        a. Routine GI assessment
        b. Oral intake and pattern for eating
        c. Indications of anorexia, dysphagia, nausea, vomiting, and/or discomfort related to and/or interfering with oral intake

    d. Height, weight, hemoglobin and hematocrit levels, and serum albumin and blood glucose concentrations

    e. Changes in the client's normal elimination patterns

4. Urinary system:
   a. Routine urologic assessment
   b. Baseline urinary patterns:
      (1) Number of times the client usually voids and at what time of day
      (2) Problems with incontinence or retention
   c. Usual fluid intake patterns and volume, including the type of fluids ingested and the time of fluid consumption
   d. Positive urine culture or abnormal findings on urinalysis

5. Neurologic system:
   a. Routine neurologic assessment
   b. Functional aspects of cognition, motor ability, and sensation
   c. Pre-existing problems, general physical condition, and communication abilities

6. Musculoskeletal system:
   a. Routine musculoskeletal assessment
   b. Impact of deficits on the client's home, work, and/or school environment

7. Integumentary system:
   a. Routine integumentary assessment
   b. Actual and potential interruptions in skin integrity
   c. Use of the facility assessment tool to predict the risk of skin breakdown
   d. Client's understanding of the cause and treatment of skin breakdown

8. Functional assessment, with various tools used to measure objectively the level at which a person is performing in any of a variety of areas:
   a. Activities of daily living
   b. Mobility
   c. Sensation
   d. Communication and cognition
   e. Social skills

9. Psychologic assessment:
   a. Changes in body image and self-esteem
   b. Defense mechanisms

c. Availability of support systems such as family and significant others

10. Vocational assessment (information on the client's current occupation, work history)

Planning and Implementation

✦ **NDx:** Impaired Physical Mobility

- The nurse
  1. Assesses for and intervenes to prevent complications of immobility
     a. Contractures:
        (1) Provides active-assist or passive range-of-motion (ROM) exercises at least daily
        (2) Provides foot support while in bed
     b. Constipation or decreased GI motility:
        (1) Assists the client to increase his or her activity level
     c. Decreased cardiac output
     d. Increased venous stasis, thrombus formation, embolism:
        (1) Applies antiembolism stockings
        (2) Avoids leg massage
        (3) Performs ROM exercises
        (4) Monitors vital signs
     e. Disorientation:
        (1) Helps the client maintain a normal sleep-wake cycle
        (2) Orients the client as needed
        (3) Controls sensory stimulation to the client
     f. Postural hypotension (avoids sudden position changes)
     g. Renal calculi:
        (1) Decreases dietary calcium
        (2) Increases fluids
        (3) Maintains acidic urine through diet or drugs
     h. Pneumonia:
        (1) Encourages the client to turn, cough, and deep breathe at least every 2 hours
        (2) Teaches respiratory exercises
     i. Pressure ulcers:
        (1) Repositions the client frequently (at least every 2 hours)
        (2) Applies pressure-relief devices as appropriate

    (3) Skin care
2. Performs ROM exercises:
   a. Exercises all joints
   b. Completes full range movement of each joint at least five or more times
   c. Performs exercises at least three times daily
   d. Does not move the joint beyond the point at which the client expresses pain or the nurse perceives stiffness or difficulty
3. Uses and teaches correct transfer techniques:
   a. Bed to wheelchair or chair:
      (1) Places the chair at an angle to the bed on the client's strong side
      (2) Locks the wheelchair brakes or secures the chair position
      (3) Helps the client to stand and to move his or her strong hand to the armrest
      (4) Keeps the client's body weight forward while the nurse and client pivot
      (5) Assists the client in sitting when the client's legs touch the chair edge
   b. Wheelchair to chair or bed:
      (1) Places the chair with the client's strong side next to the bed
      (2) Locks or secures the wheelchair brakes
      (3) Assists the client to stand and moves the client's strong hand to the armrest
      (4) Keeps the client's body weight forward while the nurse and client pivot
      (5) Assists the client in sitting and then reclining when the client's legs touch the bed edge
   c. Use of a sliding board:
      (1) Places the chair or wheelchair as close to the bed as possible
      (2) Removes the armrest from the chair (if removable) or wheelchair
      (3) Powders the sliding board
      (4) Places the sliding board under the client's buttocks
      (5) Instructs the client to reach toward his or her side
      (6) Assists the client in sliding gently to the bed or chair
4. Assists the client in gait training:
   a. Walker assisted:

  (1) Applies a gait belt around the client's waist
  (2) Assists the client to a standing position
  (3) Assists the client in placing both hands on the walker
  (4) Ensures that the client is well balanced
  (5) Assists the client repeatedly to perform the following sequence:
   — Lift the walker
   — Move the walker 2 feet forward and set it down on all legs
   — While resting on the walker, take small steps
   — Check balance

 b. Cane assisted:
  (1) Applies a gait belt around the client's waist
  (2) Assists the client to a standing position
  (3) Assists the client in placing his or her strong hand on the cane
  (4) Ensures that the client is well balanced
  (5) Assists the client repeatedly to perform the following sequence:
   — Move the cane forward
   — Move the weaker leg one step forward
   — Move the stronger leg one step forward
   — Check balance

5. Reinforces instructions from other health team members and is aware of the client's progress and abilities as he or she improves

✦ NDx: Self Care Deficit

- The nurse
  1. Collaborates with physical and occupational therapy to
     a. Identify ways to maximize the client's abilities in performing ADL
     b. Reinforce the correct use of adaptive-assistive devices
     c. Assist the client to achieve energy conservation to prevent or minimize fatigue
  2. Reinforces the correct use of assistive devices
  3. Encourages the client to eat a balanced diet

✦ NDx: Risk for Impaired Skin Integrity

- The nurse
  1. Assesses the client for risk level

2. Repositions the client every 2 hours or more and assesses the skin with each positioning
3. Encourages the client to eat a balanced diet; monitors the client's weight and serum albumin level
4. Provides frequent skin care
5. Obtains mechanical devices as appropriate:
   a. Waterbed
   b. Foam or gel mattress
   c. Air mattress
   d. Alternating-pressure mattress
   e. Air-fluidized bed (e.g., Clinitron bed)

✦ NDx: Altered Urinary Elimination

- *Reflex* or *spastic bladder* causes incontinence characterized by sudden gushing voids.
- *Flaccid bladder* results in overflow and urinary retention.
- *Uninhibited bladder* results in incontinence and incomplete emptying of the bladder.
- The nurse
  1. Initiates a bladder training program as appropriate:
     a. Intermittent catheterization and residual urine determination
     b. Consistent scheduling of toileting routines
     c. Facilitating or triggering techniques to stimulate voiding such as Valsalva's and Credé's maneuvers
  2. Administers drug therapy, as ordered:
     a. Cholinergics: bethanechol chloride (Urecholine)
     b. Antispasmodics: oxybutynin chloride (Ditropan), flavoxate hydrochloride (Urispas)
     c. Skeletal muscle relaxants: dantrolene (Dantrium), baclofen (Lioresal)
  3. Provides and teaches diet therapy:
     a. Encourages fluid intake to 2500 mL per day unless contraindicated
     b. Encourages intake of fluids that promote an acidic urine, such as tomato juice, cranberry juice, and bouillon
     c. Discourages excessive intake of milk and citrus juices, which promote alkaline urine
  4. Intervenes to prevent complications:
     a. Urinary tract infections

b. Urinary calculi or stasis

✦ **NDx:** Constipation

- The nurse designs a bowel program:
    1. Plans and implements the program based on the cause:
        a. *Upper motor neuron* disease may result in a reflex bowel pattern with defecation occurring suddenly and without warning.
        b. *Lower motor neuron* disease may result in a flaccid bowel pattern with defecation occurring infrequently and in small amounts:
            (1) Initiates a bowel program
            (2) Provides a high-fiber diet
            (3) Administers suppositories, as ordered
            (4) Maintains a consistent toileting schedule
            (5) Performs manual disimpaction as needed
        c. Uninhibited bowel pattern may result in frequent defecation, urgency, and complaints of constipation:
            (1) Maintains a consistent toileting schedule
            (2) Provides a high-fiber diet
            (3) Administers stool softeners, as ordered
    2. Modifies the bowel program if complications occur, such as constipation, diarrhea, or flatulence

---

✦ **NDx:** Ineffective Individual Coping

- The nurse
    1. Encourages the client to talk about his or her feelings
    2. Assesses the coping strategies and support systems the client used in the past and assists during rehabilitation
    3. Helps the client to use spiritual and religious beliefs to cope, as appropriate

Continuing Care

- The nurse
    1. Assists the client and family in identifying and correcting hazards in the home before discharge
    2. Ensures that the client can correctly use all adaptive-assistive devices ordered for home use
    3. Provides a detailed plan of care at the time of discharge for the client to be transferred to a long-term-care facility or rehabilitation center

4. Assesses for support systems to help the client to cope with disability
5. Refers the client to home health nursing

NURSING CARE OF THE CLIENT EXPERIENCING SENSORY DEPRIVATION

OVERVIEW

- Sensory deprivation is the reduction in variety and intensity of sensory input, with or without a change in the structure or pattern of stimulation.
- Subtypes of sensory deprivation include
  1. Absolute reduction: Stimuli in the external environment are absent.
  2. Reception deprivation: Receptor organs are impaired, and either partial or complete loss of sensation occurs.
  3. Perceptual deprivation: The client cannot recognize and interpret stimuli from the external environment.
  4. Technologic deprivation: The client is in a highly technologic environment in which the nurse focuses on the machines rather than the person.
  5. Confinement deprivation: The client is separated from significant others and familiar objects.
  6. Immobility deprivation: The client has decreased physical movement and activity.

Considerations for Elderly Clients

1. The elderly are at high risk for sensory deprivation because they *may* have decreased vision, hearing, and taste.
2. The elderly *may* be less able to process incoming stimuli as rapidly as a younger adult.

COLLABORATIVE MANAGEMENT

Assessment

- The nurse assesses for
    1. Cognitive changes, such as poor concentration, altered sequencing of thoughts, unusual ideas, bizarre thinking, impaired memory, and disorientation
    2. Emotional changes, such as anxiety, depression, crying, fear, mood swings, irritability, annoyance over trivial matters, and anger
    3. Perceptual changes, such as visual and auditory distortions, alterations in color and perceived movement of stable objects, and preoccupation with internal sensations and somatic complaints
    4. Physical changes, such as drowsiness, excessive yawning and sleep, and alterations in dexterity and hand-eye coordination movements

Planning and Implementation

✦ **NDx:** Sensory/Perceptual Alterations

- The nurse
    1. Identifies factors that contribute to sensory deprivation
    2. Increases the level of intensity of stimulation and increases the variety of patterns of incoming stimuli
    3. Tries to create an environment that resembles familiar surroundings and restores meaningful stimuli:
        a. Places pictures on the walls of the hospital room
        b. Displays personal cards and pictures on the bedside table
        c. Encourages family members to bring inexpensive personal items in from home
        d. Allows the client to wear nightgown or pajamas from home when possible
        e. Uses radio and television appropriately
        f. Has clocks and calendars easily visible
        g. Ensures that the client uses needed assistive devices such as hearing aids, eyeglasses, or contact lenses
        h. Encourages participation in self-care activities
        i. Talks with the client; explains tests and procedures

     j. Encourages the client to read, write, draw, or paint

Continuing Care

- The nurse
  1. Identifies areas in the home that may contribute to sensory deprivation
  2. Assesses the need for a community health nurse or home health aide

NURSING CARE OF THE CLIENT EXPERIENCING SENSORY OVERLOAD

OVERVIEW

- Sensory overload results from an increase in environmental stimuli—when there is multisensory bombardment of stimuli or when there is an increase in the pattern and intensity of stimuli so that the input is meaningless.
- Behavioral manifestations of sensory overload can have a health-threatening effect on the individual.

COLLABORATIVE MANAGEMENT

Assessment

- There are no clear differences between behaviors observed in sensory deprivation and those observed in sensory overload.
- The distinguishing feature of overload is that the client cannot use sleep as an escape mechanism.
- The nurse assesses for
  1. Client's status before hospitalization and reviews the medications the client is receiving to determine whether symptoms are the result of side or toxic effects or drug interactions
  2. Increased restlessness, drowsiness, sleep cycle changes, incoordination, dry mouth, heart palpitations, difficulty breathing, and lack of appetite

3. Presence of bizarre thoughts, delusions, hallucinations, irritability, mood swings, crying, fear, and depression
4. Reduced attention span, noncompliant behaviors
5. Increased level of catecholamines, 17-ketosteroids, luteinizing hormones, and increased thyroid-stimulating hormones
6. Amount and intensity of stimuli present and the degree of social isolation

Planning and Implementation

✦ NDx: Sensory/Perceptual Alterations

- The nurse
  1. Reduces the intensity of incoming stimuli and increases the meaningfulness of the stimuli
  2. Provides a consistent, predictable pattern of stimulation
  3. Keeps the noise level to a minimum
  4. Encourages the health care team to refrain from conversations at the client's bedside
  5. Maintains a normal sleep-wake cycle by dimming the lights at night and drawing curtains around the client's bed
  6. Explains all procedures, diagnostic tests, and equipment
  7. Remains calm, uses an unhurried approach, and speaks in a low, modulated voice when interacting with the client
  8. Schedules the same nurse to care for the client, when possible
  9. Develops a routine for care and activities
  10. Orients the client to reality as often as necessary
  11. Limits visitors, telephone calls, and the use of radio and television

Continuing Care

- Family or significant others should assess the home for stimuli that are potential sources of difficulties for the client.

NURSING CARE OF THE CLIENT UNDERGOING CIRCUMCISION

OVERVIEW

- Circumcision is the surgical removal of the prepuce from the penis.
- In the adult male, circumcision is usually done for medical reasons, such as to correct phimosis, a condition in which the prepuce is constricted, and to eliminate the infections that frequently occur as a result of this condition.

COLLABORATIVE MANAGEMENT

- The nurse
  1. Instructs the client to soak in a warm bath and allow the penile dressing to float off
  2. Tells the client not to replace the dressing if it falls off
  3. Informs the client that the sutures will be absorbed and do not need to be removed
  4. Instructs the client to resume normal activities within 1 week and sexual activity after 1 or 2 weeks
  5. Advises the client to take barbiturate sleeping medication, which suppresses the rapid eye movement phase of sleep, so that normal nocturnal erections do not occur
  6. Instructs the client to notify the physician for any wound complication

NURSING CARE TO PROMOTE SEXUAL HEALTH

OVERVIEW

- Sexual health includes one's freedom from physical and psychologic impairment, the awareness of open and positive attitudes toward sexual functioning, and accurate knowledge of sexuality.

- *Homosexuality* is erotic attraction to persons of the same sex.
- *Bisexuality* refers to a preference for intimate relationships with members of either sex.
- A person who is *transsexual* is completely dissatisfied with his or her gender assignment and is convinced that he or she is trapped with the wrong body; sex reassignment surgery may be performed.
- A *transvestite* wears clothes associated with the opposite sex for the sake of sexual arousal, but there is no conflict about his or her gender; cross-dressing occurs more frequently in men than women.
- *Pedophilia* is a sexual preference for children and is considered to be a psychiatric disorder.

 Transcultural Considerations

1. Cultural or religious background may influence a person's willingness to discuss sexual health.

COLLABORATIVE MANAGEMENT
Assessment

- The nurse records the client's
    1. Injury or disease of the genitourinary system
    2. Contraceptive use
    3. Development of secondary sexual characteristics
    4. Unwanted or traumatic sexual events such as rape
    5. Changes of sexual functioning related to drug or alcohol use
    6. Changes in sexual functioning since the current illness, injury, or surgery
    7. Current physical condition causing the change in body image
    8. Changes in usual activities and roles
    9. Changes in beliefs and practices about sexual functioning that have occurred as a result of illness
- The nurse assesses for
    1. Changes in external genitalia and breasts (e.g., thickening or discharge from genitalia or breasts)
    2. Dyspareunia (painful intercourse)
    3. Inhibited sexual desire: loss of interest in sexual activity or decline in libido

4. Vaginismus: muscles of the outer third of the vaginal barrel contract powerfully and prevent insertion of a tampon or other object
5. Orgasmic dysfunction: the inability to achieve orgasm (primary dysfunction) or to achieve orgasm with intercourse or at an appropriate time during intercourse (secondary dysfunction)
6. Erectile dysfunction: the inability to attain or maintain an erection of the penis of sufficient firmness to permit penetration
7. Ejaculatory dysfunction, premature: ejaculation after penetration but sooner than either partner desires
8. Retrograde ejaculation, or dry orgasm: semen discharged into the urinary bladder
9. Sexual aversion: irrational fear or phobic reaction to the thought of sexual activity or to the actual activity
10. Psychologic and social factors related to past and present functioning

Planning and Implementation

✦ NDx: Sexual Dysfunction: Dyspareunia

- In females, dyspareunia may be related to
  1. An intact hymen: The nurse refers the client to a gynecologist.
  2. Scarring from an episiotomy or pathologic conditions of the reproductive organs: The nurse refers the client to a gynecologist.
  3. Infections of the vagina or vulva: The nurse
     a. Explains methods to decrease risk of infection
     b. Administers antibiotics, as ordered
     c. Teaches the client to avoid sexual intercourse until the infection is resolved
     d. Encourages the client to rest and to increase fluid intake
  4. Insufficient vaginal lubrication: The nurse instructs the client to use a water-soluble lubricant before sexual activity or intercourse.
  5. Irritation from chemical products such as contraceptives or douches: The nurse
     a. Instructs the client to avoid excessive use of these products or to stop their use completely
     b. Encourages the use of products without scents

35

6. Psychogenic factors: The nurse refers the client to a competent therapist.

- In males, dyspareunia may be related to
    1. Inflammation or infection of the organs within the genitourinary system; the nurse
        a. Administers prescribed antibiotics
        b. Encourages the client to drink fluids and to rest
        c. Teaches the client to avoid sexual intercourse until the acute condition is resolved
    2. Exposure to vaginal contraceptive cream, jelly, or foam, or irritation from an intrauterine device: The nurse provides information and alternatives to the client and his sexual partner.
    3. Psychosocial factors: The nurse refers the client to a competent therapist.

✦ **NDx:** Sexual Dysfunction: Vaginismus and Orgasmic Dysfunction

- For the client with sexual dysfunction, the nurse
    1. Helps to identify and relieve underlying psychogenic factors, such as rape trauma syndrome, conflicts surrounding homosexual experimentation, or strong religious teachings:
        a. Encourages the client to express feelings of anxiety and conflict, if present
        b. Refers the client to a competent therapist
    2. Helps to identify and relieve underlying physical factors such as sexual activity too soon after childbirth, abnormality of the hymen, or atrophy of the vagina:
        a. Refers the client to a gynecologist
        b. Encourages the client to explore alternatives to vaginal intercourse during the healing process
        c. Explains the relationship between physical factors and involuntary muscular response
- The nurse helps the client with orgasmic dysfunction by
    1. Referring the client to a gynecologist
    2. Instructing the client in the performance of Kegel exercises
    3. Giving the client permission to talk about the problem
    4. Providing information about the relationship between stressors and the physical response of orgasm

5. Referring the client to a therapist who specializes in treating sexual disorders

✦ **NDx:** Sexual Dysfunction: Erectile Dysfunction, Premature Ejaculation, Dysfunctional or Retrograde Ejaculation

- Erectile dysfunction may be related to
  1. Spinal cord injury
  2. Diabetes mellitus
  3. Alcoholism
  4. Neurologic disease
  5. Infections of the genitourinary system
  6. Drug use or abuse
  7. Psychogenic factors
- The nurse
  1. Refers the client to a urologist or competent therapist, as appropriate
  2. Instructs the client and his partner in "sensate focus" technique
- For the client with premature ejaculation, the nurse
  1. Educates the client and his partner about the relationship between emotions and the sexual response cycle
  2. Teaches systematic relaxation exercises
- When the client's problem is retrograde ejaculation, the nurse
  1. Refers the client to a urologist
  2. Assists the client with coping skills and provides education and counseling

Continuing Care

- The nurse teaches the importance of follow-up visits with the physician(s) and other therapists.

PART II

DISEASES AND DISORDERS

ABDOMINAL TRAUMA

See Trauma, Abdominal.

ABSCESSES, ANORECTAL

OVERVIEW

- Anorectal abscesses result from obstruction of the ducts of glands in the anorectal region by feces, foreign bodies, or trauma.
- Stasis of the obstructing contents results in infection that spreads into adjacent tissue.

COLLABORATIVE MANAGEMENT

- Rectal pain is the first clinical manifestation.
- Local swelling, erythema, and tenderness on palpation appear a few days after the onset of pain.
- The diagnosis is made by physical examination and history.
- Simple perianal and ischiorectal abscesses can be excised with local anesthesia.
- Clients with more extensive abscesses require incision under regional or general anesthesia.
- The nurse
  1. Administers antibiotics, as ordered, for clients who are immunocompromised or who have diabetes, valvular disease or prostheses, or extensive cellulitis
  2. Assists the client to maintain comfort and optimal perineal hygiene by providing sitz baths, analgesics, bulk-forming agents, and stool softeners, as ordered
  3. Emphasizes the importance of on-going perineal hygiene

ABSCESSES, BRAIN

OVERVIEW

- A brain abscess is a purulent infection of the brain in which pus forms in the extradural, subdural, or intra-cerebral area.
- The number of clients with brain abscesses secondary to immunosuppression, organ transplantation, and acquired immunodeficiency syndrome (AIDS) has rapidly increased over the past two decades.
- The causative organisms are most often bacteria, such as *Streptococcus* and *Staphylococcus*.
- Most brain abscesses occur in the frontal and temporal lobes.

COLLABORATIVE MANAGEMENT

- A brain abscess is typically manifested by symptoms of a mass and of mildly increased intracranial pressure, including
  1. Headache
  2. Fever
  3. Lethargy and confusion
  4. Decreased peripheral vision
  5. Generalized weakness and possibly hemiparesis
  6. Ataxia
  7. Seizures
  8. Signs of increased intracranial pressure in late disease
  9. Elevated white blood cell (WBC) count
  10. Elevated erythrocyte sedimentation rate
- The nurse
  1. Administers antibiotics, as ordered; metronidazole (Flagyl, Novonidazol◆) may be used if an anaerobic organism is the causative agent
  2. Administers anticonvulsants, as ordered, to prevent or treat seizures
  3. Administers analgesics, as ordered, to treat the client's headache
  4. Elevates the head of the client's bed 30 to 45 degrees to promote venous drainage from the head (see also interventions for the treatment of in-

creased intracranial pressure under Tumors, Brain)
- Surgical drainage of an encapsulated abscess or a craniotomy may be performed.

ABSCESSES, HEPATIC

OVERVIEW
- Hepatic (liver) abscesses occur when the liver is invaded by bacteria or protozoa.
- Liver tissue is destroyed.
- The resulting necrotic cavity becomes filled with infected, liquefied liver cells and tissue and leukocytes.
- Liver abscess occurs infrequently and is associated with a high mortality rate.
- Pyrogenic abscesses are caused by bacteria such as *Escherichia coli, Klebsiella, Enterobacter, Salmonella, Staphylococcus,* and *Enterococcus.*
- Abscesses can result following cholangitis, liver trauma, peritonitis, sepsis, or infection extension and can occur as multiple abscesses.
- Amebic hepatic abscesses occur following amebic dysentery as a single abscess in the liver's right upper quadrant.

COLLABORATIVE MANAGEMENT
- The nurse assesses for
    1. Right upper quadrant abdominal pain
    2. Tender, palpable liver
    3. Anorexia
    4. Weight loss
    5. Nausea and vomiting
    6. Fever and chills
    7. Shoulder pain
    8. Dyspnea
- Abscess may be aspirated under ultrasonography guidance.
- Hepatic abscesses are usually diagnosed by liver scan.
- Surgical drainage is indicated only for a single, pyogenic abscess or for an amebic abscess that fails to respond to long-term antibiotic therapy.

ABSCESSES, KIDNEY

See Abscesses, Renal.

ABSCESSES, LIVER

See Abscesses, Hepatic.

ABSCESSES, PANCREATIC

- A pancreatic abscess consists of infected, necrotic pancreatic tissue.
- Pancreatic abscess usually occurs after severe acute pancreatitis, exacerbations of chronic pancreatitis, and biliary tract surgery.
- The problem may occur as a single abscess or multiloculated abscesses resulting from extensive inflammatory necrosis of the pancreas readily invaded by infectious organisms, such as *Escherichia coli, Klebsiella, Bacteroides, Staphylococcus,* and *Proteus.*
- Temperature spikes may be as high as 104° F (40° C).
- There is a 100% mortality rate if the abscess is not surgically drained; multiple drainage procedures are often required.
- Antibiotic therapy alone does not resolve the abscess.
- Pleural effusions often accompany the abscess.

ABSCESSES, PERITONSILLAR

- Peritonsillar abscess is a complication of acute tonsillitis known as *quinsy.*
- Acute infection spreads from the tonsil to the surrounding peritonsillar tissue, forming an abscess.
- The common cause is group A beta-hemolytic *Streptococcus.*
- Marked asymmetric swelling and deviation of the uvula from pus collection cause difficult swallowing, drooling, severe throat pain radiating to the ear, and voice change.
- Treatment includes
    1. Warm saline gargles or irrigations
    2. Ice collar
    3. Analgesics
    4. Antibiotics
    5. Incision and drainage of the abscess
    6. Tonsillectomy after healing

ABSCESSES, RENAL

- A renal abscess is a collection of fluid and cells resulting from an inflammatory response to bacteria in the renal parenchyma, renal fascia, or the flank.
- An abscess is suspected when fever and symptoms are unresponsive to antibiotic therapy.
- Symptoms include
    1. Fever
    2. Flank pain
    3. General malaise
    4. Local edema
- Treatment includes
    1. Broad-spectrum antibiotics
    2. Drainage by surgical incision or needle aspiration

ACHALASIA

OVERVIEW

- Achalasia is a progressively worsening dysphagia evidenced by chronic and vague complaints of difficult swallowing and of food sticking in the throat.
- The exact cause is unknown, but the accepted theory is a lack of peristalsis related to neuromuscular factors and inadequate relaxation of the lower esophageal sphincter.

COLLABORATIVE MANAGEMENT

Assessment

- The nurse records the client's
    1. Symptoms, including dysphagia, chest pain, regurgitation, and halitosis (foul mouth odor)
    2. Factors that aggravate the symptoms, such as position or diet
    3. Home treatments that relieve the symptoms, including over-the-counter drugs
    4. History of previous esophageal trauma or surgery
    5. Nutritional history, including diet habits, food intolerance, nutritional status, and weight loss
    6. Results of the barium swallow, which usually show a narrow "bird's-beak" junction at the esophageal hiatus and esophageal dilation above the junction

---

🎗 Considerations for the Elderly

Chest pain may not be the primary presenting symptom in an elderly client.

Interventions

Nonsurgical Management

- The nurse
    1. Administers anticholinergic drugs, nitrates, gastrointestinal hormones, and calcium channel blockers to lower the esophageal pressure and relax the lower esophageal sphincter, to treat symptoms

2. Teaches the client to avoid foods or habits that aggravate symptoms
3. Encourages the client to experiment with diet changes, including semisoft foods, warm foods, and liquids that may be better tolerated
4. Teaches the client to eat several small meals per day instead of three large meals
5. Advises the client to experiment with various changes in position while eating because these changes can reduce pressure sensation during meals
6. Instructs the client to sleep with the head of the bed elevated on blocks or reclining in a semisitting position

Surgical Management

- Surgery may be necessary and is aimed at facilitating food passage by dilating the unrelaxed esophageal sphincter or destroying the sphincter by esophagomyotomy.
- *Esophageal dilation* for achalasia is performed under local anesthesia with a pneumatized dilator (a pressurized bag filled with water); the nurse assesses for hemoptysis after dilation and teaches the client to drink only liquids for 24 hours after the procedure.
- An *esophagomyotomy* is performed to obliterate the sphincter and requires a thoracotomy approach to expose the esophagus; muscle fibers are cut to open the esophagus to provide less obstruction for food passage.
- Nursing care for the client undergoing esophagomyotomy is similar to that described for thoractomy under Cancer, Lung.

ACIDOSIS, METABOLIC

OVERVIEW

- Metabolic acidosis is characterized by a low pH, low bicarbonate level, normal carbon dioxide partial pressure, normal oxygen tension, elevated serum potassium level, elevated serum chloride level, and elevated anion gap.

- Common causes include
  1. Overproduction of hydrogen ions:
     a. Diabetic ketoacidosis
     b. Starvation
     c. Heavy exercise
     d. Fever
     e. Hypoxia, ischemia
     f. Ethanol, methanol, or ethylene glycol intoxication
     g. Salicylate intoxication
  2. Underelimination of hydrogen ions (renal failure)
  3. Underproduction of bicarbonate ions (decreased pancreatic and hepatic functions)
  4. Overelimination of bicarbonate ions:
     a. Diarrhea
     b. Dehydration
     c. Buffering of organic acids

COLLABORATIVE MANAGEMENT

- The nurse records the client's
  1. Age
  2. Use of prescribed and over-the-counter medications, especially those containing aspirin or alcohol
  3. Current and past medical history:
     a. Respiratory problems
     b. Renal failure
     c. Diabetes mellitus
     d. Pancreatitis
     e. Persistent diarrhea
     f. Fever
  4. Diet history, especially fasting or strict diet the week before seeking health care.
  5. Behavior and/or personality changes
- The nurse assesses for
  1. Central nervous system changes:
     a. Lethargy, confusion, stupor
     b. Depression
  2. Neuromuscular changes:
     a. Hyporeflexia
     b. Skeletal muscle weakness
     c. Flaccid paralysis
  3. Cardiac changes:
     a. Delayed electrical conduction

          (1) Bradycardia
          (2) Tall T waves
          (3) Widened QRS complex
          (4) Prolonged PR interval
       b. Hypotension
       c. Thready peripheral pulses
    4. Respiratory changes:
       a. Kussmaul's respiration (respirations deep, rapid, and not under voluntary control)
    5. Integumentary changes: warm, pink, dry skin
- Metabolic acidosis is managed by treating the underlying cause of the acid imbalance and hydration.

🕭 Considerations for Elderly Clients

- The elderly are more prone to acid-base imbalance secondary to cardiac, renal, or pulmonary problems.
- Medications that interfere with acid-base balance and fluid and electrolyte balance include diuretics, aspirin, and alcohol.

ACIDOSIS, RESPIRATORY

OVERVIEW

- An alteration in some area of respiratory function results in an inadequate exchange of oxygen and carbon dioxide resulting in retention of carbon dioxide.
- Respiratory acidosis is characterized by a low pH, elevated carbon dioxide partial pressure (PCO_2) and bicarbonate level, and decreased oxygen tension (PO_2).
- Changes in serum potassium, serum chloride, and anion gap levels vary with the duration of the acidosis and the degree of renal compensation.
- Common causes include
    1. Respiratory depression:
       a. Chemical depression: anesthetics
       b. Drugs: especially narcotics
       c. Poisons
       d. Trauma
       e. Cerebral edema
       f. Electrolyte imbalance

48

g. Guillain-Barré syndrome
      h. Myasthenia gravis
      i. Stroke, aneurysm
  2. Inadequate chest expansion:
      a. Skeletal deformities and trauma such as broken ribs, spinal cord injury
      b. Respiratory muscle weakness: muscular dystrophy
      c. Nonrespiratory conditions:
         (1) Obesity
         (2) Abdominal or thoracic masses
         (3) Ascites
         (4) Hemothorax or pneumothorax
  3. Airway obstruction that may be due to regional lymph node involvement, asthma
  4. Alveolar-capillary block:
      a. Pneumonia
      b. Pulmonary edema
      c. Atelectasis
      d. Adult respiratory distress syndrome
      e. Emphysema
      f. Tuberculosis

COLLABORATIVE MANAGEMENT

Assessment

- The nurse records the client's
  1. Age
  2. Prescribed and over-the-counter medications, especially those containing aspirin or alcohol
  3. Current and past medical history:
     a. Respiratory problems
     b. Renal failure
     c. Diabetes mellitus
     d. Pancreatitis
     e. Persistent diarrhea
     f. Fever
  4. Diet history
  5. Behavior or personality changes
- The nurse assesses for
  1. Central nervous system changes:
     a. Lethargy, confusion, stupor
     b. Depression
  2. Neuromuscular changes:
     a. Hyporeflexia
     b. Skeletal muscle weakness

49

        c. Flaccid paralysis
    3. Cardiac changes:
        a. Delayed electrical conduction
            (1) Bradycardia
            (2) Tall T waves
            (3) Widened QRS complex
            (4) Prolonged PR interval
        b. Hypotension
        c. Thready peripheral pulses
    4. Respiratory changes:
        a. Diminished respiratory efforts
        b. Shallow and rapid respirations
    5. Integumentary changes: pale to cyanotic skin
- The nurse
    1. Performs a respiratory assessment every 2 hours or more often as indicated by the client's clinical condition:
        a. Rate and depth of respirations
        b. Auscultation of breath sounds
        c. Ease with which the client moves air in and out of the lungs
        d. Presence of retractions
    2. Administers drugs to increase the diameter of the upper and lower airway and thin pulmonary secretions and improve gas exchange:
        a. Beclomethasone (Vanceril, Beclovent)
        b. Theophylline (Bronkodyl, Theo-Dur)
        c. Ephedrine, fenoterol (Berotec)
        d. Isoproterenol (Aerolone, Isuprel)
        e. Metaproterenol (Alupent)
        f. Terbutaline (Brethaire, Brethine, Bricanyl)
        g. Acetylcysteine (Airbron [black diamond], Mucomyst)
    3. Administers nebulized oxygen cautiously, particularly if the client has chronic obstructive pulmonary disease and carbon dioxide narcosis
    4. Places the client in the Fowler's or semi-Fowler's position
    5. Examines nail beds and mucous membranes for color
- The nurse
    1. Encourages the client to ingest enough calories to meet at least basal energy requirements
    2. Collaborates with the dietitian to plan small, frequent meals that have a high protein and carbohydrate content, unless contraindicated

3. Plans activities and procedures to allow the client frequent rest periods
   4. Reschedules bath, activities, and tests that are not absolutely necessary, if possible
- The nurse
   1. Ensures that the home meets the client's needs for safety and activities of daily living
   2. Instructs the client in the signs and symptoms of acidosis
   3. Refers the client to appropriate health care resources such as home health nurse, social services, and respiratory therapist

ACOUSTIC NEUROMA

See Neuroma, Acoustic.

ACQUIRED IMMUNODEFICIENCY SYNDROME

See AIDS.

ACTINIC KERATOSES

See Cancer, Skin.

51

ACUTE GLOMERULONEPHRITIS

See Glomerulonephritis, Acute.

ACUTE IDIOPATHIC POLYNEURITIS

See Guillain-Barré Syndrome.

ACUTE PANCREATITIS

See Pancreatitis, Acute.

ACUTE RENAL FAILURE

See Renal Failure, Acute.

ACUTE RESPIRATORY FAILURE

See Respiratory Failure, Acute.

ADDISON'S DISEASE

See Hypofunction, Adrenal.

ADRENAL HYPOFUNCTION

See Hypofunction, Adrenal.

ADULT RESPIRATORY DISTRESS SYNDROME

OVERVIEW

- Adult respiratory distress syndrome (ARDS) is a form of acute respiratory failure characterized by refractory hypoxemia, decreased pulmonary compliance, dyspnea, noncardiac bilateral pulmonary edema, and the presence of pulmonary infiltrates.
- It usually occurs after an acute catastrophic event in people with no previous pulmonary disease.
- The major site of injury is the alveolar capillary membrane.
- Multiple types of injury affect alveoli, which can no longer participate in gas exchange.
- Interstitial edema causes compression and obliteration of terminal airways, thereby reducing lung volume and lung compliance.
- Causes include serious nervous system injury, trauma, shock, sepsis, near-drowning, hemolytic disorders, drug ingestion, inhalation of toxic gases, pulmonary infections, pancreatitis, burns, fat and amniotic fluid emboli, pulmonary infections, pulmonary aspiration, multiple blood transfusions, and cardiopulmonary bypass.

53

- Some factors produce ARDS by direct injury to the lung such as aspiration of gastric contents, which leads to mechanical obstruction or produces an acid burn to the airway when the pH of the gastric contents is less than 2.5.
- Clients have a rapidly deteriorating respiratory status with increased work of breathing and deteriorating blood gas levels; hypoxemia persists despite high concentrations of oxygen.
- A major goal in the prevention of ARDS is early recognition of the client who is at high risk for the syndrome.

🕮 Considerations for Elderly Clients

Elderly clients who receive tube feedings are at a high risk for ARDS because aspiration of stomach contents is a major risk factor.

COLLABORATIVE MANAGEMENT
Assessment

- The nurse assesses the client for
    1. Respirations (rate and quality); usually, increased work of breathing, as indicated by hyperpnea, grunting respirations, suprasternal or intercostal retractions
    2. Cyanosis
    3. Pallor
    4. Diaphoresis
    5. Mental status changes
    6. Lung sounds (typically normal because edema is in the interstitial spaces, not the airways)
    7. Hypotension
    8. Tachycardia
    9. Dysrhythmias
    10. Lowered arterial PO_2
    11. Haziness or "whited-out" appearance on chest x-ray
    12. Normal pulmonary capillary wedge pressure (diagnostic tool to differentiate ARDS from cardiogenic pulmonary edema in which pressure is high)
    13. Positive sputum culture

Interventions

- Clients with ARDS usually require endotracheal intubation and mechanical ventilation with positive end-expiratory pressure (PEEP) and continuous positive airway pressure.
- The nurse
    1. Administers sedating drugs, antibiotics, and corticosteroids, as ordered
    2. Assesses lung sounds to monitor for the development of tension pneumothorax, a side effect of PEEP
    3. Maintains a patent airway with frequent suctioning
    4. Administers intravenous fluids; fluid volume is titrated to maintain adequate cardiac output and tissue perfusion
    5. Assesses for nutritional status and administers enteral or parenteral nutrition
    6. Collaborates with the health care team to prevent sepsis, pneumonia, and multiple organ failure

---

AIDS

OVERVIEW

- Acquired immunodeficiency syndrome (AIDS) is the late stage of a continuum of symptoms that results from infection with the human immunodeficiency virus (HIV), a retrovirus.
- AIDS is a serious, debilitating, and eventually fatal disease.
- A person with HIV infection can transmit the virus to others at all stages of the disease.
- The results of HIV infection are
    1. Lymphocytopenia with selective T4-cell depletion
    2. Abnormal T-cell function
    3. Increased production of incomplete and nonfunctional antibodies
    4. Abnormally functioning macrophages
- Epidemiologic and demographic data have shown that most people with AIDS in the United States are men

who have had homosexual and bisexual contact or persons of either sex who have used intravenous drugs.
- Women are the fastest-growing group with HIV infection and AIDS.

 Transcultural Considerations

1. AIDS has been reported in 162 countries and in each state of the United States.
2. The pattern of HIV infection and the manifestations of AIDS differ in countries such as West Africa, where HIV-2, rather than HIV-1, is the predominant viral strain.

COLLABORATIVE MANAGEMENT

Assessment

- The nurse assesses for
    1. Shortness of breath, cough
    2. Fever
    3. Night sweats
    4. Fatigue
    5. Weight loss
    6. Lymphadenopathy
    7. Diarrhea (cryptosporidiosis)
    8. Visual changes
    9. Headache
    10. Memory loss
    11. Confusion
    12. Seizures
    13. Personality changes
    14. Dry, irritated skin
    15. Rashes
    16. Skin lesions such as Kaposi's sarcoma
    17. Pain and discomfort
    18. Dyspnea on exertion, tachypnea, dry cough, fever (*Pneumocystis carinii* pneumonia [PCP])
    19. Mental changes (toxoplasmosis)
    20. Manifestations of fungal infections, such as *Candida* stomatitis
    21. Meningitis (cryptococcosis)
    22. Bacterial infections
    23. Tuberculosis
    24. Viral infections, such as cytomegalovirus (CMV) retinitis and CMV colitis
    25. Viral infections, such as herpes simplex

26. Lymphoma
27. Changes in ability to perform activities of daily living (ADL)
28. Availability of a support system, such as family and significant others
29. Current employment status and occupation
30. Social activities and hobbies
31. Self-esteem and body image changes
32. Suicidal ideation, depression
33. Involvement with community resources or support groups
34. Leukopenia
35. Decreased T4 cells
36. Positive ELISA and Western blot analysis
37. Positive quantitative RNA analysis

Planning and Implementation

✦ NDx: Risk for Infection

- Clients with HIV are at high risk for *opportunistic* infections.
- Drug therapy includes azidothymidine (AZT) or zidovudine (Retrovir). Side effects include macrocytic anemia, mild headache, nausea, abdominal pain, diarrhea, and less commonly changes in white blood cell count or liver function tests.
- DDI (Videx) is used for clients who are unable to tolerate AZT or who have continued loss of immune function despite AZT therapy. Side effects include pancreatitis and peripheral neuropathy.
- Drug therapy continues to change as the result of intense research.

✦ NDx: Impaired Gas Exchange

- The nurse
    1. Assesses respiratory status frequently
    2. Monitors arterial blood gases
    3. Provides oxygen and room humidification
    4. Performs chest physiotherapy
    5. Encourages fluid intake as tolerated
    6. Elevates the head of the bed to facilitate breathing
    7. Helps the client pace activities to minimize shortness of breath
    8. Administers antipyretics to reduce fever
    9. Assists with ADL as needed

10. Administers trimethoprim-sulfamethazole (Bactrim, Protrin◆) or pentamidine (Pentam, Lomidine◆), as ordered, for PCP

✦ NDx: Altered Nutrition: Less than Body Requirements

- The nurse
  1. Collaborates with the health care team to determine the exact cause of the nutritional problem(s)
  2. Obtains a calorie count
  3. Weighs the client daily
  4. Provides small frequent meals or snacks with high caloric and nutritional value; offers high-calorie supplements (in collaboration with a dietitian)
  5. Assesses the client's food preferences and dietary, cultural, and religious practices and helps the client select foods to meet these needs
  6. Gives enteral or parenteral feedings if needed
  7. Provides a soft or bland diet
  8. Provides meticulous mouth care and assists the client to rinse the mouth with sodium bicarbonate and normal saline; provides the client with a soft toothbrush, and intervenes to treat mouth pain
  9. Administers supplemental vitamins, as ordered
  10. Administers ketoconazole (Nizoral) or fluconazole (Diflucan) or amphotericin B, as ordered

✦ NDx: Diarrhea

- The nurse
  1. Administers diphenoxylate hydrochloride (Lomotil, Diarsed◆), as ordered, to control diarrhea
  2. Collaborates with the dietitian to provide a diet low in roughage and fat; spicy or very sweet food, alcohol, dairy products, and caffeine are also avoided
  3. Provides the client with a bedside commode or bedpan as needed

✦ NDx: Altered Thought Processes

- The nurse
  1. Establishes baseline neurologic and mental status
  2. Observes for and reports changes in behavior that may be related to the loss and psychologic stress experienced by the client

3. Assists with ADL, as needed
4. Reorients the client to the environment; uses calendars, clocks, and radios; puts the bed near the window if possible
5. Paces the client's activities; gives simple directions and uses short and uncomplicated sentences
6. Teaches the family and significant others techniques to use to help orient the client
7. Administers anticonvulsants as ordered, for seizures

✦ NDx: Impaired Skin Integrity

- The nurse
    1. Monitors for progression of lesions
    2. Avoids pressure (uses egg crate, air, or water mattress)
    3. Uses careful hygienic measures
    4. Provides meticulous skin care
    5. Gives analgesics, as ordered, if needed
- Kaposi's sarcoma is the most common skin lesion.
- Rapidly progressive Kaposi's sarcoma is treated with chemotherapy.
- Radiation therapy is transiently effective.
- Interferon-alpha is effective, especially in clients with better immune function.
- Changes in appearance can be minimized by the use of make-up, long-sleeved shirts, and hats.
- Herpes simplex virus abscess is also a commonly seen skin lesion in clients with HIV infection.
- The nurse
    1. Cleans the abscess with a diluted solution of povidone-iodine and leaves it open to the air or uses a heat lamp to help it dry
    2. Administers drug therapy as ordered with acyclovir (Zovirax), which is potentially toxic to the kidney; thus, the client must maintain adequate hydration
    3. Implements wound and skin precautions

✦ NDx: Self-Esteem Disturbance

- Self-esteem is affected by changes in appearance, in relationships with others, in day-to-day activity, and in job performance and possibly by guilt about lifestyle.
- The nurse
    1. Provides a climate of acceptance
    2. Allows for privacy

3. Offers a safe environment
4. Encourages self-care, independence, control, and decision making
5. Helps formulate attainable short-term goals
6. Is honest with his or her feelings

✦ **NDx:** Social Isolation

- The nurse
    1. Explains the rationale for Standard Precautions to the client and visitors
    2. Visits the client frequently and provides for diversional activities
    3. Encourages the client to verbalize feelings about self, coping skills, and sense of ability to control the situation
    4. Educates the client, family, and significant others about prevention of HIV transmission

Continuing Care

- The nurse
    1. Identifies the actual and potential need for care, such as a visiting nurse, Meals on Wheels, a home health aide, 24-hour supervision, community mental health agencies
    2. Identifies and corrects any hazards in the home before discharge
    3. Refers the client to a support group
- The nurse teaches the client and family
    1. The mode of transmission of HIV infection
    2. The need to notify sexual contacts
    3. Signs and symptoms of infections
    4. Importance of not changing pet litter boxes
    5. Self care strategies such as good hygiene, balance of rest and exercise, skin and oral care
    6. How to safely administer medications
    7. Importance of good nutrition, proper food handling
    8. The importance of follow-up visits with the physician(s)

AIRWAY OBSTRUCTION, UPPER

See Obstruction, Upper Airway.

ALKALOSIS, METABOLIC

OVERVIEW

- Metabolic alkalosis is characterized by a high pH, elevated bicarbonate (above 28 mEq/L), normal oxygen tension, rising carbon dioxide partial pressure, decreased serum potassium level, decreased serum calcium level.
- Common causes include
    1. Increase of base components:
        a. excessive use of antacids, bicarbonates
        b. Milk-alkali syndrome
        c. Blood transfusion
        d. Total parenteral nutrition (TPN)
    2. Decrease of acid components:
        a. Prolonged vomiting
        b. Nasogastric suctioning
        c. Cushing's syndrome
        d. Hyperaldosteronism
        e. Use of thiazide diuretics

COLLABORATIVE MANAGEMENT

- The nurse assesses for
    1. Central nervous system changes:
        a. Lightheadedness
        b. Changes in the ability to concentrate
        c. Anxiety, irritability, agitation
        d. Tetany, seizures
        e. Positive Chvostek's sign
        f. Positive Trousseau's sign
        g. Paresthesia

2. Neuromuscular changes:
   a. Hyperreflexia
   b. Muscle cramping and twitching
   c. Skeletal muscle weakness
3. Cardiac changes:
   a. Increased heart rate
   b. Normal or low blood pressure
   c. Increased digitalis toxicity
4. Respiratory changes: decreased respiratory effort associated with skeletal muscle weakness

- Metabolic alkalosis is managed by treating the underlying cause of the alkalosis and restoring normal fluid, electrolyte, and acid-base balance.

ALKALOSIS, RESPIRATORY

OVERVIEW

- Respiratory alkalosis results from the excessive loss of carbon dioxide through hyperventilation, direct stimulation of the respiratory centers.
- Common causes include
  1. Hyperventilation
  2. Anxiety and fear
  3. Improperly set ventilators
  4. Drugs:
     a. Salicylates
     b. Catecholamines
     c. Progesterone
  5. Hypoxemia
  6. Asphyxiation
  7. High altitudes
  8. Shock
  9. Pneumonia
  10. Asthma
  11. Pulmonary emboli

COLLABORATIVE MANAGEMENT

- The nurse assesses for
  1. Central nervous system changes:
     a. Memory changes
     b. Changes in the ability to concentrate

    c. Anxiety, irritability
    d. Tetany, seizures
    e. Positive Chvostek's sign
    f. Positive Trousseau's sign
    g. Paresthesia
  2. Neuromuscular changes:
    a. Hyperreflexia
    b. Muscle cramping and twitching
    c. Skeletal muscle weakness
  3. Cardiac changes:
    a. Increased heart rate
    b. Normal or low blood pressure
    c. Increased digitalis toxicity
  4. Respiratory changes (increased rate and depth of ventilation)

- Respiratory alkalosis is managed by treating the underlying cause of the alkalosis usually with drug therapy.

ALS

See Amyotrophic Lateral Sclerosis.

ALZHEIMER'S DISEASE

OVERVIEW

- Alzheimer's disease, also known as senile dementia, Alzheimer's type (SDAT), is a chronic, progressive, degenerative disease that accounts for 60% of the dementias occurring in persons older than 65 years.
- Alzheimer's disease is also seen in people in their 40s and 50s, which is referred to as early dementia, or *presenile dementia, Alzheimer's type.*
- The disease is characterized by memory loss and progressive cognitive impairment caused by neurofibrillary tangles and senile plaques in the brain.

63

- The exact cause of Alzheimer's disease is unknown; genetic predisposition, chemical changes, environmental agents, and immunologic causes are theories and risk factors.

COLLABORATIVE MANAGEMENT

Assessment

- The nurse records the client's
    1. Age
    2. Current employment status and work history
    3. Ability to fulfill household responsibilities: grocery shopping, laundry, and meal planning
    4. Driving ability
    5. Ability to handle routine financial transactions
    6. Communication skills
    7. Behavior
    8. Family history of Alzheimer's disease
    9. Past medical history, with particular attention to head trauma, viral illness, or exposure to metal or toxic waste
- The nurse assesses the client for
    1. Indicators of the stages of the disease:
        a. Early or stage I Alzheimer's is characterized by forgetfulness, mild memory loss, decreased performance, loss of judgment and subtle changes in personality and behavior.
        b. Mild or stage II is characterized by severe impairments in all cognitive functions, gross intellectual impairments, physical impairment, loss of ability to care for self, visual-spacial deficits, and speech-language problems.
        c. Severe or stage III is characterized by severe physical and cognitive deterioration and total dependence for activities of daily living (ADL).
    2. Cognitive changes, such as deficits in attention, concentration, judgment, and perception
    3. Alterations in communication abilities
    4. Indications of tremors, myoclonus, and seizure activity
    5. Reaction to changes in routine and environment
    6. Impaired social interaction, disinterest in hobbies, loss of interest in current affairs
    7. Behavioral changes such as aggressiveness, sexual acting out, rapid mood swings, and increased confusion at night or when fatigued

8. Wandering
9. Hoarding of other's or own belongings
10. Paranoia, delusions, hallucinations
11. Depression
12. Dependency in self-care
- Genetic testing, specifically for apolipoprotein E (apo E), may be helpful as an ancillary test

Planning and Implementation

✦ NDx: Altered Thought Processes

- The nurse
  1. Provides a structured, consistent environment
  2. Establishes a daily routine; explains changes in routine before they occur and again immediately before they take place
  3. Places familiar objects, clocks, and single-date calendars in easy view of the client
  4. Reorients the client to the environment frequently (early stages)
  5. Uses validation therapy for later stages of the disease to prevent agitation
  6. Assists the client to maintain independence in ADL as long as possible; places complete clothing outfits on a single hanger (if client is able to dress)
  7. Allows the client to participate in meal planning, grocery shopping, and other household routines as able
  8. Suggests adaptive devices for the home, such as grab bars in the bathroom
  9. Develops an individualized bowel and bladder program for the client
  10. Attracts the client's attention before conversing
  11. Keeps the environment free of distractions
  12. Speaks slowly and distinctly in short, clear sentences
  13. Allows sufficient time for the client to respond
  14. Administers ergoloid mesylates (Hydergine, Niloric) or tacrine (Cognex), as ordered
  15. Tetrahydroaminoacridine (THA) (Tactrine), Aricept, and physostigmine (Antilirium) have improved cognitive function in some clients for short periods of time
  16. Administers amitriptyline (Elavil, Levate◆), doxepin (Sinequan, Triadapin◆), or imipramine (Tofranil, Impril◆) to treat depression, as ordered

65

✦ NDx: Risk for Injury

- The nurse
    1. Ensures that the client always wears an identification bracelet
    2. Ensures that alarms or other distractions for outside doors are working properly at all times
    3. Checks the client frequently
    4. Takes the client for walks several times per day and encourages the client to participate in activities to decrease his or her restlessness
    5. Talks calmly and softly, redirecting the client as needed and using diversion
    6. Implements seizure precautions if there is a history of seizures
    7. Administers phenytoin (Dilantin) or carbamazepine (Tegretol, Mazepine◆) to treat seizures, as ordered
    8. Administers psychotropic agents (Haldol, Mellaril), as ordered, to treat specific emotional or psychotic behaviors, such as hallucinations or delusions
    9. Observes for side effects of psychotropic agents, including increased confusion and extrapyramidal symptoms

✦ NDx: Ineffective Family Coping

- The nurse
    1. Advises the family to seek legal counsel regarding the client's competency and the need to obtain guardianship or durable power of attorney
    2. Refers the family to a local support group affiliated with the Alzheimer's Disease and Related Disorders Association
    3. Encourages the family to maintain its own social network and to obtain respite care periodically
    4. Assists the family to identify and develop strategies to cope with the long-term consequences of the disease

✦ NDx: Sleep Pattern Disturbance

- The nurse
    1. Establishes prebedtime ritual:
        a. Personal hygiene
        b. Quiet environment
        c. Back rub or small snack

2. Keeps the client active during the day with a balance between active and passive activities; discourages the client from taking a nap, if possible
3. Administers chloral hydrate, as ordered, for sleep

Continuing Care

- Whenever possible, the client should be assigned to a case manager who can assess their need for health care resources and facilitate appropriate placement throughout the continuum of care
- The nurse teaches the client and family
  1. How to assist the client with ADL
  2. How to use assistive-adaptive equipment
  3. How to select and prepare food that the client is able to chew and swallow, with dietary consultation
  4. How to prevent wandering
  5. What to do in the event of seizure
  6. How to prevent the client from injury
  7. Drug information, if prescribed
  8. How to implement the prescribed exercise program
  9. The importance of follow-up visits with the physician and other therapists
- The nurse refers the client's family and significant others to the local chapter of the Alzheimer's Disease and Related Disorders Association.

AMENORRHEA

OVERVIEW

- *Amenorrhea* is the absence of menstrual periods.
- *Primary amenorrhea,* menstruation that has failed to occur by age 16, is associated with anomalies of the reproductive tract; hypothalamic and pituitary disorders, such as delayed puberty; systemic diseases such as thyroid and adrenal dysfunction, diabetes, and malnutrition; ovarian disease; and malformations of the reproductive tract.
- *Secondary amenorrhea,* menstruation that has started but has stopped and has not recurred for 3 months, is

associated with functional disorders such as pregnancy; menopause; lactation; cervical stenosis; Asherman's syndrome; polycystic ovary disease; pituitary tumor or insufficiency; psychogenic stress; excessive physical activities; medications such as antihypertensives, birth control pills, and phenothiazines; nutritional conditions such as obesity, anorexia nervosa, and sudden weight loss; and ovarian disease, failure, or destruction.

COLLABORATIVE MANAGEMENT
Assessment
- The nurse assesses for
    1. Family history of menstruation
    2. Family history of genetic abnormalities
    3. Ambiguous genitalia at birth
    4. Development of secondary sex characteristics
    5. Nutritional habits
    6. Past surgery
    7. Emotional stress
    8. Physical characteristics of primary amenorrhea:
        a. Anomalies of the genital tract, including external genitalia
        b. Short stature
        c. Lack of breast development
        d. Lack of pubic and axillary hair
    9. Factors involved in secondary amenorrhea:
        a. Menstrual history
        b. Obstetric history
        c. History of sexual activity
        d. Symptoms of pregnancy
        e. Current and past eating habits and dieting
        f. Physical activity
        g. Hormonal deficiencies
        h. Drug history
        i. Galactorrhea (watery or milky breast secretions in non-breastfeeding or nulliparous women)
        j. Hirsutism (unusual hair growth in women)

Interventions
- Management is directed at correcting the underlying cause:
    1. Hormone replacement
    2. Corrective surgery
    3. Stimulation of ovulation

68

4. Periodic progesterone withdrawal
5. Counseling and emotional support

AMPUTATION

OVERVIEW

- Amputation is a removal of a part of the body.
- The psychologic ramifications of the procedure are often more devastating than the physical impairment that results.
- *Traumatic* amputation occurs when a body part is severed unexpectedly, such as by a saw; attempts to replant it may be made.
- *Prehospital care* of a severed digit or other body part includes
    1. Wrapping the body part in a cool, dry cloth, moistened with saline, if possible.
    2. Placing the body part in a sealed plastic bag and placing the bag in ice water
- Methods of *surgical* amputation include
    1. *Open,* or guillotine, amputation, used for clients who have or are likely to develop an infection; the wound remains open, with drains to allow drainage to escape from the site until the infection clears
    2. *Closed,* or flap, amputation, in which skin flaps are pulled over the bone end and are sutured in place as part of the amputation procedure
- Loss of all or any of the small toes presents minor disability.
- Loss of the great toe is significant because it affects balance, gait, and "push-off" ability during walking.
- Midfoot amputations (e.g., LisFranc and Chopart procedures) and the Syme procedure (most of the foot is removed, but the ankle remains intact) are performed for peripheral vascular disease.
- Other lower extremity amputations are below-knee amputation (BKA), above-knee amputation (AKA), hip disarticulation (removal of the hip joint), and hemicorporectomy (hemipelvectomy and translumbar amputation).

- *Upper extremity* amputations are generally more incapacitating because the arms and hands are needed for activities of daily living (ADL).
- Complications of elective or traumatic amputations include hemorrhage, infection, phantom limb pain, problems associated with immobility, neuroma, and flexion contractures.

➤ Transcultural Considerations

The incidence of lower extremity amputations is greater in the African-American population because the incidence of peripheral vascular disease is greater in this population.

COLLABORATIVE MANAGEMENT
Assessment

- The nurse assesses for
    1. Skin color, temperature, sensation, and pulses in both the affected and unaffected extremities
    2. Capillary refill
    3. Concurrent medical problems
    4. The client's psychologic preparation for an amputation
    5. Self-concept, self-esteem, and body image disturbance
    6. The family's reaction to the surgery
    7. Ankle/brachial index by dividing ankle systolic pressure by brachial systolic pressure (should be greater than or equal to 1.00)
    8. Results of blood flow studies, such as ultrasound, plethysmography, and laser Doppler flowmetry

Interventions

- The nurse
    1. Assists the client to perform range-of-motion (ROM) and muscle-strengthening exercises
    2. Teaches the client to use assistive-adaptive devices (e.g., crutches, walker) before surgery, if appropriate
    3. Arranges for the client to see a prosthetist before surgery to begin planning for postoperative needs; some clients are fitted with temporary prostheses at the time of surgery

4. Initiates special measures for lower extremity amputations:
   a. Ensures that the bed is equipped with a firm mattress and a trapeze and overhead frame
   b. Assists the client into a prone position every 3 to 4 hours for 20 to 30 minutes to prevent hip contractures
   c. Instructs the client to push the residual limb down toward the bed while supporting it on a pillow (for BKAs)
   d. Elevates the limb on a pillow for 24 hours after surgery (this is controversial; follow hospital policy)
   e. Inspects the limb daily to ensure that it lies flat on the bed surface
5. Takes measures to prevent complications of immobility, such as atelectasis, pneumonia, confusion, or thromboembolism

- Using the word "stump" when referring to the remaining portion of the limb is controversial.
- The nurse
  1. Assesses the client's verbal and nonverbal references to the affected area
  2. Asks the client to verbalize his or her feelings about changes in body image and self-esteem; the client may verbalize acceptance but refuse to look at the area during a dressing change
  3. Provides realistic information about potential changes in lifestyle, job, and recreational activities; however, many clients are able to return to previous activities because of advances in prosthetic devices
  4. Refers to a vocational counselor for evaluation as appropriate
  5. Helps the client set realistic goals and objectives
  6. Stresses the client's personal strengths
  7. Reassures the client and his or her sexual partner that an intimate relationship is possible; assists them to adjust to changes; refers them to a sexual counselor as needed
- The nurse provides relief measures for postoperative or post-traumatic stump pain.
- The nurse recognizes that phantom limb pain is real.
  1. The client complains of pain in the removed body part.

2. The pain is described as burning, crushing, or cramping or as a numbness or tingling; the client feels that the missing part is in a distorted position.
3. Pain is triggered by touching the stump and increased stress, anxiety, or depression.
4. Opioids may not be as effective for phantom limb pain but are effective for stump pain.
5. Beta-blocking agents, anticonvulsants, and antispasmodics may be prescribed for phantom limb pain.
6. Other treatment measures include ultrasound, massage, exercises, biofeedback, distraction therapy, hypnosis, and psychotherapy.

- The nurse
  1. Recognizes that initial pressure dressings and drains are removed 48 to 72 hours after surgery
  2. Inspects the wound for signs of inflammation, such as redness and swelling
  3. Records the characteristics of drainage
  4. Follows hospital procedure for wrapping the stump; a stump shrinker or heavy stockinette may be used in place of an elastic bandage
  5. Monitors the skin flap for adequate tissue perfusion
  6. Recognizes that the area should be warm, not hot
  7. Assesses for the presence of proximal pulses and compares to the other extremity

- The nurse teaches care of the prosthesis, if worn:
  1. Refinish a wooden prosthesis once every 6 months.
  2. Clean it with mild soap and water, and dry it completely.
  3. Replace worn inserts and liners when heavily soiled.
  4. Check all mechanical parts periodically for unusual sound or movements.
  5. Grease mechanical parts as instructed by the prosthetist.
  6. Use garters to keep stockings or socks in place.

- The nurse emphasizes the importance of follow-up visits with the physician(s) and other therapists.

ℰ Considerations for Elderly Clients

1. Hip disarticulation and higher amputations are not done for elderly clients because the prostheses are

cumbersome and increased energy is required for ambulation.

2. Complications of immobility may be more common in elderly clients.
3. Capillary refill testing may be done using the skin near the nail bed if nails are too thick.

Amyotrophic lateral sclerosis

- Amyotrophic lateral sclerosis (ALS), also known as Lou Gehrig's disease, is a progressive degenerative disease involving the motor system.
- Mental status changes do not occur.
- The disease is characterized by fatigue, muscle atrophy, weakness, tongue atrophy, dysphagia, nasal quality to speech, and dysarthria.
- As the disease progresses, flaccid quadriplegia develops and respiratory muscles become involved, leading to pneumonia and death.
- There is no known cure.
- Treatment is symptomatic and directed toward the following: impaired physical mobility, total self-care deficit, altered nutritional status, ineffective breathing pattern and airway clearance, impaired gas exchange, and urinary and bowel incontinence.
- Riluzole (Rilutek) has been approved for use for clients with ALS and is associated with increased survival time.

Anal fissure

See Fissure, Anal.

ANAL FISTULA

See Fistula, Anal.

ANAPHYLAXIS

OVERVIEW

- Anaphylaxis is the rapid, systemic, simultaneous occurrence of a type I hypersensitivity reaction in multiple organs.
- Anaphylaxis occurs within seconds to minutes of exposure to a causative allergen, such as a drug, foreign protein, insect venom, or food.

COLLABORATIVE MANAGEMENT

Assessment

- The nurse assesses for
  1. Apprehension
  2. Weakness
  3. Anxiety (the client may complain of a feeling of impending doom)
  4. Generalized pruritus and urticaria
  5. Erythema
  6. Angioedema of the eyes, lips, or tongue
  7. Cutaneous wheals or urticarial eruptions that are intensely pruritic and sometimes coalesce
  8. Bronchoconstriction and spasm, as well as mucosal edema and hypersecretion of mucus
  9. Respiratory assessment that reveals congestion, rhinorrhea, dyspnea, wheezing, crackles, and diminished breath sounds
  10. Laryngeal edema (hoarseness, stridor)
  11. Hypotension
  12. Rapid, weak, and possibly irregular pulse
  13. Diaphoresis
  14. Confusion
  15. Dysrhythmias

16. Shock
17. Cardiac arrest

Interventions

- The nurse
  1. Establishes an airway *immediately* and has a tracheostomy set available (emergency care)
  2. Administers supplemental oxygen through a nasal cannula or face mask
  3. Elevates the head of bed unless contraindicated secondary to hypotension
- Medications that may be administered include:
  1. Epinephrine (1:1000), 0.2 to 0.5 mL as soon as the client displays symptoms of systemic anaphylaxis; may repeat every 15 to 20 minutes if needed
  2. Diphenhydramine (Benadryl) Allerdryl, 25 to 100 mg, to treat angioedema and urticaria
  3. Aminophylline, 6 mg/kg intravenously for severe bronchospasm then initiates maintenance therapy at 0.3 to 0.5 mg/kg/hr
  4. Inhaled beta-adrenergic agonist such as metaproterenol (Alupent) or albuterol (Proventil) every 2 to 4 hours
  5. Corticosteroids for persistent symptoms
- The nurse
  1. Monitors arterial blood gases
  2. Suctions fluids as needed
  3. Performs frequent respiratory assessments
  4. Monitors cardiac rhythm (dysrhythmias can occur secondary to anaphylaxis or treatment)
  5. Carefully observes the client for fluid overload from rapid administration of medications, IV fluids
- The nurse consults with the physician about the need for the client to carry an emergency anaphylaxis kit.

ANEMIA, APLASTIC

OVERVIEW

- Aplastic anemia is a deficiency of circulating erythrocytes (red blood cells [RBCs]) because of arrested development of RBCs within the bone marrow. It is usually accompanied by agranulocytosis (decreased leukocytes) and thrombocytopenia (decreased platelets).
- Deficiency of all three types of cells is called *pancytopenia.*
- The cause is often unknown but may be associated with exposure to myelotoxic agents and viral infection.

COLLABORATIVE MANAGEMENT

- Blood transfusions are the mainstay of treatment.
- Drugs to treat underlying disease may be given in addition to general immunosuppressive agents.
- Splenectomy and bone marrow transplantation may be necessary for client survival.

ANEMIA, FOLIC ACID DEFICIENCY

OVERVIEW

- Folic acid deficiency is often produced by vitamin B_{12} deficiency; primary folic acid deficiency may also occur.
- Causes of folic acid deficiency include poor nutrition (especially in clients with alcoholism); malabsorption syndromes, such as Crohn's disease; and drugs such as methotrexate, some anticonvulsants, and oral contraceptives, which block folic acid conversion to its active form.

COLLABORATIVE MANAGEMENT

- Clinical manifestations are similar to those for vitamin B_{12} deficiency without the accompanying nervous system manifestations.

76

- Prevention of folic acid deficiency is aimed at identifying high-risk clients, such as alcoholics, the elderly, and others susceptible to malnutrition.
- The nurse
  1. Teaches the client to consume foods high in folic acid, such as green leafy vegetables, liver, yeast, citrus fruits, dried beans, and nuts
  2. Administers folic acid supplements

Anemia, Iron Deficiency

OVERVIEW

- Iron deficiency anemia is the most common type of anemia; if a person has an iron deficiency, depletion of iron stores occurs first, followed by a reduction in hemoglobin. As a result, the red blood cells (RBCs) are small (microcytic).
- Iron deficiency anemia can result from blood loss, increased metabolic energy demands, gastrointestinal malabsorption, and dietary inadequacy.

COLLABORATIVE MANAGEMENT

- Weakness and pallor are typical mild manifestations.
- The nurse
  1. Teaches the client to increase oral intake of iron by reviewing the common sources obtained from food, such as liver and other organ meats, red meat, kidney beans, whole wheat breads and cereals, green leafy vegetables, carrots, egg yolks, and raisins and other dried fruit
  2. Administers iron orally or parenterally
  3. Explains that iron preparations often change the color of stools to black

ANEMIA, SICKLE CELL

OVERVIEW

- Sickle cell anemia is an autosomal codominant hereditary disorder that causes a single amino acid change in
  the beta chain of the hemoglobin molecule, creating
  an abnormal type of hemoglobin, hemoglobin S (Hb
  S), instead of hemoglobin A. Insufficient oxygen causes
  the red blood cells (RBCs) containing Hb S to become
  sickle-shaped. As a result, they clump together and form
  clusters that obstruct capillary blood flow. In addition,
  the cells live 20 days rather than the usual 120-day life
  span of normal RBCs.

 Transcultural Considerations

Sickle cell anemia occurs frequently in African-Americans as well as in African, Mediterranean, Asian, Caribbean, Middle Eastern, and Central American populations.

COLLABORATIVE MANAGEMENT

Assessment

- The nurse
  1. Questions the client about previous crises, includ-
     ing precipitating events, severity, and ususal treat-
     ments
  2. Reviews all activities and events during the previ-
     ous 24 hours with the client to obtain information
     about fatigue, activity tolerance, and participation
     in activities of daily living (ADL)
- The physical assessment reveals
  1. Pain (the most common symptom during sickle
     cell crisis)
  2. Extremities distal to blood vessels occlusion that
     are cool to the touch with slow capillary refill
  3. Skin that is pale or cyanotic. With cyanosis the
     lips, and tongue are gray and the palms, soles, con-
     junctiva, and nail beds have a bluish tinge
  4. Jaundice
  5. Stasis ulcers or pressure ulcers may be present on
     the lower extremities

6. Abdominal organs are usually the first to be damaged as a result of multiple episodes of hypoxia and ischemia
7. Joints may be damaged and undergo necrotic degeneration. Range of motion in all joints may be limited
8. Seizure activity or clinical manifestations of a stroke secondary to central nervous system infarct or hypoxia
9. Behavioral changes from hypoxia

- Laboratory findings indicative of sickle cell disease include large percentage of Hb S present on electrophoresis, low hematocrit, elevated reticulocyte, elevated white cell count.
- Bone changes may be seen on x-ray.

Interventions

- Pain management in sickle cell crisis
  1. Meperidine (Demerol), morphine, hydromorphone (Dilaudid) are administered IV on a *routine* schedule until relief is obtained; dose is then tapered
  2. Moderate pain is treated with oral doses of codeine, morphine sulfate or NSAIDs
- Hydroxyurea (Hydrea) may be used for pain management in adults.
- Nonpharmacologic pain management
  1. Relaxation techniques
  2. Proper positioning
  3. Aromatherapy, warm room
  4. Warm soaks or compresses
- The nurse assesses the client for infection.
  1. Monitors CBC with differential white count
  2. Inspects the oral mucosa for lesions indicating a fungal or viral infection
  3. Inspects the urine for odor, cloudiness and asks the client about sensation of urgency, burning or pain on urination
  4. Prophylactic antibiotic therapy may be given
- Management of sickle cell anemia focuses on prevention and treatment of crises.
- The nurse
  1. Teaches the client the early signs and symptoms of hypoxia and hypoxemia, and sickle cell crisis
  2. Explains the hereditary nature of the disease, especially as related to childbearing

1. Clients who show evidence of damage to vital organs are advised against becoming pregnant.
2. The use of oral contraceptives is controversial.

- Treatment of crises includes pain management, fluid replacement, oxygen therapy, and correction of the condition contributing to hypoxia.
- Bone marrow transplantation may be undertaken to permanently correct the problem of abnormal hemoglobin.

ANEMIA, VITAMIN B$_{12}$ DEFICIENCY

OVERVIEW

- A deficiency of vitamin B$_{12}$ indirectly causes anemia by inhibiting folic acid transportation and limiting DNA synthesis in red blood cell precursor cells; the immature precursor cells increase in size (macrocytic).
- Anemia caused by failure to absorb vitamin B$_{12}$ is called *pernicious* anemia.

COLLABORATIVE MANAGEMENT

- Anemia as a result of vitamin B$_{12}$ deficiency may be mild or severe, usually develops slowly, and produces few symptoms.

Assessment

- The nurse assesses the client for
  1. Severe pallor
  2. Jaundice
  3. Glossitis (smooth, red, "beefy" tongue)
  4. Fatigue
  5. Weight loss
  6. Paresthesias in the feet and hands
  7. Disturbances of balance and gait

Interventions

- The nurse
    1. Teaches the client to eat foods high in vitamin B_{12}, such as animal proteins, eggs, and dairy products
    2. Administers vitamin supplements
    3. Administers vitamin B_{12} parenterally on a regular basis, for pernicious anemia
    4. Encourages the client to rest as needed

ANEURYSMS

OVERVIEW

- An aneurysm is a permanent localized dilation of an artery, which enlarges the artery to at least one and a half times its normal diameter.
- An aneurysm forms when the media, or the middle layer of the artery, is weakened, producing a stretching effect in the intima (the inner layer) and adventitia (the outer layer of the artery).
- The effect of blood pressure on the artery wall produces further weakness in the media and enlarges the aneurysm.
- The most common cause is arteriosclerosis; atheromatous plaque forms and weakens the intimal surface.
- Hypertension and cigarette smoking are contributing factors.
- The types of aneurysms include
    1. *Saccular,* an outpouching from a distinct portion of the artery wall
    2. *Fusiform,* the diffuse dilation involving the total circumference of the artery
    3. *Dissecting,* a cavity formed when blood separates the layers of the artery wall
- The most common aneurysm site is the aorta.
- Abdominal aneurysms arise below the level of renal arteries but above the iliac bifurcation.
- Thoracic aneurysms develop between the origin of the left subclavian artery and the diaphragm.
- The thoracic aorta is the most common site for dissecting aneurysms.

- Femoral and popliteal aneurysms are relatively uncommon.
- Aneurysms can thrombose, embolize, or rupture (the most frequent and life-threatening complication).

COLLABORATIVE MANAGEMENT

Assessment

- The nurse assesses for clinical manifestations of abdominal aortic aneurysms:
    1. Prominent pulsation in the upper abdomen (do not palpate)
    2. Abdominal bruit
    3. Abdominal, flank, or back pain
    4. Severe sudden pain (which may radiate), abdominal distention, and hypovolemic shock, *if* rupture occurs
- The nurse assesses for clinical manifestations of thoracic aneurysms:
    1. Hoarseness
    2. Shortness of breath
    3. Difficulty swallowing
    4. Visible mass above the suprasternal notch (occasional)
    5. Sudden and excruciating back or chest pain, *if* rupture occurs
- The nurse also assesses for
    1. Presence of mass on x-ray
    2. Results of ultrasonography

Interventions

Nonsurgical Management

- Antihypertensive drugs are prescribed to maintain normal blood pressure and to decrease stress on the aneurysm.
- The nurse
    1. Teaches the client the importance of keeping scheduled CT scan appointments to monitor growth of the aneurysm
    2. Reviews with the client the clinical manifestations of aneurysms, which need to be promptly reported

Surgical Management

- Surgical removal of the aneurysm and replacement of the excised portion with graft placement may be performed as an elective or emergency procedure. Ruptures always require emergency surgery.

- The nurse provides preoperative care:
  1. Administers large volumes of intravenous fluids if the aneurysm has ruptured to maintain tissue perfusion and blood pressure
  2. Assesses all peripheral pulses to serve as a baseline for comparison after surgery
  3. Provides routine preoperative care
- Postoperative care varies with the type of aneurysm repair.
- Care of the client with an abdominal aneurysm repair is similar to that provided for clients with other abdominal surgeries. The client is admitted to the critical care unit and is often maintained on a mechanical ventilator overnight.
- The nurse provides specific postoperative care, in addition to providing routine postoperative care:
  1. Assesses vital signs every hour
  2. Assesses circulation by checking pulses distal to the graft site
  3. Reports signs of occlusion immediately to the physician, such as pulse changes, severe pain, cool to cold extremities below the graft, and white or blue extremities
- Abdominal aortic aneurysm repair requires assessment of renal function because the aorta is clamped during the repair, potentially compromising the blood flow to the kidneys.
- The nurse additionally
  1. Assesses hourly urinary output and urine color
  2. Monitors daily blood urea nitrogen and creatinine levels
  3. Limits elevation of the head of the bed to 45 degrees to avoid flexion of the graft
  4. Assesses the client's respiratory rate and depth, and breath sounds hourly
  5. Administers opioid analgesics for pain, as ordered
  6. Maintains nasogastric tube suction for 3 or 4 days until bowel sounds return
  7. Monitors for complications such as myocardial infaction, graft occlusion or rupture, hypovolemia or renal failure, respiratory distress, and paralytic illeus

- Care of the client undergoing thoracic aneurysm repair is similar to other thoracic surgeries. (See Cancer, Lung.)
- The nurse additionally
    1. Assesses for signs of bleeding by monitoring chest tube drainage for excess drainage
    2. Monitors for cardiac dysrhythmias, paraplegia, and respiratory distress
    3. Teaches the client with abdominal aortic aneurysms to report abdominal fullness, pain or back pain
    4. Instructs the client with thoracic aneurysm repair to report back pain, shortness of breath, difficulty swallowing, or hoarseness

Continuing Care

- The nurse emphasizes the importance of compliance with the schedule of CTs to monitor the size of the aneurysm in clients who have not had surgery.
- The nurse
    1. Teaches the client to restrict activities (if surgery was performed)
        a. Avoid lifting heavy objects for 6 to 12 weeks postoperatively
        b. Use discretion in activities that involve pulling, pushing, or straining, such as vacuuming, changing bed linens, moving furniture, mopping or sweeping, raking leaves, mowing grass, and chopping wood
        c. Defer driving a car for several weeks
    2. Provides written and oral wound care instructions, if needed
    3. Provides pain management instructions, as ordered

ANORECTAL ABSCESSES

See Abscesses, Anorectal.

ANOREXIA NERVOSA

OVERVIEW

- Anorexia nervosa is a serious eating disorder that takes the form of indirect self-destructive behavior and can become life-threatening; it is the clinical syndrome of self-induced starvation.
- The anorexic person refuses to eat because of an intense fear of losing control of eating and becoming fat.
- The disorder occurs primarily in females, and onset occurs during early adolescence.
- Medical sequelae occur from the effects of starvation and unhealthy behaviors, such as purging by vomiting or abuse of laxatives or diuretics.
- *Diagnostic and Statistical Manual of Mental Disorders,* Fourth Edition (*DSM-IV*) diagnostic criteria include

    1. Refusal to maintain body weight at or above a minimally normal weight for age and height (e.g., weight loss leading to maintenance of body weight less than 85% of that expected; or failure to make expected weight gain during period of growth, leading to body weight less than 85% of that expected).
    2. Intense fear of gaining weight or becoming fat, even though underweight.
    3. Disturbance in the way in which one's body weight or shape is experienced, undue influence of body weight or shape on self-evaluation, or denial of the seriousness of the current low body weight.
    4. In postmenarcheal females, amenorrhea, i.e., the absence of at least three consecutive menstrual cycles. (A woman is considered to have amenorrhea if her periods occur only following hormone, e.g., estrogen, administration.)

Specify type:

> **Restricting Type:** during the current episode of anorexia nervosa, the person has not regularly engaged in binge-eating or purging behavior (i.e., self-induced vomiting or the misuse of laxatives, diuretics, or enemas).

85

Binge-Eating/Purging Type: during the current episode of anorexia nervosa, the person has regularly engaged in binge-eating or purging behavior (i.e., self-induced vomiting or the misuse of laxatives, diuretics, or enemas).

 Transcultural Considerations

1. Anorexia nervosa is most commonly diagnosed in females from the middle and upper classes in the Western culture.
2. Anorexia nervosa occurs less often in African-American women than in Caucasian women.

COLLABORATIVE MANAGEMENT
Assessment

- The nurse records the client's
  1. Demographic data, including age, sex, socioeconomic status, education, and occupation
  2. History of medical problems, including gastrointestinal symptoms such as nausea, vomiting, esophagitis, irritable bowel syndrome, and constipation
  3. Concerns about physical functioning, such as weakness, fatigue, intolerance to cold, changes in sleep habits, swelling in body part, or seizures
  4. Weight history and data on current weight, height, and body build
  5. Sexual history, including onset of breast development; age, weight, and height at onset of menarche; menstrual history and details about amenorrhea, if present
  6. Attitudes and behaviors related to food and weight
  7. Reports of changes in appetite or denial of appetite, use of appetite-suppressant drugs, self-induced vomiting, and frequency of weighing self
  8. Typical pattern of eating
  9. Use of laxatives and diuretics and habits of hiding or throwing away food
  10. History of psychiatric illness and treatment
  11. Family history of psychiatric illness and treatment
  12. Activity level
  13. Use of cigarettes, alcohol, or drugs
- The nurse assesses for
  1. Weight loss (may be severely emaciated)

2. Amenorrhea

   3. Hypothermia (decreased core body temperature) to 95° F (35° C)

   4. Decreased blood pressure, heart rate, and respiratory rate

   5. Loss of muscle mass and subcutaneous fat

   6. Fine lanugo hair

   7. Hypokalemic metabolic acidosis from vomiting, laxatives, and diuretics

   8. Edema (resulting from decreased plasma proteins)

   9. Discolored tooth enamel from exposure to gastric acid

  10. Psychosocial factors, such as high academic achievement, motivation, and compliance; sense of ineffectiveness and low self-esteem; desire for parental approval and striving for perfection; and poor sexual adjustment

  11. Profound anemia (decreased hemoglobin, hematocrit, red blood cell count)

  12. Decreased serum albumin and serum transferrin levels

  13. Electrolyte imbalances (decreased potassium, chloride, magnesium, and calcium levels)

  14. Hypoglycemia

  15. Elevated BUN (in presence of dehydration)

  16. Elevated serum amylase level

  17. Hormone imbalances (decreased reproductive hormones and thyroxine)

- The nurse pays special attention to reports of a tendency toward

   1. Perfectionism

   2. Self-criticism

   3. Compulsiveness

   4. Low mood or fluctuations

   5. Anxiety

   6. Phobias

Planning and Implementation

   ✦ **NDx:** Altered Nutrition: Less than Body Requirements

- The nurse

   1. Provides a diet of 1200 to 1600 calories per day, in collaboration with the dietitian, with foods selected by the client

2. Increases calories gradually to ensure steady weight gain of 2 to 4 pounds (0.9 to 1.8 kg) per week and to avoid abdominal distention with gastric dilation
3. Administers intravenous (IV) fluids or liquid feedings by nasogastric tube, as ordered, if the client persistently refuses food

✦ NDx: Pain

- Opioid analgesics are *never* indicated because of potential decreased stomach and bowel motility.
- The nurse
    1. Administers acetaminophen (Tylenol), as ordered, for minor abdominal discomfort
    2. Administers antacids, as ordered, for the discomfort of indigestion
    3. Provides a low-lactose, low-lipid diet; milk products and fats are slowly introduced during the second or third week of refeeding and are withdrawn if cramping is severe

✦ NDx: Fluid Volume Deficit

- The nurse
    1. Provides hourly oral fluids, including water, juice, soda, coffee, and tea, but avoiding milk
    2. Administers isotonic IV fluids, as ordered, if oral fluids are refused or volume replacement is needed
    3. Maintains a strict record of intake and output
    4. Assesses blood pressure, urinary output and concentration, and skin and mucous membrane moisture

✦ NDx: Risk for Fluid Volume Excess

- Diuretics are not recommended for refeeding edema; they are indicated in heart failure.
- Refeeding edema responds well to low-salt diets.
- Fluid restriction is limited to 1000 to 1500 mL/day.
- The nurse
    1. Keeps the client's legs elevated to decrease dependent edema
    2. Cautions the client to remove restrictive jewelry, clothes, and shoes

✦ **NDx:** Constipation

- The nurse
    1. Initiates a bowel regimen, as ordered, including a bulk laxative such as psyllium (Metamucil) and a stool softener such as docusate (Colace)
    2. Administers a cathartic suppository such as bisacodyl (Dulcolax, Bisacolax◆) or a sodium phosphate (Fleet) enema for persistent constipation, as ordered
    3. Provides high-fiber foods and adequate fluids, in collaboration with the dietitian

✦ **NDx:** Anxiety

- Extremely anxious clients may require an antianxiety agent before meals (e.g., a short-acting anxiolytic agent such as lorazepam [Ativan, Novolorazem◆])
- The nurse
    1. Allows the client to control decisions and give input into non–food-related issues
    2. Provides emotional support and encouragement during mealtimes and after meals and snacks
    3. Teaches relaxation techniques and guided imagery

✦ **NDx:** Body Image Disturbance

- The nurse
    1. Encourages the client to express feelings about body size and function and points out misconceptions to the client without arguing
    2. Provides positive feedback for accurate perception of body size and function and helps the client to accept changes

✦ **NDx:** Ineffective Individual Coping

- The nurse
    1. Administers antidepressants, as ordered, if a diagnosis of depression is made
    2. Arranges individual therapy with a psychiatrist, psychologist, or psychiatric liaison nurse as an inpatient and after discharge, as ordered
    3. Teaches that support groups organized by recovering anorexics and families provide education and support during periods of stress for the client and family

- The nurse
    1. Monitors behavior and provides support combined with client motivation
    2. Instructs the client and family on specific information related to the illness and treatment plan, emphasizing the consequences of noncompliance

✦ **NDx:** Altered Family Processes

- The nurse
    1. Assists family members to understand the illness and the treatment approach
    2. Consults with the social worker or family therapist for referral and follow-up

Continuing Care

- Educational efforts are focused on teaching the client and family to recognize and understand the physical, behavioral, and emotional characteristics of the disease.
- The teaching plan is individualized to identify client-specific problems.
- The nurse teaches the client and family
    1. Use of food patterns and exchanges (consult with a dietitian)
    2. Avoidance of family conflicts at mealtimes
    3. The importance of follow-up visits with the physician(s)
    4. The importance of the recommended type and amount of exercise
- The nurse encourages the client and family to discuss their fears and concerns.
- The nurse provides appropriate information about health care resources, including the National Anorexic Aid Society.

Aortic Dissection

See Dissection, Aortic.

AORTIC INSUFFICIENCY (AORTIC REGURGITATION)

See Insufficiency, Aortic (Aortic Regurgitation).

AORTIC REGURGITATION

See Insufficiency, Aortic (Aortic Regurgitation).

AORTIC STENOSIS

See Stenosis, Aortic.

APHAKIA

See Refractive Errors.

APLASTIC ANEMIA

See Anemia, Aplastic.

APPENDICITIS

OVERVIEW

- Appendicitis is an acute inflammation of the vermiform appendix, the small, finger-like pouch attached to the cecum of the colon.
- Appendicitis occurs when there is ulceration of the mucosa or when the lumen of the appendix is obstructed with calculi composed of fecal material (fecaliths), calcium-phosphate–rich mucus, and inorganic salts.
- Inflammation leads to infection as bacteria invade the wall of the appendix.
- Appendicitis is the most common cause of acute inflammation in the right lower abdominal quadrant.
- Appendicitis may occur at any age, but the peak incidence is between the ages of 20 and 30 years.

⏳ Considerations for Elderly Clients

1. Appendicitis is not common in the elderly, but perforation occurs frequently as a complication of appendicitis.
2. The diagnosis of appendicitis is difficult to establish for the elderly because they have a decreased response to the usual pain signals and have vague or mild symptoms.

COLLABORATIVE MANAGEMENT

Assessment

- The nurse assesses for
  1. Sudden onset of abdominal pain originating in the epigastric or periumbilical area and shifting to the right lower quadrant
  2. Nausea and vomiting
  3. Anorexia after the initial diagnosis of pain
  4. Urge to defecate or pass flatus
  5. Abdominal tenderness, which may be absent in early stages or diffuse with localization to the right lower quadrant in later stages of inflammation (McBurney's point)
  6. Muscle rigidity and rebound tenderness

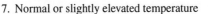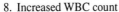

7. Normal or slightly elevated temperature
8. Increased WBC count

Interventions

- The nurse keeps the client on nothing-by-mouth status and administers fluids intravenously, as ordered, before emergent surgical appendectomy (removal of the appendix).
- Appendectomy may be performed as a *traditional* procedure through a small incision or by means of *laparoscopy.*
- If abscess is present, surgical drains are inserted during surgery.
- If peritonitis is present, the client will have a nasogastric tube in place to prevent gastric distention.
- The nurse provides routine postoperative care for a *traditional* appendectomy:
  1. Assesses the abdominal drains for excess drainage
  2. Maintains the client's nasogastric tube or other drainage devices if inserted intraoperatively for peritonitis
  3. Administers intravenous antibiotics
  4. Assists the client out of bed on the evening of surgery
  5. Administers opioid analgesia
- After a *laparoscopic* procedure, the nurse
  1. Monitors vital signs and puncture sites
  2. Prepares the client for discharge on the day of surgery or the next day

ARDS

See Adult Respiratory Distress Syndrome.

ARF

See Renal Failure, Acute.

ARTERIAL DISEASE, PERIPHERAL

OVERVIEW

- Peripheral arterial disease (PAD) is a chronic condition in which partial or total arterial occlusion deprives the lower extremities of oxygen or nutrients.
- Tissue damage generally occurs below the arterial destruction, and the location of the occlusion determines the location of tissue damage.
- Obstructions are characterized as inflow or outflow according to the arteries involved and their relationship to the inguinal ligament.
- Clients with chronic PAD seek treatment for the characteristic leg pain known as intermittent claudication.
- Four stages of PAD include
    1. Stage I: Asymptomatic:
        a. No claudication is present.
        b. Bruit or aneurysm may be present.
        c. Physical examination may rarely reveal decreased pulses.
    2. Stage II: Claudication:
        a. Muscle pain, cramping, or burning is exacerbated by exercise and relieved by rest.
        b. Symptoms are reproducible with exercise.
    3. Stage III: Rest pain:
        a. Pain while resting commonly wakes the client at night.
        b. Pain is described as a numbness, burning, toothache-type of pain.
        c. Pain usually occurs in the distal portion of the extremity (toes, arch, forefoot, or heel) and only rarely the calf or ankle.
        d. Pain is relieved by placing the extremity in a dependent position.
    4. Stage IV: Necrosis/gangrene:
        a. Ulcers and blackened tissue occur on the toes, forefoot, and heel.
        b. A distinctive gangrenous odor is present.
- Acute peripheral vascular disease occurs when there is an acute obstruction by a thrombus or embolus, caus-

ing severe, acute pain below the level of the obstruction.

- Risk factors for acute disease include hypertension, hyperlipidemia, diabetes mellitus, cigarette smoking, obesity, and familial predisposition.

💇 Women's Health Considerations

1. 25% of women ages 55 to 74 develop peripheral vascular disease.
2. Estrogen replacement therapy and cholesterol lowering drugs may slow the development of arteriosclerosis in women.
3. Women appear to be at increased risk for amputation when compared to men.

COLLABORATIVE MANAGEMENT
Assessment

- The nurse records the client's
    1. Leg pain with exercise or rest
    2. Discomfort in the lower back, buttocks, or thighs (inflow disease)
    3. Burning or cramping in the calves, ankles, feet, and toes (outflow disease)
    4. History of acute or chronic pain
* The nurse assesses for
    1. Ischemic changes of the extremity:
        a. Loss of hair on the lower calf, ankle, and foot
        b. Dry, scaly skin
        c. Thickened toenails
        d. Color changes (elevation pallor or dependent rubor)
        e. Mottled and cool or cold extremity
    2. Pulses present or absent
    3. Ulcer formation:
        a. Arterial ulcers develop on the toes, between the toes, or on upper aspect of the foot. They are painful.
        b. Diabetic ulcers develop on the plantar surface of the foot, over metatarsal heads, on the heel, or on pressure areas. They may not be painful.
        c. Venous stasis ulcers occur at the ankles, with discoloration of the lower extremity at the ulcer. They cause minimal pain.

Planning and Implementation

Nonsurgical Management

- The nurse teaches methods of increasing arterial blood flow in chronic arterial disease:
    1. Exercise, which promotes collateral circulation
    2. Position changes, which promote circulation and decrease swelling
    3. Improvement of vasodilation by providing warmth to the affected extremity, such as wearing socks or insulated bedroom shoes and maintaining a warm home environment; the nurse cautions the client not to apply direct heat to the lower limbs, which may cause burns due to decreased sensitivity
    4. Prevention of vasoconstriction by decreasing exposure to cold and avoiding nicotine, caffeine, and emotional stress
    5. Drug therapy, including vasodilators, defibrination agents, and antiplatelet therapy
    6. Control of hypertension
- *Percutaneous transluminal angioplasty* (PTA) dilates arteries that are occluded or stenosed with a balloon catheter.
- *Laser-assisted angioplasty* may be used to open an occluded artery.
- *Mechanical rotational abrasive atherectomy* is used to improve blood flow to ischemic limbs for scraping plaque while minimizing danger to the vessel wall.
- The nurse prepares the client for PTA or laser-assisted angioplasty by giving the client nothing by mouth after midnight and scrubbing the groin area with an aseptic soap, as ordered.
- After PTA, the nurse
    1. Observes the puncture site for bleeding
    2. Closely monitors vital signs
    3. Checks the distal pulses of both limbs
    4. Encourages the client to maintain bed rest for 6 to 8 hours, as ordered, with the limb in a straight position
    5. Administers anticoagulation therapy, such as heparin, for 3 days, as ordered; then administers dipyridamole for 3 to 6 months, as ordered
    6. Encourages the client to take aspirin on a permanent basis, as ordered

96

Surgical Management

- An emergency surgical *embolectomy* is performed on clients who experience an acute peripheral artery occlusion by an embolus.
- Surgery for clients with chronic PAD is usually elective.
- Arterial revascularization surgery is used to increase arterial blood flow in an affected limb and includes *inflow* procedures, such as aortoiliac bypass, aortofemoral bypass, and axillofemoral bypass; and *outflow* procedures, including femoropopliteal bypass and femorotibial bypass.
- Grafting materials for bypass surgeries include the autogenous saphenous vein and synthetic graft material, such as polytetrafluoroethylene.
- The nurse provides routine preoperative care.
- The nurse provides postoperative care:
    1. Monitors for the patency of the graft by checking for changes in the extremity:
        a. Color
        b. Temperature
        c. Pulse intensity
        d. Pain intensity (pain changes from a throbbing pain, which occurs from increased blood flow to the affected limb, to ischemic pain, as experienced before surgery)
    2. Marks the site of the distal pulses, which are best palpated or auscultated with Doppler ultrasonography
    3. Monitors the client's blood pressure, notifying the physician for increases and decreases beyond desired ranges
    4. Avoids bending the knee and hip of the affected limb
    5. Monitors for signs and symptoms of infection at or around the graft and incision sites, such as hardness, tenderness, redness, or warmth
- Thrombectomy (removal of the clot) is the most common treatment for acute graft occlusion; thrombolytic therapy may be used.
- Compartment syndrome occurs when tissue pressure within a confined body space becomes elevated and restricts blood flow.
    1. The nurse assesses the extremity for worsening pain, fullness, swelling, and tenseness.

2. Notifying the physician, removal or loosening of the dressing, and placing the extremity at the level of the heart is done when the nurse suspects compartment syndrome.

Continuing Care

- The client would benefit from a case manager who can follow the patient across the continuum of care.
- The nurse
    1. Reinforces the need for individualized positioning and an exercise plan
    2. Teaches the client to avoid raising the legs above the level of the heart unless he or she also has venous stasis
    3. Provides written and oral foot care instructions
        a. Keep the feet clean by washing with a mild soap in room-temperature water
        b. Keep the feet dry, especially between the toes and ankles
        c. Avoid injury or extended pressure to the feet and ankles
        d. Always wear comfortable, well-fitting shoes
        e. Keep the toenails clean, and cut them straight across
        f. Prevent dry, cracked skin
        g. Prevent exposure to extreme heat or cold
        h. Avoid heating pads
        i. Avoid constricting garments
    4. Provides dressing change and incision care instructions, if necessary
    5. Provides instructions concerning discharge medications
    6. Encourages the client to avoid smoking and to limit daily intake of fat to less than 30% of total calories

ARTERIOSCLEROSIS AND ATHEROSCLEROSIS

OVERVIEW

- Arteriosclerosis is a thickening or hardening of the arterial wall of the vascular system.
- Atherosclerosis, a type of arteriosclerosis, involves the formation of a plaque within the arterial wall.
- Atherosclerosis is the most common type of arterial obstruction; the process results in coronary artery disease (CAD), cerebrovascular disease (CVA), and peripheral vascular disease (PVD).
- The exact pathophysiologic mechanism of atherosclerosis is unknown.
- Atherosclerosis begins as a fatty streak on the intimal surface of an artery and develops into a fibrous plaque that partially or completely occludes the artery's blood flow.
- The final stage of atherosclerosis occurs when the fibrous lesion becomes calcified, hemorrhagic, ulcerated, or thrombosed.
- The rate of progression of this process is thought to be influenced by genetic factors; certain diseases, such as diabetes mellitus; and certain behaviors, including smoking, diet, and exercise.

𝒲 Women's Health Considerations

Coronary artery disease is much less common in premenopausal women than in age-matched men because of the lipid-lowering effect of estrogen.

COLLABORATIVE MANAGEMENT

Assessment

- The nurse assesses for
  1. Dry skin
  2. Atrophic changes, such as hair loss and thickened or clubbed nails
  3. Pallor around the lips and nail beds
  4. Rubor of the skin

5. Hypertension
6. Arterial pulsation, including rate and intensity (often diminished or absent)
7. Arterial bruits
8. Temperature differences in lower extremities
9. Prolonged capillary refill
10. Elevated serum cholesterol (elevated low-density lipoprotein [LDL] and low or normal high-density lipoprotein [HDL]) and triglyceride levels

Interventions

- The nurse
   1. Encourages the client to stop smoking (cigarette smoking lowers levels of HDL cholesterol)
   2. Teaches the client to limit dietary fat to 30% of total calories per day, in collaboration with the dietitian
   3. Teaches the client to limit cholesterol intake, as prescribed, following the Step One or Step Two American Heart Association diet
   4. Reinforces the need for a routine exercise program
   5. Administers cholesterol-lowering agents such as nicotinic acid (Nicobid) or clofibrate (Atromid-S, Claripex◆), as ordered, for clients who do not respond to diet therapy and other nondrug measures
   6. Teaches the client to seek a smoking cessation group such as the American Cancer Societ''s Fresh Start program, if needed

Transcultural Considerations

- African Americans have a higher prevalence of smoking than other ethnic groups.
- African American women are less likely to stop smoking than Caucasian women.

ARTHRITIS, RHEUMATOID

OVERVIEW

- Rheumatoid arthritis (RA) is a chronic, progressive, systemic inflammatory process that affects primarily synovial joints. It occurs three times more often in women than in men.
- RA is considered to be a probable autoimmune disease.
- Other areas of the body can be affected; vasculitis can cause malfunction and eventual failure of an organ or system.

 Transcultural Considerations

Prevalence rates among northern Native Americans are three to seven times higher than in non–Native Americans.

COLLABORATIVE MANAGEMENT

Assessment

- The nurse assesses the joints for
    1. Inflammation, tenderness, and stiffness; bilateral and symmetric joint involvement
    2. Deformities
    3. Moderate to severe pain and morning stiffness (lasting more than 30 minutes)
    4. Softness or a spongy feeling because of synovitis and effusions
    5. Muscle atrophy
    6. Decreased range of motion
- The nurse assesses for systemic involvement
    1. Low-grade fever
    2. Fatigue
    3. Weakness
    4. Anorexia, weight loss
    5. Paresthesia (particularly in elderly clients)
    6. Osteoporosis
    7. Anemia
    8. Vasculitis

9. Peripheral neuropathy
10. Pericarditis
11. Fibrotic lung disease
12. Renal disease
13. Sjogren's syndrome
14. Subcutaneous nodules
15. Respiratory compromise, including pleurisy, pneumonitis, diffuse interstitial fibrosis, and pulmonary hypertension
16. Ocular involvement, such as iritis or scleritis
17. Body image disturbance, poor self-esteem
18. Positive rheumatoid factor:
    a. Positive Rose-Waaler test
    b. Positive latex agglutination test
19. Elevated erythrocyte sedimentation rate
20. Positive antinuclear antibody test

Interventions

- The nurse administers drug therapy, as ordered:
    1. Salicylates (ASA, Ancasal◆):
       a. The initial dose is 12 to 18 tablets each day in four divided doses, until a therapeutic serum salicylate level of 20 to 25 mg/dL is achieved.
       b. When symptoms are relieved, the dosage is adjusted to a maintenance level of 15 to 20 mg/dL.
       c. Elderly clients are at high risk for side effects and toxic effects.
    2. Nonsteroidal anti-inflammatory drugs (NSAIDs):
       a. NSAIDs may be used in combination with salicylates if pain and inflammation are not decreased within 6 to 12 weeks.
       b. They may cause retention of fluids and sodium; observation is needed for hypertension, changes in renal function, and fluid retention.
    3. Gold therapy:
       a. Gold therapy is used in combination with salicylates and NSAIDs.
       b. It may induce remission as well as decrease pain and inflammation.
       c. Weekly injections of 25 to 50 mg of gold or sodium thiomalate (Myochrysine) are administered until improvement is seen or a cumulative total dosage of 1000 mg is administered.

d. Weekly injections are tapered slowly to once a month if they are effective; if remission is not seen after a total of 1000 mg has been given, the drug is discontinued.

   e. Toxic effects include rash, blood dyscrasias, and renal involvement.

   f. Oral gold preparation such as auranofin (Ridaura) may be used in place of injections; side effects include nausea, vomiting, and diarrhea.

  4. Antineoplastic agents:

   a. Antineoplastic agents are used in clients with life-threatening RA.

   b. Agents include azathioprine (Imuran) and methotrexate.

- Other analgesics include acetaminophen (Tylenol, Exdol◆, Datril), propoxyphene (Darvon, Novoropoxyn), and propoxyphene with acetaminophen (Darvocet-N 100).
- Other pain-relief measures include rest, positioning, ice and heat, imagery, music therapy, and stress management.
- If pain is not controlled, synovectomy, osteotomy, or total joint replacement may be necessary.
- The nurse
  1. Collaborates with the occupational therapist to obtain needed assistive-adaptive devices
  2. Teaches the client alternative strategies to activities of daily living, such as using the palm of the hand to squeeze toothpaste onto the toothbrush; collaborates with the dietary department to have the tray set up so the client can easily manipulate items
- The nurse identifies factors that contribute to fatigue:
  1. Anemia:
     a. Anemia is treated with iron, folic acid, vitamin supplements, or a combination of these.
     b. The client is assessed for drug-related blood loss, such as that caused by salicylate therapy, by testing the stool for occult blood.
  2. Muscle atrophy: daily exercise program
  3. Inadequate rest: quiet environment; warm beverage before bed
- The nurse teaches the principles of energy conservation:
  1. Pacing activities

2. Setting priorities
3. Allowing rest periods
4. Obtaining assistance when possible; delegating activities to the family
- The nurse
  1. Determines the client's reaction to changes
  2. Communicates acceptance of the client by establishing a trusting relationship
  3. Encourages the client to wear street clothes and his or her own night clothes or bathrobe
  4. Assists with grooming, such as shaving and make-up
  5. Emphasizes the client's strengths
  6. Treats the client with patience and understanding, since the client often appears to be manipulative and demanding

Continuing Care

- The nurse
  1. Assists the client and family to identify structural changes needed in the home before discharge
  2. Ensures that the client can correctly use all adaptive-assistive devices ordered for home use
  3. Provides a detailed plan of care at the time of discharge for clients to be transferred to a rehabilitation or long-term-care facility
  4. Provides drug information
  5. Reviews energy conservation measures
  6. Reviews the prescribed exercise program
  7. Teaches joint protection measures
  8. Refers the client to the dietitian, counselor, home health nurse, rehabilitation therapist, and local and state support groups as needed
  9. Emphasizes the importance of follow-up visits with the physician(s) and other therapists

ASBESTOSIS

See Pulmonary Disease, Occupational.

ASTIGMATISM

See Refractive Errors.

ATHEROSCLEROSIS

See Arteriosclerosis and Atherosclerosis.

ATOPIC ALLERGY

See Allergy, Atopic.

AUTOIMMUNE THROMBOCYTOPENIC PURPURA

See Thrombocytopenic Purpura, Autoimmune.

Back Pain

See Pain, Back.

Bacterial Endocarditis

See Endocarditis, Infective.

Bartholin's Cysts

See Cysts, Bartholin's.

Basal Cell Carcinoma

See Cancer, Skin.

Bell's Palsy

See Paralysis, Facial.

BENIGN PROSTATIC HYPERPLASIA

See Prostatic Hyperplasia, Benign.

BENIGN PROSTATIC HYPERTROPHY

See Prostatic Hypertrophy, Benign.

BERYLLIOSIS

See Pulmonary Disease, Occupational.

BLADDER TRAUMA

See Trauma, Bladder.

BLEEDING, DYSFUNCTIONAL UTERINE

OVERVIEW

- Dysfunctional uterine bleeding (DUB) is abnormal bleeding that is excessive or abnormal in amount or frequency without predisposing anatomic or systemic conditions.
- DUB occurs in the absence of ovulation related to ovarian function.
- DUB is associated with polycystic ovary disease, stress, extreme weight changes, and long-term use of drugs, including anticholinergics, morphine, and oral contraceptives.

COLLABORATIVE MANAGEMENT

Assessment

- The nurse assesses for
  1. Symptoms of anemia
  2. Symptoms of systemic disease, such as renal or hepatic disease
  3. Obesity
  4. Undernutrition
  5. Abnormal hair growth
  6. Abdominal pain
  7. Abdominal masses
  8. Abnormalities in external genitalia

Interventions

Nonsurgical Management

- The nurse
  1. Provides reassurance and comfort
  2. Administers hormone therapy for women with anovulatory DUB, which includes medroxyprogesterone or combination oral contraceptives, as ordered
- Treatment for women with ovulatory DUB who have inadequate progesterone levels includes progesterone supplements.

Surgical Management

- Surgical management includes diagnostic dilation and curettage (D&C), which involves scraping of the endometrial tissue to assess for possible causes of bleeding or to remove bleeding tissue; laser endometrial ablation; and hysterectomy.
- The nurse
    1. Prepares the client for surgery and provides routine postoperative care, including assessment of vaginal bleeding
    2. Reviews postoperative instructions after D&C:
        a. Avoid sexual intercourse, tub bathing, and the use of tampons for 2 weeks
        b. Understand that slight bleeding is normal, but if bleeding is as heavy as the normal menstrual period or persists for 2 weeks, notify the physician
        c. Use a hot water bottle or heating pad to relieve abdominal cramping
        d. Take mild analgesics, such as acetaminophen, for abdominal pain

Blindness

OVERVIEW

- Blindness may be total or diminished vision in one or both eyes.
- Types of blindness include
    1. Color: unable to distinguish certain colors; primary colors seen as gray
    2. Legally blind: best visual acuity with corrective lenses in the better eye 20/200 or less or if the widest diameter of the visual field in that eye is no greater than 20 degrees
    3. Loss of peripheral vision
    4. Loss of central vision

COLLABORATIVE MANAGEMENT

- The nurse
    1. Orients the client to the immediate environment
        a. Describes the approximate size of the room

109

    b. Describes a focal point in the room to serve as a point of reference, such as a chair or the bed, and then describes all other objects in relation to the focal point

    c. Accompanies the client to other important areas in the room (bathroom)

    d. Never leaves the client in the middle of an unfamiliar room

2. Assists the client in establishing the locations of personal objects, such as the call light, clock, and water pitcher
3. Never changes the location of objects without the client's consent
4. Sets up the meal tray and uses an imaginary clock placement to orient the client to food placement
5. Instructs the client to grasp her or his elbow while keeping the elbow close to the body and alerts the client to hazards such as steps or a narrow doorway when assisting with ambulation
6. Monitors the client's use of a cane (held in the client's dominant hand) to help detect obstacles
7. Knocks before entering the client's room; identifies self and the purpose of the visit
8. Provides for diversional activities

• Newly blind clients may experience a brief period of physical or psychologic immobility, hopelessness, anger, or denial.

BOILS

See Infections, Skin.

BONE CANCER

See Cancer, Bone.

BONE TUMORS, BENIGN

See Tumors, Benign Bone.

BONE TUMORS, MALIGNANT

See Cancer, Bone.

BPH

See Prostatic Hyperplasia, Benign.

BRAIN ABSCESSES

See Abscesses, Brain.

BRAIN TUMORS

See Tumors, Brain.

BREAST CANCER

See Cancer, Breast.

BREAST DISEASE, FIBROCYSTIC

OVERVIEW

- Fibrocystic breast disease (FBD), also called cystic disease or dysplasia, is the most common breast problem in women in their 20s.
- The *first stage* is characterized by premenstrual bilateral fullness and tenderness, especially in the outer upper quadrant; symptoms resolve after menstruation and recur before the next menstrual cycle.
- In the *second stage,* which occurs in women in their late 20s and 30s, bilateral, multicentric nodular areas appear that feel like small marbles, with fullness and soreness.
- The *third stage* occurs in clients between the ages of 35 and 55, when microscopic or macroscopic cysts develop.
- The cysts, which occur suddenly and are associated with pain, tenderness, or burning, are usually three-dimensional, smooth, mobile, and well delineated.
- The cause of FBD is unknown but appears to be related to normal fluctuations in progesterone and estrogen levels during the menstrual cycle.

COLLABORATIVE MANAGEMENT

- Hormonal manipulation is the primary means of intervention and includes oral contraceptives to suppress oversecretion of estrogen; tamoxifen (Nolvadex, TamofenR) may be used to decrease estrogen levels.
- Other interventions include
  1. Administration of vitamins C, E, and B complex
  2. Administration of diuretics to prevent premenstrual breast engorgement
  3. Avoidance of caffeine (but not scientifically proven)
  4. Avoidance of excess salt intake before menses
  5. Administration of mild analgesics
  6. Practice of regular breast self-examination
  7. Application of ice or heat
  8. Use of a well-padded, supportive brassiere

112

BREAST FIBROADENOMA

See Fibroadenoma, Breast.

BUERGER'S DISEASE

OVERVIEW

- Buerger's disease, or thromboangiitis obliterans, is an uncommon occlusive arterial vascular disease limited to medium and small arteries and veins in the body; larger arteries become involved in the late stages of disease.
- The distal upper and lower limbs are most frequently affected.
- The disease often extends to the perivascular tissue, resulting in fibrosis and scarring that binds the artery, vein, and nerve firmly together.
- The cause of the disease is unknown.
- There is a strong association with smoking, familial or genetic predisposition, and autoimmune causes.
- Smoking cessation usually arrests the disease process; persistence in smoking causes occlusion in more-proximal vessels.

COLLABORATIVE MANAGEMENT

- Clinical manifestations include
    1. Claudication (pain in muscles resulting from an inadequate blood supply) of the arch of the foot
    2. Intermittent claudication in the lower extremities
    3. Ischemic pain occurring in the digits while at rest
    4. Increased sensitivity to cold
    5. Complaints of coldness and numbness
    6. Diminished pulses in the distal extremities
    7. Cool extremities
    8. Red or cyanotic extremities in dependent position
    9. Ulcerations and gangrene in the digits
- Interventions include
    1. Complete abstinence from alcohol and smoking

113

2. Prevention of extreme or prolonged exposure to cold
3. Vasodilator drugs, such as nifedipine (Procardia, Adalat)

BULIMIA NERVOSA

OVERVIEW

- Bulimia nervosa is an eating disorder characterized by episodes of binge-eating that recur, are uncontrolled, and involve the ingestion of large amounts of food in a short time; women are typically affected in their late teens.
- Binge-eating is usually followed by some form of purging behavior, such as vomiting or the excess use of laxatives or diuretics.
- Purging behavior is an attempt to regain a sense of control and to eliminate the ingested calories; it may be precipitated by a variety of factors, such as hunger, boredom, anger, anxiety, or depression.
- An intense fear of fatness distinguishes the bulimic from people who binge-eat for pleasure or stress reduction.
- The *Diagnostic and Statistical Manual of Mental Disorders,* Fourth Edition (*DSM-IV*) diagnostic criteria include
    1. Recurrent episodes of binge eating. An example of binge eating is characterized by both of the following:
        a. Eating, in a discrete period of time (e.g., within any 2-hour period), an amount of food that is definitely larger than most people would eat during a similar period of time and under similar circumstances.
        b. A sense of lack of control over eating during the episode (e.g., a feeling that one cannot stop eating or control what or how much one is eating).
    2. Recurrent inappropriate compensatory behavior in order to prevent weight gain, such as self-induced vomiting; misuse of laxatives, diuretics, enemas,

or other medications; fasting; or excessive exercise.

3. The binge-eating and inappropriate compensatory behaviors both occur, on average, at least twice a week for 3 months.
4. Self-evaluation is unduly influenced by body shape and weight.
5. The disturbance does not occur exclusively during episodes of Anorexia Nervosa.

Specify type:

1. **Purging Type:** during the current episode of Bulimia Nervosa, the person has regularly engaged in self-induced vomiting or the misuse of laxatives, diuretics, or enemas.
2. **Nonpurging Type:** during the current episode of Bulimia Nervosa, the person has used other inappropriate compensatory behaviors, such as fasting or excessive exercise, but has not regularly engaged in self-induced vomiting or the misuse of laxatives, diuretics, or enemas.

Women's Health Considerations

- Sexual abuse is a risk factor for an eating disorder.

Transcultural Considerations

Bulimia nervosa occurs more often in Chinese men than Chinese women.

COLLABORATIVE MANAGEMENT

Assessment

- The nurse records the client's
    1. Sequelae of vomiting and laxative abuse, including cardiac, renal, and gastrointestinal tract problems
    2. History of seizures
    3. Use of ipecac syrup to induce vomiting
    4. Weight history, including highest, lowest, and fluctuations
    5. Sexual activity and/or abuse
    6. Attitudes and behaviors related to food and weight
    7. Specific information about binges
    8. Method of purging

115

9. Activity
10. Previous episodes of psychiatric illness
11. Family history
- Also see Anorexia Nervosa ("Assessment")
- The nurse assesses for
    1. Normal, healthy body (usually)
    2. Weakness and tiredness
    3. Constipation
    4. Depression
    5. Irregular heartbeat
    6. Signs of urinary tract infection
    7. Seizures and peripheral paresthesias
    8. Dry mouth and swelling of the parotid glands
    9. Loss of tooth enamel and color change
    10. Gastrointestinal tract disturbances, such as esophagitis, gastric dilation, or loss of bowel reactivity
    11. Dehydration alternating with rebound fluid retention
    12. Irregular menses or amenorrhea
    13. Chronic hypokalemia (may cause metabolic alkalosis)
    14. Anemia
    15. Decreased serum magnesium level
    16. Elevated serum amylase level
    17. Decreased levels of reproductive hormones
    18. Abnormal electrocardiogram (ECG)

Interventions

- Tranylcypromine sulfate (Parnate), a monoamine oxidase inhibitor, or a serotonergic agonist, such as fluoxetine (Prozac) or sertraline hydrochloride (Zoloft), isapirone, may be used to decrease the client's urge to binge.
- Other antidepressants, such as nortriptyline (Aventyl), may also be ordered.
- Based on the client's basal metabolic rate, caloric requirements may be low for the bulimic (1000 to 1200 kcal/day).
- The nurse
    1. Stresses that correct food portions and eating patterns are emphasized rather than calorie counting
    2. Encourages the client to eat slowly
    3. Teaches the importance of increased activity level and a regular exercise program

4. Cautions the client to avoid exercise extremes
5. Provides a low-sodium diet (2 g/day) to minimize fluid retention
6. Limits the client's fluid intake to 1000 mL/day when edema is severe

- The nurse
    1. Administers oral potassium supplements, as ordered, to treat potassium levels of 3.0 to 3.4 mEq/L; decreased potassium levels may cause cardiac dysrhythmias, which can lead to sudden cardiac arrest
    2. Administers intravenous sodium chloride and potassium, as ordered, for more serious electrolyte imbalances
    3. Monitors vital signs and assesses for irregular pulse rate and rhythm
    4. Monitors cardiac status
    5. Monitors for recurrent purging behaviors
- The nurse
    1. Arranges for the client to have individual therapy with a psychiatrist, psychologist, or psychiatric nurse specialist as an inpatient and after discharge
    2. Teaches the client and family about groups that provide support during periods of stress and on an ongoing basis

BURNS

OVERVIEW

- A burn is an injury to the skin and other epithelial tissues caused by exposure to temperature extremes, radiation, electrical current, mechanical abrasion, or chemical abrasion. Clients who have burns experience a variety of physiologic, metabolic, and psychologic changes.
- Burns are classified according to their depth:

1. *Superficial-thickness* injuries produce the least destruction of all types because the epidermis is the only portion of the skin affected. These injuries are sometimes referred to as *first-degree* burns. This type of burn frequently occurs from sunburn or short (flash) exposure to high intensity heat.
2. *Partial-thickness* injuries damage only part of the skin, with remaining tissue capable of stimulating regeneration and successful wound healing. Second-degree burns are partial-thickness injuries. If the burn is superficial, a vesicle (blister) forms. Deep partial-thickness or second-degree burns reach the deeper layers of the dermis and destroy structures within the dermis, such as nerves and hair follicles. Blisters are rare in deep partial-thickness burns.
3. *Full-thickness* burns involve damage to all layers of the skin and do not heal spontaneously.
   a. *Third-degree* burns damage the entire dermal layer down to and sometimes including the subcutaneous fat; all dermal appendages are destroyed, and the regeneration function of the skin is absent.
   b. *Fourth-degree* burns occur when damage extends beyond the subcutaneous level and includes muscle and bone; usually the wounds contain a thick, dry, charred eschar, which is black and always without sensation.

- Compensatory responses to burns depend on the depth of the injury. Responses include
  1. Inflammation (immediate response)
  2. Sympathetic nervous system response (stress response)
  3. Vascular changes, including a shift of fluid from the intravascular space into the interstitial space ("third spacing"), which causes hypovolemia, metabolic acidosis, hyperkalemia, and hypernatremia (lasts up to 24 to 36 hours); the fluid shifts back into the intravascular space after 24 to 36 hours, causing hyponatremia and hypokalemia
  4. Respiratory insufficiency
  5. Gastrointestinal (GI) changes, such as Curling's ulcer and decreased peristalsis
  6. Metabolic changes, which result in body temperature changes

7. Immune system compromise
8. Decreased cardiac output until 18 to 36 hours after the burn

- Common types of burns and emergency interventions limiting the extent of injury include

  1. *Dry heat (flame) or moist heat (hot liquids):* The client should stop, drop, and roll to smother flames; clothes that are on fire or saturated with hot liquids should be removed.
  2. *Chemical:* Treatment depends on the type of chemical involved but generally should be flushed with copious amounts of water; agents containing sodium or potassium are covered with mineral oil and are not flushed with water.
  3. *Electrical:* The client should be separated from the electric current by shutting off the source of electricity or using a nonconductive implement, such as wooden poles or ropes made of plant fiber.
  4. *Radiation:* Treatment depends on whether the source is sealed or not sealed (self-contained).

Considerations for Elderly Clients

1. The skin of elderly persons is thinner and more easily damaged than that of younger persons; therefore, burns tend to be more extensive in the elderly.
2. Healing time is slower in the elderly, increasing the risk for infection and other complications.
3. Cardiac changes in elderly clients limit the amount and types of fluids used in resuscitation; they are also more likely to experience shock and renal failure.
4. The immune responses of older clients may be reduced, increasing the risk of infection and sepsis. In addition, elderly clients may not have a fever when an infection is present.
5. The elderly are more likely to have a pre-existing medical condition that may further compromise vital organ function or interfere with fluid resuscitation and treatment.

COLLABORATIVE MANAGEMENT

Assessment

- The nurse records
    1. Time of injury
    2. Source of heat or injurious agent
    3. Detailed description of how the burn occurred
    4. Whether the influence of alcohol or drugs may have been a factor
    5. A description of the place or environment where the burn occurred
    6. Events occurring from the time of the burn to admission
    7. Any other events or circumstances contributing to the injury
- The nurse records the client's
    1. Medical history
    2. Current medications
    3. Smoking history and history of drug or alcohol use
    4. Weight
- The nurse assesses for
    1. Direct airway injury:
        a. Changes in the appearance and function of the mouth, nose, pharynx, trachea, and pulmonary mechanisms
        b. Facial injury or singed hair on the head, eyebrows, eyelids, and nasal mucosa
        c. Blisters and soot on the lips and oral mucosa
        d. Alterations in breathing patterns (progressive hoarseness, expiratory wheeze, crowing, and stridor)
    2. Carbon monoxide poisoning:
        a. Headache
        b. Decreased cerebral function and visual acuity, coma
        c. Tinnitus
        d. Nausea
        e. Irritability
        f. Pale to reddish-purple skin
    3. Smoke poisoning:
        a. Atelectasis and pulmonary edema
        b. Hemorrhagic bronchitis 6 to 72 hours after injury

4. Pulmonary fluid overload:
    a. Shortness of breath, hypoxia
    b. Moist breath sounds and crackles

5. Cardiovascular dysfunction:
    a. Hypovolemic and cardiogenic shock
    b. Rapid, thready pulse
    c. Hypotension and a wide pulse pressure
    d. Diminished peripheral pulses
    e. Slow or absent capillary refill
    f. Edema
    g. Complications that generally develop 48 hours after injury, such as fluid overload, heart failure, and pulmonary edema
6. Renal dysfunction:
    a. Decreased urinary output
    b. Renal failure
7. Integumentary changes:
    a. Depth of injury
    b. Color and appearance of skin
    c. Estimation of injury size compared with the total body surface area (TBSA)
8. GI dysfunction:
    a. Paralytic ileus
    b. Gastric dilation and vomiting
    c. GI ulceration
    d. Occult blood in the stool
9. Electrolyte changes
10. Increased white blood cell (WBC) count, followed by a decrease
11. Neuroendocrine dysfunction:
    a. Hypothermia
    b. Weight loss and subsequent negative nitrogen balance
    c. Pseudodiabetes, which causes hyperglycemia and ketosis
12. Immune system dysfunction:
    a. Infections
    b. Sepsis
13. Musculoskeletal dysfunction:
    a. Problems that develop secondary to immobility, healing process, treatment, and other injuries
    b. Decreased range of motion (ROM)
14. Body image changes
15. Grieving
16. Anxiety and fear

Planning and Implementation

✦ **NDx:** Decreased Cardiac Output; Fluid Volume Deficit; Altered Tissue Perfusion

- The client receives extensive infusion of intravenous fluids; commonly used fluids include Ringer's lactate, normal saline, colloids, and glucose in water.
- The nurse
    1. Follows facility fluid resuscitation formula and protocol
    2. Monitors vital signs to determine adequate fluid resuscitation, including
        a. Clear mentation
        b. Normal blood pressure and pulse for the client
        c. Central venous pressure (CVP) between 6 and 9 cm H_2O
        d. Urinary output equal to 1 mL of urine per kilogram of body weight (30 to 100 mL) per hour
    3. Records strict measurement of intake and output
    4. Adjusts fluid intake to maintain urinary output between 30 and 100 mL/hr
    5. Does not administer diuretics as they decrease circulating volume and cardiac output and may lead to a dangerous reduction in perfusion to other vital organs; however, diuretics may be given to the client with an electrical burn, as ordered
    6. Provides intensive cardiac monitoring such as CVP, pulmonary artery pressures, and cardiac output
    7. Monitors for cardiac dysrhythmias such as atrial fibrillation
- An escharotomy may be performed to incise but not remove the eschar, if present.

✦ **NDx:** Ineffective Breathing Pattern

- The nurse
    1. Performs a respiratory assessment every hour
        a. Auscultates the lung fields for quality and depth of respirations
        b. Loosens tight dressings if necessary to facilitate chest expansion
    2. Turns and encourages the client to cough and deep breathe at least every 2 hours
    3. Has intubation equipment readily available (crowing, stridor, and dyspnea are indications for immediate intubation)

122

4. Assists the physician with bronchoscopy to examine the vocal cords, respiratory tract accurate diagnosis, deep suctioning of the lungs, and/or removal of sloughing necrotic material

5. Suctions client as clinically indicated; obtains sputum culture to determine whether an infection is contributing to breathing problems

6. Performs chest physiotherapy and incentive spirometry

7. Administers aerosol treatments, as ordered

8. Obtains arterial blood gases and chest x-rays, as indicated

9. Administers oxygen therapy; intubation and mechanical ventilation are indicated if the PaO_2 is less than 60 mmHg; a tracheostomy may be necessary for long-term intubation

10. Administers antibiotics, as ordered, for pneumonia or other pulmonary infections

✦ NDx: Pain

- The nurse
  1. Assesses the client's pain tolerance, coping mechanisms, and physical status
  2. Administers opioid and nonopioid analgesics, such as morphine, meperidine (Demerol), and nalbuphine (Nubain)
  3. Monitors the client receiving anesthetic agents, such as ketamine (Ketalar), pentobarbital sodium (Nembutal), and nitrous oxide
  4. Teaches relaxation techniques, meditative breathing, guided imagery, and music therapy
  5. Increases the client's sleep and rest periods to reduce the adverse effects of sleep deprivation, to replenish catecholamine stores, and to restore the diurnal effects of endorphins
  6. Provides tactile stimulation through frequent position changes and massages; maintains a comfortable room temperature
  7. Allows the client participation in pain control (e.g., patient-controlled analgesia)

✦ NDx: Potential for Pulmonary Edema

- The nurse administers
  1. Digoxin or another inotropic agent to improve left ventricular function

2. Diuretics may or may not be given based upon the client's vascular hydration status and renal function

✦ NDx: Potential for Adult Respiratory Distress Syndrome (ARDS)

- Positive end-expiratory pressure (PEEP) is combined with intermittent mandatory ventilation (IMV).
- The nurse assesses and documents the client's response so appropriate ventilator changes can be made.
- Neuromuscular blocking agents can be used in clients requiring mechanical ventilation to reduce or eliminate spontaneous breathing efforts and to reduce oxygen consumption.

✦ NDx: Impaired Skin Integrity

- The health care team performs an in-depth assessment of burned and nonburned skin areas to determine the degree of skin integrity, adequacy of circulation, presence of infection, and effectiveness of therapy.
- Wound debridement procedures can be
    1. *Mechanical:* using hydrotherapy (immersion in tub, shower on a specially designed table, successively washing only small areas of the wound); forceps and scissors are used to remove loose, nonviable tissue
    2. *Enzymatic:* can occur naturally by autolysis (spontaneous disintegration of tissue by the action of the client's own cellular enzymes) or artificially by application of proteolytic agents such as sutilains (Travase)
    3. *Surgical:* excising the burn wound by either a tangential or a fascial excision technique and covering it with a skin graft or temporary covering. The procedure, performed within the first 5 days after injury, reduces the number of hydrotherapy treatments that are needed, but risks include massive blood loss and complications associated with anesthesia
- Types of dressings usually used are
    1. *Standard:* involve the application of topical antibiotics on the burn wound, followed by sterile application of multiple layers of gauze. The number of gauze layers used depends on the depth of the injury, the amount of drainage expected, the client's mobility, and the frequency of dressing changes

2. *Biologic:* contain some amount of viable tissue or are derived from once-living tissue

   a. The biologic dressing is used to debride untidy wounds after eschar separation, to promote reepithelialization of deep second-degree burns, to cover a burn temporarily after wound excision, and to protect granulation tissue between autographs.

   b. *Heterograft* is skin from another species, such as a pig. Rejection occurs after 24 to 72 hours, and the heterograpt is replaced on a continuous basis until closure with an autograft is complete.

   c. *Homograft* is skin from another human, usually a cadaver. Rejection can occur after 24 hours, but in some cases the graft remains adherent for up to 90 days.

   d. *Amniotic membrane* is used because it has a low cost, ready accessibility, and large size.

   e. *Artificial skin* is a relatively new approach to skin closure; it gradually dissolves as new, healthy skin replaces it.

   f. *Cultured skin* can be grown in a laboratory for grafting.

3. *Synthetic* and *biosynthetic:* such as Op Site, Vigilon, Biobrane, and Tegaderm; usually in place for 2 to 5 days

✦ NDx: Risk for Infection

- The nurse
  1. Monitors for signs of sepsis, including altered sensorium, increased respiratory rate, hypothermia or hyperthermia, oliguria, elevated serum glucose, glycosuria, decreased platelet count, and increased WBC count with a left shift
  2. Observes the wound for pervasive odor, exudate, changes in texture, purulent drainage, color changes, and redness at the wound edges
- Aggressive surgical debridement of the wound may be necessary if the colony count approaches 105 colonies per gram of tissue.
- Tetanus toxoid is given; additional administration of tetanus immune globulin is recommended when the history of tetanus immunity is questionable.
- Topical antibiotics or antimicrobials are administered using the open technique (ointment is applied without further dressing of the wound) or closed technique

(burn is covered with a dressing after the ointment is applied).

- Topical agents commonly used in the treatment of burns include
    1. Silver sulfadiazine (Silvadene, Flamazine◆):
        a. Causes adverse side effects, including local allergic reactions and leukopenia
        b. Is not consistently effective for burns covering more than 60% of the client's body
    2. Mafenide acetate (Sulfamylon):
        a. Causes severe pain if used on partial thickness burns
        b. Causes adverse side effects, including metabolic acidosis and superinfection
        c. Is effective against Pseudomonas organisms
    3. Collagenase (Santyl with polysporin powder):
        a. Painless and easy to apply
        b. Change dressing every day
        c. Expensive; used only on partial-thickness injuries
    4. Povidone-iodine (Betadine):
        a. Is effective against many infections not well controlled by silver sulfadiazine
        b. May cause electrolyte imbalance and metabolic acidosis and form crust if burns are not properly cleaned
    5. Nitrofurazone (Furacin):
        a. Is effective against *Staphylococcus aureus* and some antibiotic-resistant organisms
        b. May cause contact dermatitis; messy to apply
        c. May cause renal problems if used in clients with extensive burns
    6. Gentamicin sulfate (Garamycin, Gentamar◆)
        a. Is effective against many organisms, including Pseudomonas; does not cause pain when applied
        b. Causes adverse reactions, including ototoxicity and nephrotoxicity
    7. Bacitracin with polymyxin B sulfate (Polysporin):
        a. Is bactericidal for gram-positive and gram-negative organisms; aesthetically suitable for use on face
        b. May cause itching, burning, or inflammation; cannot be used for full-thickness burns

- Drugs with systemic effects used to treat infections include the aminoglycosides and cephalosporins:
    1. A higher dose than normal is required to maintain therapeutic serum levels; dosage is determined by peak and trough serum levels.
    2. Adverse reactions include ototoxity and nephrotoxicity.
- The nurse ensures isolation therapy:
    1. Proper and consistent hand washing is the single most effective technique to prevent the transmission of infection.
    2. The client is isolated according to the specific organism and facility procedure.
    3. Special isolation procedures may be needed if the organism becomes resistant to antibiotic therapy.
    4. Visitors are restricted while the client is immunosuppressed; ill persons and small children should be restricted.
- The nurse
    1. Wears gloves whenever coming in contact with the burn; changes gloves when handling wounds on different areas of the body
    2. Uses disposable equipment as much as possible and does not share equipment between clients

✦ **NDx:** Altered Nutrition: Less than Body Requirements

- Total parenteral nutrition (TPN) may be needed until the client has sufficient gastric motility for oral or tube feedings.
- The nurse
    1. Provides a high-calorie and high-protein diet and offers supplemental feedings as needed
    2. Collaborates with the dietitian and client to plan alternatives to conventional nutritional patterns
    3. Encourages the client to order food whenever the client says that he or she can eat, not just at the scheduled mealtime

✦ **NDx:** Impaired Physical Mobility

- The nurse
    1. Maintains the client in a neutral body position with minimal flexion

127

2. Uses splints and other conforming devices according to the prescribed schedule
3. Performs range-of-motion (ROM) exercises at least three times a day
4. Assists the client to ambulate as soon as possible
5. Applies pressure dressings to prevent formation of contractures and tight hypertrophic scars, including
   a. Ace bandages
   b. Custom-fitted elasticized clothing items (Jobst garments), which are worn 23 hours per day, every day, until the scar tissue is mature

✦ **NDx:** Body Image Disturbance

- The nurse
  1. Reassures the client that feelings of grief, loss, anxiety, anger, fear, and guilt are normal
  2. Collaborates with other health team members (e.g., psychiatrist, social worker) to address these problems
  3. Accepts the client's physical and psychologic characteristics
  4. Provides information and support
  5. Engages the client in decision-making and independent activities
  6. Provides information on and resources for reconstructive and cosmetic surgery, if needed

Continuing Care

- The nurse begins the discharge process early by assessing the client's and family's readiness for discharge and care requirements.
- Needs to be addressed before discharge include
  1. Financial assessment
  2. Evaluation of family resources
  3. Psychological referral
  4. Designation of principal learners (specific family members or significant others who will help with care)
     a. Teaches wound care and dressing changes, including use of correct technique, how to dispose of soiled dressings, methods to prevent contamination and signs and symptoms of infection

b. Teaches the proper use of prosthetic and positioning devices
c. Teaches how to apply pressure garments correctly

5. Rehabilitation referral
6. Home assessment
7. Medical equipment needed in the home
8. Evaluation of community resources and referral as needed
9. Referral to home health care as needed
10. Reentry programs for school or work environment
11. Nursing home/transition care placement
12. Prosthetic rehabilitation

- The nurse
    1. Helps the client to deal with the reactions of others to the sight of healing wounds and disfigurement

Byssinosis

See Pulmonary Disease, Occupational

CAD

See Coronary Artery Disease.

CAL

See Airflow Limitation, Chronic.

Calculi, Urinary

See Urolithiasis.

Calculous Cholecystitis

See Cholelithiasis.

Cancer

OVERVIEW

- A diagnosis of cancer causes psychological distress and has the potential to disrupt personal and professional relationships, finances, role identity, self esteem, body image, and normal physiologic functioning.
- The danger of cancer is that it invades and destroys normal tissue, compromising physiologic function in that tissue.
- Pathologic alterations can occur as a result of treatment regimens and are referred to as secondary effects.
- Physiologic dysfunction due to cancer may lead to
    1. Impaired immune and hematopoietic function:
        a. Occurs most often in clients with leukemia and lymphoma
        b. Makes the client susceptible to infection (decreased white blood cells [WBCs]), anemia (decreased red blood cells [RBCs]), and a tendency to bleed (decreased platelets)
    2. Altered gastrointestinal (GI) structure and function:
        a. Affects the client's nutritional status
        b. Contributes to anorexia
        c. Leads to the development of *cachexia,* a profound nutritional deficit

130

d. Makes the role of nutritional support for clients with cancer, especially those undergoing treatment, complex and controversial; a diet high in protein and carbohydrates helps the client maintain weight but can contribute to cancer progression

3. Motor and sensory deficits:
   a. These result from cancers that invade bone and compress nerves
   b. Bone metastasis can cause fractures, spinal cord compression, and hypercalcemia
   c. Pain from the effects of cancer is caused by bone involvement, nerve compression, soft-tissue infiltration, visceral (organ) involvement, muscle spasm, lymphedema, increased intracranial pressure, and myopathy; pain also results from cancer treatment, immobility, or concurrent disorders, such as musculoskeletal disease
4. Decreased respiratory function:
   a. Results from airway obstruction with tumor, lung tissue involvement, or blockage of blood flow through the chest and lungs
   b. Dyspnea and pulmonary edema are common

- Therapies for cancer include
  1. *Surgery* to remove cancerous tissue:
     a. Surgery may be performed for prophylaxis, diagnosis, cure, control, palliation, determination of therapy effectiveness, or reconstruction
     b. Nursing care depends on the type of procedure performed
     c. How much function after surgery is lost and how the loss affects the client depends on the location and extent of the surgery
  2. *Radiation* to destroy malignant cells with minimal exposure of normal cells to the cell-damaging actions of the radiation:
     a. The therapeutic radiation dose varies according to the tumor's size, location, and degree of radiation sensitivity as well as radiation sensitivity of the surrounding normal tissues.
     b. *Teletherapy:* the actual radiation source external to the client and remote from the tumor site. This type of therapy is called external beam radiation.
     c. *Brachytherapy* is delivered by direct contact with the tumor through unsealed radiation

sources (oral, intravenous, or intracavitary) or as sealed radiation sources (implants, interstitial needles, or seeds).

d. Side effects of radiation therapy vary according to site; skin changes and alopecia are the most common effects. Some changes are permanent, depending on the dose of the radiation and location of the site.

e. Nursing care for clients receiving external radiation includes education:

    (1) Wash the irradiated area gently each day with either water alone or a mild soap and water

    (2) Use your hand rather than a washcloth

    (3) Do not remove the markings that indicate where the radiation beam is to be focused

    (4) Use no powders, ointments, lotions, or creams on the skin unless directed to do so by the radiologist

    (5) Wear soft clothing over the skin at the radiation site

    (6) Avoid wearing belts or any other constrictive clothing over the radiation site

    (7) Keep the irradiated area from being exposed to the sun

    (8) Avoid heat exposure

    (9) Schedule activities to allow for frequent rest periods

    (10) Altered taste sensation and aversion to red meat is a common side effect

f. Nursing care for clients with sealed radioactive implants includes the following (although hospital protocols vary):

    (1) Assign the client to a private room with a private bath

    (2) Place a "Caution: Radioactive Material" sign on the door of the client's room

    (3) Wear a dosimeter film badge at all times while caring for the client to measure the exposure to radiation

    (4) Do not care for the client if you are pregnant; do not allow children under 16 or pregnant women to visit

    (5) Limit each visitor to 30 minutes a day and keep visitors at least 6 feet from the radiation source

  (6) Never touch the radiation source with bare hands; if it is dislodged, use long-handled forceps to place it into the lead container kept in the client's room

  (7) Save all dressings and bed linens until after the radiation source is removed, then properly dispose of them

3. Chemotherapy—the treatment of cancer through the use of chemical agents:

 a. Chemotherapy is used to cure, to increase mean survival time, and to decrease the chance of specific life-threatening complications.

 b. Chemotherapeutic agents are administered systemically and exert their cytotoxic (cell-damaging) effects against both healthy and cancerous cells.

 c. The normal cells that undergo frequent cell division are the most profoundly affected—skin, hair, epithelial GI tract lining, spermatocytes, and hematopoietic cells.

 d. Classifications of chemotherapeutic agents include antimetabolites, antitumor antibiotics, alkylating agents, antimiotic agents, and miscellaneous agents, such as asparaginase (Elspar, Kidrolase◆) and procarbazine (Matulane, Natulanar).

 e. Chemotherapy often involves the administration of a combination of agents.

 f. Chemotherapeutic dosing is typically based on the client's total body surface area and the type of cancer.

 g. Although the intravenous route is the most common for drug administration, chemotherapy may also be given by the oral, intra-arterial, isolated limb perfusion, and intracavitary routes.

 h. Extravasation is a major complication of IV administration.

  (1) Usually resolves without extensive treatment if less than 0.05 mL of the drug has infiltrated; surgical intervention may be necessary to treat more severe infiltration.

  (2) Immediate treatment depends on the specific agent extravasated.

  (3) Document the event according to institution protocol.

i. The major role of the nurse in caring for clients receiving chemotherapy is management of the symptoms that the client experiences as a result of the therapy; the major side effects include alopecia, nausea and vomiting, mucositis, and immunosuppression.

(1) For clients with *alopecia,* the nurse
  — Reminds the client that hair loss will occur but is temporary
  — Suggests scarves, turbans, hats, or wigs
  — Cautions the client that when hair grows back, its color, texture, and thickness may be different

(2) For clients with *nausea* and *vomiting,* the nurse
  — Administers antiemetics and monitors the client response; drug combinations must be individualized for best effect
  — Promotes comfort through anxiety-reducing techniques, such as progressive relaxation and imagery
  — Monitors the client for dehydration and electrolyte imbalances

(3) For clients with *mucositis,* the nurse
  — Performs frequent mouth assessments; documents finding
  — Teaches the client to avoid traumatizing the oral mucosa
    • use a soft-bristled toothbrush or sponge for mouth care
    • avoid using dental floss and water pressure gum cleaners such as a water pic
    • avoid alcohol- or glycerin-based mouthwashes
  — Assists the client in menu choices to avoid spicy or hard foods
  — Applies petroleum jelly to the client's lips as needed
  — Suggests that the client use a solution of half peroxide and half normal saline for rinsing every 12 hours
  — Administers antimicrobial and analgesic topical medications, as ordered
  — Administers "artificial saliva," as needed

— Cleans toothbrush with a bleach or peroxide solution or runs it through a dishwasher daily
— Assists the patient with mouth care before and after every meal and at bedtime

(4) For clients with *immunosuppression,* a potential life-threatening side effect, the nurse
— Places the client in a private room if possible
— Uses good hand-washing techniques and teaches the client to do the same
— Wears a mask in the client's room
— Uses strict aseptic technique for all invasive procedures
— Avoids the use of indwelling urinary catheters
— Monitors the WBC count daily
— Keeps fresh flowers and potted plants out of the client's room
— Teaches the client to eat a low-bacteria diet by avoiding salads, raw fruit and vegetables, raw and undercooked meat, pepper, and paprika
— Teaches other infection-control measures for the client at home, including avoiding crowds and people who are sick, bathing every day, not sharing personal toilet articles, not drinking water that has been standing for more than 15 minutes, not changing pet litter boxes or animal cages, and taking temperature daily

4. Other drugs used for treating cancer include hormones, hormone antagonists, and biologic response modifiers (immunotherapy).

- Oncologic emergencies include

   1. *Sepsis* and *disseminated intravascular coagulation* (DIC):
      a. Sepsis, or septicemia, occurs when pathogens enter the bloodstream; septic shock is a life-threatening result of sepsis.
      b. DIC is a clotting problem that is triggered by many severe illnesses, including cancer. In clients with cancer, DIC is caused by sepsis

through release of thrombin or thromboplastin (clotting factors). Abnormal clot formation occurs in small vessels and is followed by extensive bleeding.

   c. Treatment includes anticoagulants (heparin) followed by cryoprecipitated clotting factors.

2. *Syndrome of inappropriate antidiuretic hormone* (see Syndrome of Inappropriate Antidiuretic Hormone)

3. *Spinal cord compression* (see Tumors, Spinal Cord)

4. *Hypercalcemia* (see Hypercalcemia)

5. *Superior vena cava* (SVC) syndrome

   a. SVC syndrome occurs when the SVC is compressed or obstructed by tumor growth.

   b. Early signs and symptoms include upper body edema, followed by dyspnea, cyanosis, mental status changes, decreased cardiac output, and hemorrhage.

   c. Treatment is high-dose radiation.

6. *Tumor lysis syndrome*

   a. In tumor lysis syndrome, large quantities of tumor cells are destroyed rapidly.

   b. Serum potassium levels increase rapidly, and purine release causes hyperuricemia, resulting in cardiac and renal failure.

   c. The best treatment is prevention through hydration with 3 to 5 L of fluid a day, if possible.

   d. Drugs such as allopurinol (Zyloprim, Alloprin◆) are used to reduce uric acid levels.

   e. Intravenous administration of glucose and insulin may be used to decrease serum potassium levels.

   f. In severe cases, the client may require dialysis.

CANCER, BONE

OVERVIEW

- There are several types of *primary* tumors.

   1. *Osteosarcoma,* or osteogenic sarcoma, is the most common and is most frequently found in the distal

femur, proximal tibia, and humerus; the lesion typically metastasizes to the lungs within 2 years of treatment and occurs more often in males than in females (2:1) between ages 10 and 30 years and in older clients with Paget's disease.

2. *Ewing's sarcoma* is the most malignant, often extending into soft tissue and metastasizing to the lungs and other bones; it occurs most often in children and adults in their 20s, affecting men more than women.
3. *Chondrosarcoma* typically affects the pelvis and proximal femur near the diaphysis; it strikes people who are middle-aged and older.
4. *Fibrosarcoma* is an uncommon, slow-growing tumor that can metastasize to the lungs; it typically occurs in middle-aged men.

- The source of the primary tumor includes the prostate, the kidney, the thyroid, and the lungs (bone-seeking cancers).
- Secondary tumors originate in other tissues, metastasize to bone, and are found most often in the older age group.
- Secondary tumors metastasize primarily to the vertebrae, the pelvis, and the ribs.

COLLABORATIVE MANAGEMENT

Assessment

- The nurse records the client's
    1. History of radiation therapy for cancer
    2. General health status
    3. Family history of neoplasms
- The nurse assesses for
    1. Pain
    2. Swelling
    3. Tender, palpable mass
    4. Ability to perform activities of daily living (ADL)
    5. Low-grade fever, fatigue, and pallor (seen in Ewing's sarcoma)
    6. Level of support system to help the client cope with the diagnosis and treatment
    7. Anxiety and fear
    8. Elevated serum alkaline phosphatase
    9. Possible elevations of serum calcium level and erythrocyte sedimentation rate

137

- Bone biopsy determines tumor type, grade, and stage.

Planning and Implementation

✦ NDx: Pain

Nonsurgical Management

- Analgesics and nondrug pain relief measures are used.
- Chemotherapeutic agents, given alone or in combination with radiation therapy and surgery, work best for small, metastatic lesions. The drugs selected are determined in part by the primary source of the tumor.
- Radiation therapy is as effective as surgery for Ewing's sarcoma in reducing the size of the tumor and thereby decreasing pain; radiation is palliative for metastatic bone disease.

Surgical Management

- *Wide excision* is the removal of the lesion surrounded by an intact cuff of normal tissue; it leads to cure of low-grade tumors only.
- *Radical resection* includes the removal of the lesion and of the entire muscle, bone, and other tissues directly involved; bone deficits may be corrected with grafts.
- *Percutaneous cordotomy* may be done to treat intractable pain.
- The nurse provides preoperative care:
    1. Provides psychologic support; answers questions and explains routines and procedures
    2. Administers chemotherapy, as ordered
- The nurse provides postoperative care:
    1. Assesses neurovascular status
    2. Observes and records wound drainage
    3. Maintains pressure dressing and suction as ordered
    4. Encourages muscle-strengthening and range-of-motion exercises as soon as permitted; a continuous passive motion (CPM) machine may be used
    5. Assists with ADL as needed

✦ NDx: Anticipatory Grieving

- The nurse
    1. Allows the client and family to verbalize their feelings

2. Refers questions outside the scope of nursing practice to the physician, spiritual counselor, or other appropriate professional
3. Encourages the client and family to write down their questions and have them available when the physician visits

✦ **NDx:** Body Image Disturbance

- The nurse
  1. Recognizes and accepts the client's view about body image alteration
  2. Develops a trusting relationship with the client
  3. Allows the client to verbalize his or her feelings
  4. Emphasizes the client's strengths and remaining capabilities
  5. Assists the client to set realistic goals regarding lifestyle

✦ **NDx:** Potential for Fractures

- The nurse
  1. Maintains a hazard-free environment to prevent falls and to minimize trauma (pathologic fracture)
  2. Teaches strengthening exercises

Continuing Care

- The nurse
  1. Collaborates with the health care team to ensure that the client can correctly use all assistive-adaptive devices ordered for home use
  2. Instructs the client on the complications and side effects of radiation therapy, such as dry skin
  3. Explains the complications and side effects of chemotherapy, such as nausea and vomiting
  4. Teaches wound care, as needed
  5. Develops and reinforces a pain management program:
     a. Drug information, including the importance of taking the correct dosage at the right time
     b. Progressive relaxation techniques and music therapy
  6. Reviews the prescribed exercise regimen
  7. Emphasizes the importance of follow-up visits with the physician(s) and other members of the health care team

8. Refers the client to a local cancer support group

CANCER, BREAST

OVERVIEW

- Breast cancer is the leading cause of death among women 35 to 54 years of age in the United States; less than 1% of all cases of breast cancer occur in men.
- The most common type of breast cancer is *infiltrating ductal carcinoma,* which originates in the epithelial cells lining the mammary ducts; the cancer remaining in the duct is noninvasive.
- Cancer is classified as invasive when it penetrates the tissue surrounding the duct and grows in an irregular pattern.
- The mass is irregular and poorly defined; fibrosis develops around the cancerous tumor and contributes to dimpling, which is characteristically seen in advanced disease.
- The tumor invades the lymphatic channels, blocking skin drainage and causing edema and an orange peel appearance of the skin (peau d'orange).
- Invasion of the lymphatic channels carries tumor cells to the lymphatic nodes in the axilla.
- The tumor replaces the skin, and ulceration of the overlying skin occurs.
- Common sites of metastatic disease are bone, lungs, brain, and liver.
- The stages of breast cancer are
    1. Stage I: smaller than 2 cm without lymph node involvement
    2. Stage II: 2 to 5 cm without lymph node involvement
    3. Stage III: larger than 5 cm with no lymph node involvement; smaller than 2 cm with axillary node involvement or 2 to 5 cm with supraclavicular or intraclavicular node involvement
    4. Stage IV: any size, with or without lymph node involvement, but distant metastasis is present
- Risk factors for breast cancer include increased age,

family history of breast cancer, exposure to ionizing radiation, early menarche, history of benign breast disease, nulliparity, first birth after age 30, and late menopause. A high alcohol and fat intake may increase the risk of breast cancer.

Considerations for Elderly Clients

- By age 85, each American woman faces a 1-in-9 risk of being diagnosed with breast cancer.

→ Transcultural Considerations

- Although the incidence of breast cancer is higher in Caucasians, death rates are higher for African-American women at every stage of the disease.
- Latino/Hispanic women have a lower incidence of breast cancer than Caucasians, but have a higher death rate.
- It is the most common cause of cancer among Asian and Pacific Island women.

COLLABORATIVE MANAGEMENT
Assessment

- The nurse records the client's
    1. Age, sex, and race
    2. Marital status
    3. Height and weight
    4. Personal and family history of breast cancer
    5. Hormonal history
    6. Age at first menarche
    7. Age at menopause
    8. Age at first child's birth
    9. Number of children
    10. History of breast mass discovery and medical care intervention
    11. Health maintenance, including regularity of breast self-examination and mammography history
    12. Diet history, including alcohol and fat intake
    13. Medications
- The nurse assesses for
    1. Mass location, size, shape, consistency, and fixation to surrounding tissues
    2. Skin changes, such as dimpling, peau d'orange, increased vascularity, nipple retraction, or ulceration

141

3. Enlarged axillary and supraclavicular lymph nodes
4. Breast pain or soreness
- Mammography, ultrasonography, and biopsy are used to diagnose breast cancer.
- Women with estrogen receptor-positive tumors respond best to adjuvant therapy and have a better overall survival rate.
- Three major issues the woman has to fear are:
  1. Fear of cancer
  2. Threats to body image and sexuality, intimate relationships, and survival
  3. Decisional conflict related to treatment options

Planning and Implementation

✦ NDx: Anxiety

- The nurse
  1. Assesses the client's perceptions and level of anxiety concerning the possible diagnosis
  2. Allows the client to ventilate feelings, even if a diagnosis has not been established
  3. Encourages the client to seek information and outside resources
  4. Contacts resource groups, such as Reach to Recovery

✦ NDx: Potential for Metastasis

Nonsurgical Management

- Radiation may be used in conjunction with chemotherapy for late-stage breast cancer.

Surgical Management

- Conservative surgical management of breast cancer is used for early disease and usually involves *lumpectomy with lymph node dissection,* in which only the tumor and lymph nodes are removed, leaving the breast tissue intact, or a *simple mastectomy,* in which breast tissue and usually the nipple are removed, but the lymph nodes are left intact, followed by radiation.
- In a *modified radical mastectomy,* the breast tissue, nipple, and lymph nodes are removed, but muscles are left intact.
- In a *Halsted radical mastectomy,* the breast tissue, nipple, underlying muscles, and lymph nodes are removed (not commonly performed).

- Preoperative care focuses on psychologic preparation, as well as usual preoperative measures.
- The nurse provides postoperative care
  1. Places the client on the back with the head of the bed elevated at least 30 degrees or on the unaffected side, with the arm on the surgical side elevated on a pillow
  2. Assesses drains and dressings for constriction, position, and functioning
  3. Records amount of postoperative drainage and reports excess
  4. Assesses operative site for swelling or presence of fluid collection under skin flaps
  5. Consults with the physical therapist to recommend and teach the client appropriate postmastectomy exercises (with the physician's consent)
  6. Reviews the exercise program with the client
  7. Assesses for signs and symptoms of infection
  8. Provides routine postoperative care
- The nurse instructs the client to
  1. Avoid having blood pressures taken on, blood drawn from, or injections in the affected arm
  2. Avoid injury to the affected arm, such as burns, scratches, and scrapes
  3. Treat injuries immediately to avoid infection
- The decision to follow the original surgical procedure with chemotherapy, radiation, or hormonal therapy is based on the stage of the breast cancer, the age and menopausal state of the client, client preference, pathologic examination, and hormone receptor status.
- Women who have estrogen receptor-positive tumors are given tamoxifen (Nolvadex, Tamofen◆).
- Breast reconstruction may begin during the original surgery or may be done later in one or more stages using skin flaps or prostheses.

Continuing Care

- The nurse refers the client to home health service for care of drains and dressings and assistance with ADLs.
- The nurse instructs the client and family on
  1. Measures to optimize positive body image after mastectomy
  2. Information to enhance interpersonal relationships and roles

143

3. Postmastectomy exercises to regain full range of motion
4. Measures to prevent infection of the incision
5. Measures to prevent injury, infection, and swelling of the affected arm, including avoidance of blood pressure measurements, injections, or venipunctures; wearing mitts or gloves for protection when appropriate; and treating cuts and scrapes quickly
6. The importance of avoiding the use of deodorant, lotion, and ointment on the affected arm
7. The importance of reporting signs of swelling, redness, increased heat, and tenderness to the physician
8. The importance of monthly breast self-examination

- The nurse refers the client to community resources, including Reach for Recovery and ENCORE.

Cancer, Cervical

OVERVIEW

- Cervical cancer, the third most frequently occurring reproductive cancer, can be preinvasive or invasive.
- Preinvasive cancer is limited to the cervix and usually originates in the area called the transformation zone.
- Invasive cancer is in the cervix and other pelvic structures.
- Squamous cell cancers spread by direct extension to the vaginal mucosa, the lower uterine segment, the parametrium, the pelvic wall, the bladder, and the bowel.
- Metastasis is usually confined to the pelvis, but distant metastases occur through lymphatic spread.
- Premalignant changes can be described from dysplasia, the earliest change, to carcinoma in situ (CIS), the most advanced premalignant change.
- Preinvasive cancers can also be described using the term *cervical intraepithelial neoplasia* (CIN) and can be classified according to their severity.

- Risk factors associated with cervical cancer include
    1. Low socioeconomic status
    2. Early age at first sexual contact or first pregnancy
    3. Multiple sexual partners
    4. Intrauterine exposure to diethylstilbestrol (DES)

 Transcultural Considerations

The occurrence of cervical cancer is twice as high in African-American women as in Caucasian women.

COLLABORATIVE MANAGEMENT
Assessment

- The nurse assesses for
    1. Painless vaginal bleeding (the classic symptom)
    2. Watery, blood-tinged discharge that may become dark and foul smelling as the disease progresses
    3. Leg pain or unilateral leg swelling (a late sign)
    4. Weight loss
    5. Pelvic pain
    6. Dysuria
    7. Hematuria
    8. Rectal bleeding
    9. Chest pain
    10. Coughing
    11. Abnormal Papanicolaou's stain test (Pap smear) results

Interventions

Nonsurgical Management (of CIN)

- Laser therapy is used when all boundaries of the lesion are visible during colposcopic examination.
- Cryosurgery involves placing a probe against the cervix to cause freezing of the tissues and subsequent necrosis.

Nonsurgical Management (of Invasive Cervical Cancer)

- The intracavitary and external radiation therapy is used in combination, depending on the extent and location of the lesion.
- For nursing management of clients undergoing radiation therapy, refer to Cancer.
- Chemotherapy has generally performed poorly for cervical cancers.

145

Surgical Management

- Conization may be used therapeutically for CIN in women who desire childbearing; it is the definitive treatment for microinvasive cervical cancer.
- A vaginal hysterectomy is commonly performed.
- A radical hysterectomy and bilateral lymph node dissection is as effective as radiation for cancer that extends beyond the cervix but not to the pelvic wall.
- For preoperative and postoperative care, see "Surgical Management" under Leiomyoma, Uterine.
- *Pelvic exenteration* is a radical surgical procedure used for recurrent cancers if there is no lymph node involvement:
    1. *Anterior exenteration* is the removal of the uterus, ovaries, fallopian tubes, vagina, bladder, urethra, and pelvic lymph nodes.
    2. *Posterior exenteration* is the removal of the uterus, ovaries, fallopian tubes, descending colon, rectum, and anal canal.
    3. *Total exenteration* is a combination of the anterior and posterior procedures, with urinary diversion created by an ileal conduit and a colostomy for passage of feces.
- The nurse provides preoperative care:
    1. Assesses anxiety, concerns about sexual functioning, and the ability to adjust to altered body image
    2. Assists in selection of stoma sites
    3. Provides extensive bowel preparation
    4. Provides routine preoperative care
- The nurse informs the client what to expect after surgery:
    1. Transfer to a critical care unit
    2. Multiple intravenous lines
    3. Other invasive lines and monitoring, such as an arterial line
    4. Nasogastric tube
- Refer to Cancer, Colorectal, for preoperative and postoperative care for the client undergoing colostomy and Cancer, Urothelial, for preoperative and postoperative care for the client undergoing ileal conduit.
- After surgery, the nurse assesses for
    1. Cardiovascular complications, such as hemorrhage and shock

    2. Pulmonary complications, such as atelectasis and pneumonia
    3. Fluid and electrolyte imbalances, such as metabolic acidosis or alkalosis
    4. Renal complications
    5. Gastrointestinal complications, such as paralytic ileus
    6. Pain
    7. Wound infection, dehiscence, or evisceration

- The nurse provides postoperative care:
  1. Assists with coughing and deep-breathing
  2. Observes for dehydration
  3. Monitors urinary output
  4. Administers opioid analgesics, as ordered
  5. Administers and monitors total parenteral nutrition, as ordered
  6. Administers prophylactic heparin and applies antiembolism stockings, as ordered, to prevent deep venous thrombosis
  7. Administers antibiotics, as ordered
  8. Performs perineal irrigations
  9. Provides sitz baths

Continuing Care

- The nurse implements a teaching plan for the client undergoing exenteration:
  1. Colostomy and/or ileal conduit care
  2. Care for perineal drainage (for several months to a year)
  3. Use of sanitary pads
  4. Dietary adjustment to maintain high nutritional intake
  5. Medication effects, dosages, and side effects
  6. Sexual counseling about alternatives to intercourse
  7. Activity modification; walking
  8. Information about complications, including infection and bowel obstruction
  9. Emotional support about changes in body image
  10. Importance of follow-up visits with the physician(s)

CANCER, COLORECTAL

OVERVIEW

- Colorectal cancer is the most common cancer in the United States.
- The malignant process begins in cells lining the bowel wall.
- Tumors occur in all areas of the colon, and most cancers develop from adenomatous polyps, the primary risk factor.
- Other risk factors include
    1. High intake of red meat and animal fat
    2 High intake of fatty foods, refined carbohydrates, or fried or broiled meats and fish
- Foods recommended for prevention of colorectal cancer include
    1. Fruits and vegetables, especially cruciferous vegetables from the cabbage family (e.g., cabbage, broccoli, cauliflower, brussels sprouts)
    2. Whole grain products
    3. Adequate fluids, especially water

🐾 Women's Health Considerations

1. Colon cancer is the third most common type of cancer in women.
2. Women with histories of breast, endometrial, or ovarian cancer have an increased risk of the disease.

➔ Transcultural Considerations

1. The incidence of colorectal cancer in the United States appears to be declining for all groups except African-American men.
2. There is a high incidence of colorectal cancer in Western industrialized countries and a low incidence in Japan, Finland, and Africa, probably related to diet.

- Tumors spread by direct invasion and through the lymphatic and circulatory systems.

148

- Complications include bowel perforation with peritonitis, abscess or fistula formation, frank hemorrhage,
and complete intestinal obstruction.

COLLABORATIVE MANAGEMENT

C

Assessment

- The nurse records the client's
    1. Diet history
    2. Family history of colorectal cancer
    3. Personal history of ulcerative colitis, familial poly-
    posis, or adenomas
    4. Change in bowel habits with or without blood in
    stool
    5. Weight loss, pain, abdominal fullness (late find-
    ings)
    6. Results of barium enema and colonoscopy
- The nurse assesses for
    1. Rectal bleeding (the most common manifestation)
    2. Change in stool
    3. Anemia (low hematocrit and hemoglobin; stool
    positive for occult blood)
    4. Cachexia (a late sign)
    5. Guarding or abdominal distention (a late sign)
    6. Abdominal mass (a late sign)

Planning and Implementation

✦ **NDx:** Grieving

- The nurse observes and identifies:
    1. The client's and family's current method of cop-
    ing
    2. The client's and family's present perceptions of
    the client's health problem
    3. Effective sources of support used in the past
- The nurse encourages the client to verbalize feelings
about the ostomy and to look at and touch the stoma.
- When the client is physically able, the nurse encourages the client's participation.

✦ **NDx:** Potential for Metastasis

Nonsurgical Management

- Preoperative radiation therapy aids in creating more
definite tumor margins, facilitating surgical resection.

- Radiation is also used postoperatively to decrease the risk of recurrence or palliatively to reduce pain, hemorrhage, bowel obstruction, or metastasis.
- Chemotherapy is used postoperatively to assist in control of metastatic symptoms and spread of the disease or is used to treat stage III cancer.
- The chemotherapeutic drug typically used is 5-fluorouracil (5-FU) in conjunction with levamisole (Ergamisol).
- Intrahepatic arterial chemotherapy is given with liver metastasis (usually 5-FU).

Surgical Management

- Colon resection, with or without formation of a colostomy, and abdominal-perineal (A-P) resection are the most common surgical procedures for tumors located in the colon or rectum.
- The bowel segment containing the tumor is resected (removed) along with several inches of bowel beyond the tumor margin, and an end-to-end anastomosis is performed; a temporary or permanent colostomy may be performed.
- In an A-P resection, the entire rectum and support structures are removed, and the anus is closed with permanent colostomy.
- The nurse provides preoperative care
    1. Reinforces the physician's explanation of the procedure
    2. Consults the enterostomal therapist (ET) if a colostomy is planned, to assist in identifying optimal placement of the ostomy and to instruct the client about the rationale and general principles of ostomies
    3. Instructs the client to consume only clear liquids for a day or longer before bowel surgery to minimize colonic contents
    4. Prepares the client for general anesthesia
    5. Administers laxatives, enemas, or GoLYTELY, if ordered, the morning of surgery or the day before surgery to mechanically clean the bowel ("bowel prep")
    6. Administers antibiotics preoperatively, as ordered
- The nurse provides postoperative care
    1. Places petroleum gauze over the stoma to keep it moist, followed by a dry, sterile dressing, if a pouch system is not in place immediately postoperatively

2. Places a pouch system on the stoma as soon as possible, in collaboration with the enterostomal therapist
3. Observes the stoma for
   a. Necrotic tissue
   b. Unusual amount of bleeding
   c. Color changes (the normal color is red-pink, indicating high vascularity; pale pink indicates low hemoglobin and hematocrit levels, and purple-black indicates compromised circulation)
4. Checks the pouch system for proper fit and signs of leakage
5. Assesses for functioning of the colostomy 2 to 4 days postoperatively; stool is liquid immediately postoperatively but becomes more solid
6. Empties the pouch when excess gas has collected or when it is one third to one half full of stool
7. Irrigates the perineal wound, if present, as ordered
8. Changes the perineal wound dressing, as directed
9. Assesses perineal wound; copious serosanguineous drainage is expected
10. Provides comfort measures for perineal itching and pain, such as antipruritic medications (benzocaine) and sitz baths
11. Assesses for signs of infection, abscess, or other complications
12. Instructs the client regarding activities such as assuming a side-lying position, avoiding sitting for long periods, and using a foam pad or pillow when in a sitting position
13. Administers cephalosporin antibiotics intravenously, as ordered
14. Administers pain medication, as ordered

Continuing Care

- The nurse provides verbal and written postoperative instructions:
  1. Inspection of the abdominal incision (and perineal wound if an A-P resection was done) for redness, tenderness, swelling, and drainage
  2. Dressing change and wound care procedures
  3. Colostomy care, including care of the stoma, application of the pouch system, skin protection, irrigation, and gas and odor control
  4. Pain management, including medications

5. Dietary control and avoidance of foods that cause excess gas formation and odor
6. Tips on how to resume normal activities, including work, travel, and sexual intercourse
7. Signs and symptoms of complications, such as intestinal obstruction and perforation

- The nurse provides contacts for community and health resources as needed:
  1. Social services
  2. ET
  3. United Ostomy Association
  4. American Cancer Society
  5. Home health services
  6. Pharmacy or other medical supply source

CANCER, ENDOMETRIAL

OVERVIEW

- Endometrial cancer (cancer of the uterus) is the most frequently occurring reproductive organ cancer.
- It is a slow-growing tumor associated with menopause and arises from the glandular component of the endometrial mucosa.
- Its initial growth is within the uterine cavity, followed by extension into the myometrium and cervix.
- The spread occurs through the lymphatics to the ovaries and parametrial, pelvic, inguinal, and para-aortic lymph nodes; by hematogenous metastasis to the lungs, liver, or bone; and by transtubal or intra-abdominal spread to the peritoneal cavity.
- Risk factors associated with endometrial cancer include
  1. Obesity
  2. Diabetes mellitus
  3. History of uterine polyps
  4. History of infertility
  5. Nulliparity
  6. Polycystic ovarian disease
  7. Estrogen stimulation, including unopposed menopausal estrogen replacement therapy (ERT)
  8. Late menopause
  9. Family history of uterine cancer

Transcultural Considerations

Endometrial cancer occurs more frequently in Caucasian women than in African-American women and typically in postmenopausal women aged 50 to 65 years.

COLLABORATIVE MANAGEMENT

Assessment

- The nurse records the client's
    1. Family history of endometrial cancer
    2. History of uterine cancer, diabetes, and hypertension
    3. Age
    4. Race
    5. History of obesity
    6. Childbearing status
    7. Prolonged estrogen use
- The nurse assesses for
    1. Postmenopausal bleeding (the primary symptom)
    2. Watery, serosanguineous vaginal discharge
    3. Low back pain
    4. Abdominal pain
    5. Low pelvic pain
    6. Enlarged uterus

Interventions

Nonsurgical Management

- Radiation therapy (external and internal) is used alone or in combination with surgery, depending on the stage of the cancer.
- If intracavity radiation therapy (IRT) is performed, an applicator is positioned within the uterus through the vagina.
- The nurse
    1. Maintains strict isolation and radiation precautions
    2. Provides bed rest, lying the client on her back, with the head either flat or elevated less than 20 degrees
    3. Restricts active movement to prevent dislodgment
    4. Inserts a Foley catheter
    5. Assesses for skin breakdown
    6. Provides a low-residue diet
    7. Encourages fluid intake

8. Administers antiemetics, broad-spectrum anti-infectives, tranquilizers, analgesics, heparin, and antidiarrheal medications
9. Restricts visitors

- Nurses who are pregnant or attempting pregnancy are usually not assigned clients undergoing IRT.
- The nurse instructs the client undergoing external radiation to
    1. Observe for signs of skin breakdown
    2. Avoid sunbathing
    3. Avoid bathing over the markings that outline the treatment site
    4. Recognize the complications of treatment, including cystitis, diarrhea, and nutritional alterations
- Chemotherapy is used to treat advanced and recurrent disease. Agents used include doxorubicin (Adriamycin), cisplatin, cyclophosphamide (Cytoxin, Proxytox◆). (See discussion of nursing care under Cancer.)
- Progesterone therapy may be used for stage I and II cancers, which are estrogen-dependent, and for stage IV cancer as palliative treatment. Hormones frequently used are medroxyprogesterone (Depo-Provera) and megestrol acetate (Megace).

Surgical Management

- Total abdominal hysterectomy and bilateral salpingo-oophorectomy are performed for stage I tumors, and a radical hysterectomy is performed for stage II.
- Refer to preoperative and postoperative care for the client undergoing hysterectomy under Cancer, Cervical.
- The nurse
    1. Provides emotional support
    2. Creates an atmosphere that encourages the client to ask questions and express fears and concerns
    3. Recognizes that reactions to radiation therapy vary among clients and that some may feel unclean or radioactive after treatments
    4. Provides information about alopecia (loss of hair) with chemotherapy and suggests that wigs, hats, scarves, or turbans be worn until regrowth occurs

Continuing Care

- The nurse provides the following information

1. Side effects that should be reported to the physician include vaginal bleeding, rectal bleeding, foul-smelling discharge, abdominal pain or distention, and hematuria
2. High-dose radiation causes sterility
3. Vaginal shrinkage occurs
4. Sexual partners cannot "catch" cancer
5. The client is not radioactive
6. Vaginal douching may decrease inflammation
7. A normal diet may be resumed

- The nurse teaches the client the following information if the client undergoes an abdominal hysterectomy:
    1. Avoid or limit stair climbing for 1 month
    2. Avoid tub baths and sitting for long periods
    3. Avoid strenuous activity or lifting anything weighing more than 10 to 20 pounds
    4. Expect physical changes
    5. Participate in moderate exercise, such as walking
    6. Consume foods that aid in healing, such as those high in protein, iron, and vitamin C
    7. Avoid sexual intercourse for 3 to 6 weeks
    8. Observe for signs of complications, including infection
    9. Expect emotional reactions
    10. Keep follow-up visits with the physician(s)

- The nurse refers the client to the local chapter of the American Cancer Society.

CANCER, ESOPHAGEAL

See Tumors, Esophageal.

CANCER, GASTRIC

See Cancer, Stomach.

CANCER, HEAD AND NECK

OVERVIEW

- Head and neck cancer is a curable disease when discovered early.
- Prognosis for those with more advanced disease depends on the extent and location of the tumor.
- Most of these tumors are squamous cell carcinomas, which may present as malignant ulcerations with underlying ulceration.
- Spread is predominantly to adjacent anatomic areas, such as mucosa, muscle, and bone.
- The two most important risk factors for the development of head and neck cancer are tobacco and alcohol use. Other factors include chewing tobacco use, pipe smoking, marijuana use, voice abuse, chronic laryngitis, exposure to industrial chemicals or hardwood dust, and complete neglect of oral hygiene.

Transcultural Considerations

1. Death rates in the non-Caucasian population from cancer of the larynx have increased 110% in the past 30 years.
2. Death rates in women with oral or laryngeal cancers have increased for all races during the past 30 years.

COLLABORATIVE MANAGEMENT

Assessment

- The nurse records the client's
    1. Risk factors for head and neck cancer
    2. Diet
    3. Impact of a history of chronic lung disease on the client's breathing pattern
    4. Family history of cancer
    5. Occupation and whether the job requires continual oral communication
    6. Interests
- The nurse assesses for
    1. Pain

2. Lump in the mouth, neck, or throat
3. Difficulty in swallowing
4. Color changes in the mouth or tongue to red, white, gray, dark brown, or black

5. Oral lesions that do not heal
6. Persistent or unexplained oral bleeding
7. Numbness of the mouth, lips, or face
8. Change in the fit of dentures
9. Burning sensation when drinking citrus juices or hot liquids
10. Persistent unilateral ear pain
11. Hoarseness or change in voice quality
12. Persistent or recurrent sore throat
13. Dyspnea
14. Anorexia or weight loss
15. Denial, guilt, blame, or shame
16. Ability to perform activities of daily living

Planning and Implementation

✦ NDx: Ineffective Breathing Pattern

- When planning treatment, the physician considers the client's general physical condition, nutritional status, and age, as well as the effects of the tumor on body function and the client's personal choice of therapy.
- Specific treatment depends on the extent and location of the lesion.

Nonsurgical Management

- The nurse
  1. Monitors the client's respiratory status by assessing respiratory rate, breath sounds, pulse oximetry, arterial blood gas values, and pulmonary function tests
  2. Positions the client to obtain optimal air exchange, and educates the client and family about the use of the Fowler's and semi-Fowler's position
  3. Monitors the client receiving radiation therapy for side effects, hoarseness, sore throat, difficulty swallowing, pain, skin irritation
  4. Provides adequate nutrition and hydration to lessen the effects of radiation therapy
- Chemotherapy is used alone and in combination with radiation therapy and surgery.
- Multiple-drug regimens may produce a higher response rate.

Surgical Management

- Surgical procedures include
    1. Laryngectomy with cordectomy, cordal stripping, partial laryngectomy, or complete laryngectomy
    2. Tracheostomy
    3. Oropharyngeal cancer resection
- Preoperatively, the nurse explains and instructs the client on
    1. Self-care activities for maintaining the airway
    2. Compensatory methods of communication
    3. Suctioning
    4. Pain control methods
    5. Critical care environment
    6. Nutritional support
    7. Feeding tubes
    8. Outcome goals for discharge
- Postoperatively, the nurse
    1. Monitors the client's airway for patency, vital signs, hemodynamic status, and level of comfort
    2. Monitors the client for complications of the surgical procedure
        a. Airway obstruction
        b. Hemorrhage
        c. Wound breakdown
        d. Tumor recurrence
    3. Provides wound, flap, and reconstructive tissue care, as ordered
    4. Provides tracheostomy or laryngectomy tube care, as needed:
        a. Checks the cuff pressure
        b. Provides humidification and warm air, as ordered
        c. Suctions, as needed, and monitors the client for hypoxia and tissue trauma
        d. Changes tracheostomy ties, per institution policy
    5. Monitors the client for complications of the tracheostomy tube:
        a. Obstruction with secretions
        b. Dislodgment and/or accidental decannulation
        c. Pneumothorax
        d. Subcutaneous emphysema
        e. Bleeding
        f. Infection

6. Turns and repositions the client frequently
7. Encourages the client to cough and suctions the mouth and airway, as needed
8. Provides nutritional support initially through intravenous feedings and then through tube feedings
9. Assesses the client's ability to swallow before removing the feeding tube and beginning oral feedings
10. Collaborates with the speech/language pathologist to develop and implement the speech rehabilitation program:
    a. Writing
    b. Use of artificial larynx followed by learning esophageal speech
    c. Use of electrolarynges
11. Provides frequent oral hygiene

✦ **NDx:** Risk for Aspiration

- A dynamic swallowing study evaluates the client's ability to protect the airway from aspiration and helps determine the appropriate method of swallow rehabilitation.
- For the client with a nasogastric tube, the nurse
    1. Elevates the head of the bed
    2. Adheres to tube-feeding regimens
    3. Checks residual feeding amounts every 4 to 6 hours or before bolus feeding
    4. Evaluates the client's tolerance of tube feeding
    5. Inflates the tracheostomy tube before feeding
    6. Collaborates with the speech/language pathologist to teach the client alternative methods of swallowing

✦ **NDx:** Anxiety

The nurse
1. Explores with the client the reasons for anxiety and fear
   a. Unknown
   b. Pain
   c. Airway compromise
   d. Hospitalization
   e. Loss of control
2. Refers the client to home care nurses or community support organizations
3. Administers antianxiety medication, as ordered

159

- The nurse
    1. Provides encouragement and support
    2. Assists the client to integrate into the home and social environment
    3. Refers the client and family to counseling, as needed
    4. Suggests clothing and accessories that can be used to cover the areas of disfigurement

Continuing Care

- The nurse
    1. Collaborates with the case manager to ensure that the client or family can provide the needed support:
        a. Care of the stoma, tracheostomy, or laryngectomy tube
        b. Incision and airway care
        c. Observation for signs of infection
        d. Activities of daily living
        e. Maintenance of humidity in the home
        f. Communication devices and techniques
    2. Refers the client to community health agencies familiar with the care of clients with head and neck cancer
    3. Coordinates the referrals made by the interdisciplinary team:
        a. Home care agencies
        b. Nutritionists
        c. Nurses
        d. Physical and occupational therapists
        e. Speech/language pathologist
        f. Social workers
    4. Encourages the client to return to a normal social life

CANCER, HEPATIC

See Cancer, Liver.

CANCER, KIDNEY

See Cancer, Renal.

CANCER, LIVER

- Primary hepatic carcinoma is rare in the United States.
- The most common form is hepatoma, and signs include jaundice, ascites, bleeding, and encephalopathy.
- Liver cancer usually develops as a metastatic process from primary cancer sites, such as the esophagus, stomach, colon, rectum, breasts, lungs, or skin (malignant melanoma).
- Elevated serum alkaline phosphatase levels are common, and a needle biopsy confirms metastasis.
- Surgery is indicated for the client with a single metastatic lesion; a hepatic lobe resection is performed.
- High-dose hepatic chemotherapy may be given, and hepatic artery ligation deprives the metastatic lesion of oxygen.

CANCER, LUNG

OVERVIEW

- Lung cancer is the leading cause of cancer-related deaths worldwide
- Bronchogenic carcinoma spreads through direct extension and lymphatic dissemination.
- The four major types of lung cancer are
    1. Small cell (oat cell)
    2. Epidermal (squamous cell)
    3. Adenocarcinoma
    4. Large cell anaplastic carcinoma

Women's Health Considerations

- Deaths from lung cancer in women exceed deaths from all other cancers including breast cancer.

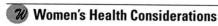 **Transcultural Considerations**

1. Lung cancer occurs more often and with higher mortality in non-Caucasians than in Caucasians.
2. Most common newly diagnosed cancer in African-Americans.
3. Mortality rates are higher in countries with significant paper and petroleum industries.

COLLABORATIVE MANAGEMENT

Assessment

- The nurse records the client's
  1. Smoking history
  2. Environmental exposure to carcinogens
  3. Hoarseness
  4. Complaints of pain or vague discomfort
  5. Shoulder, arm, or chest wall pain
  6. Dyspnea and related respiratory symptoms
- The nurse assesses for
  1. Sputum quantity and quality
  2. Breathing patterns
  3. Abnormal retractions, stridor, and/or use of accessory muscles
  4. Asymmetry of diaphragmatic movement
  5. Chest wall tenderness
  6. Decreased tactile fremitus over areas of consolidation
  7. Tracheal deviation
  8. Dullness or obvious masses on percussion of the chest wall
  9. Decreased or absent breath sounds over the tumor
  10. Increased vocal fremitus, which indicates consolidation
  11. Pleural friction rub
  12. Distant heart sounds
  13. Cardiac dysrhythmias
  14. Cyanosis of the lips or fingertips, or clubbing
  15. Lethargy and somnolence
  16. Pain radiating to the shoulder

Planning and Implementation

✦ NDx: Impaired Gas Exchange

Nonsurgical Management

- The nurse
    1. Provides symptomatic relief with medications, especially bronchodilators and steroids to decrease bronchospasm, inflammation, and edema
    2. Positions the client in an upright position for ease of breathing
    3. Provides supplemental oxygen
    4. Administers chemotherapy to promote tumor regression
        a. Understands the mode of action of each agent
        b. Takes measures to control side effects
        c. Educates the client and family and explains how they can manage potential side effects
    5. Administers immunotherapy, as ordered, with tumor extracts, irradiated whole tumor cells, or cells killed by other methods; and/or nonspecific immune therapy with bacille Calmette-Guérin vaccine and levamisole
- Radiation therapy may be used for localized intrathoracic lung cancers; it is also used as a palliation for hemoptosis, bronchial obstruction, dysphagia, and bone pain.
- Thoracentesis may be performed to relieve pleural effusion.
- A chest tube and sclerosing agent may be inserted to create a pleurodesis, which causes adherence of the pleura to the chest wall, eliminating the potential space and preventing effusion accumulation.

Surgical Management

- Surgical management includes
    1. *Laser therapy,* to relieve endobronchial obstructions
    2. *Thoracotomy,* an opening into the thoracic cavity to locate tumors, perform a biopsy, or identify sites of bleeding or injury
        a. *Thoracotomy with pneumonectomy* (removal of the lung), for bronchogenic carcinoma, involvement of a mainstem bronchus, or invasion of the main pulmonary artery
        b. *Thoracotomy with simple lobectomy* (removal of a lobe), for tumors confined to a single lobe

163

c. *Thoracotomy with sleeve lobectomy* (removal of the affected lobe and adjacent lobe) is done when carcinomas are within or compress a lobar bronchus

3. *Resection* is any surgical removal of part of the lung that does not involve a complete lobectomy.
   a. *Limited resection* is done for clients unable to tolerate lobectomy or pneumonectomy.
   b. *Segmental resection* (segmentectomy) is a pulmonary resection that includes the bronchus, pulmonary artery and vein, and lung parenchyma of the involved lung segment(s).
   c. *Wedge resection* is the removal of the peripheral portion of small localized area of disease.

- The nurse provides routine preoperative care and instructions on what to expect postoperatively.
- The nurse provides postoperative care:
   1. Provides routine postoperative care
   2. Maintains chest tubes and the closed chest drainage systems, which drain air and blood that accumulate in the pleural space
   3. Monitors for excess bleeding in the drainage system
   4. Monitors for an air leak in the underwater seal chamber
   5. Checks for the rise and fall of fluid in the column as the client breathes in and out
   6. Assesses for the absence or presence of lung sounds
   7. Does *not* turn postoperative pneumonectomy clients onto the operative side. Positioning on the operative side can place increased stress on the bronchial stump incision and risk disruption of the suture line

✦ **NDx:** Pain

- The nurse
   1. Performs a complete pain assessment and questions the client about factors that intensify and relieve the pain
   2. Administers analgesics (parenteral, oral, transdermal opioids)
   3. Intervenes with nonpharmacologic measures such as positioning, hot or cold compresses, distractions, and guided imagery

Continuing Care

- The nurse provides health teaching:
  1. Physical activity limitations
  2. Coping with dyspnea
  3. Pain relief measures, including prescription medication
  4. Importance of minimizing exposure to others with infections
  5. Signs and symptoms that should be reported to health care professionals
  6. Psychosocial preparations, depending on prognosis
- The client is referred to community health agencies, as needed.

Cancer, Mouth

See Cancer, Oral.

Cancer, Nasal and Sinus

OVERVIEW

- Tumors of the nose and sinuses are uncommon; they may be benign or malignant.
- Symptoms mimic sinusitis and include persistent nasal obstruction, drainage, bloody discharge, and pain.

 Transcultural Considerations

The incidence of nasopharyngeal cancer is higher in Asian-Americans than in other groups; the cause may be environmental.

COLLABORATIVE MANAGEMENT

- Treatment includes
  1. Radiation therapy (primary treatment)

2. Surgical resection (possible nasal prosthesis)
3. Chemotherapy (rare)
- The nurse
    1. Provides routine postoperative care if surgery was performed
    2. Maintains a patent airway (tracheostomy care may be required)
    3. Provides wound care and strict attention to the client's nutritional needs
    4. Provides meticulous mouth care and maxillary cavity care using saline irrigations
    5. Manages pain and monitors the client for infection

CANCER, ORAL

OVERVIEW

- Tumors of the oral cavity are classified as premalignant, malignant, or benign; this focuses on premalignant and malignant lesions.
- *Premalignant* lesions include
    1. *Leukoplakia*—a white spot or patch in the mouth that is usually asymptomatic. It can be caused by mechanical factors, such as poorly fitting dentures, cheek nibbling, malocclusion, or smoking (sometimes referred to as "smoker's patch"); by familial factors; or by poor nutrition.
    2. *Erythroplakia*—a red, velvety-appearing patch in the mouth that is usually asymptomatic; 90% of all lesions are early squamous cell carcinoma.
- The types of oral cancer include
    1. Squamous cell carcinoma, which grows slowly and is associated with the use of tobacco and alcohol, as well as poor nutrition
    2. Basal cell carcinoma, which occurs primarily on the lips and which usually does not metastasize
    3. Kaposi's sarcoma, which appears as painless red-purple oral plaques and is associated with acquired immunodeficiency syndrome (AIDS) (see AIDS)

Transcultural Considerations

1. The relative survival rate for Caucasians with oral cancer and pharyngeal cancer is 55% compared to a relative 5-year survival rate of 33% for African Americans with oral cancer.

2. The 30-year trend in death rates due to oral cancers in men shows a decrease among Caucasians but a 70% increase in the non-Caucasian population.

3. Clients who work outdoors are more likely to have basal cell carcinomas, especially Caucasians with fair skin.

COLLABORATIVE MANAGEMENT

Assessment

- The nurse records the client's
    1. Employment history and history of exposure to known carcinogens or irritants, such as tobacco and alcohol
    2. Family history of cancer, especially oral cancer
    3. Oral hygiene practices
    4. Past and current nutritional status
- The nurse assesses the client for
    1. Lesions in the oral cavity
    2. Evidence of mouth pain
    3. Alteration in speech
    4. Enlarged cervical lymph nodes (indicate metastasis)
    5. Fear of cancer
    6. Body image disturbance

Planning and Implementation

✦ **NDx:** Risk for Ineffective Breathing Pattern

Nonsurgical Management

- Maintaining airway patency is the goal of nursing interventions and is centered on decreasing the tenacity of oral secretions, enabling the client to expectorate secretions, and decreasing edema of the head and neck.
- The nurse
    1. Suggests modifications in oral hygiene practice, such as use of a water pic or gauze sponges, because of oral pain, bleeding, or edema

2. Instructs the client to avoid the use of commercial mouthwashes, which contain alcohol; use a solution of a half teaspoon of baking soda in 8 ounces of water or a solution of half hydrogen peroxide and half normal saline
3. Provides oral suction with a Yankauer catheter as needed
4. Promotes fluid intake to thin secretions
5. Elevates the head of the bed at least 30 degrees
6. Administers steroids and antibiotics, as ordered

Surgical Management

- A tracheostomy may be needed for the client to sustain normal breathing.

✦ NDx: Altered Oral Mucous Membrane

Nonsurgical Management

- The two standard nonsurgical therapies for clients with cancer of the oral cavity are radiation therapy and chemotherapy:
  1. Radiation therapy can be administered by external beam to the tumor site or by implantation of radioactive substances directly into the tumor area (interstitial radiation therapy).
  2. Methotrexate, bleomycin, cisplatin, cyclophosphamide, and doxorubicin are some of the chemotherapeutic agents that may be used to treat oral cancers.
- The nurse instructs the client to use foam toothbrushes soaked in chlorheide to reduce bacteria and control candidiasis.

Surgical Management

- Small, noninvasive lesions can be excised using carbon dioxide laser therapy or cryotherapy (extreme cold application) in a surgical center. Clients with more invasive or extensive lesions require more radical surgical excision.
- The nurse provides preoperative care:
  1. Assesses the client's understanding of the surgical procedure
  2. Reviews preoperative and postoperative expectations with the client and family or other support persons:
     a. For small lesion excision: liquid to soft food diet after surgery, no activity limitations, and analgesic therapy

b. For large lesion excision (composite resection): probable tracheostomy, oxygen therapy, temporary speech loss (from the tracheostomy), frequent vital sign monitoring, nothing-by-mouth (NPO) status for 7 to 10 days, and placement of intravenous lines

- The nurse provides postoperative care:
  1. After local excision, teaches the client routine gentle oral hygiene and advises him or her to avoid extremely hot food and beverages, spicy foods, hard or crisp foods, and alcohol until the area is completely healed
  2. Maintains airway patency after extensive excision or composite resection (the most important intervention)
  3. Assesses the need for a speech/language pathologist
  4. Avoids performing oral hygiene or suction or taking the client's oral temperature until ordered by the physician
  5. Provides gentle mouth care when permitted
  6. Elevates the head of the bed to at least 30 degrees
  7. Administers analgesics for pain, as ordered
  8. Maintains enteral or parenteral nutrition while the client is on NPO status
  9. Monitors for difficulty in swallowing, aspiration, or leakage of saliva or fluids from the suture line

Continuing Care

- The nurse
  1. Assesses the client's need for equipment, such as that required for oral suctioning and nasogastric (enteral) feedings at home
  2. Provides instructions regarding medications, diet or feedings, dressing changes, early symptoms of infection, and special treatments, such as tracheostomy care
  3. Collaborates with the dietitian to meet the client's nutritional needs
  4. Refers the client and family to home health services, if needed, for treatments, pain control, nutritional support, and emotional support
  5. Assesses the client for body image disturbance
  6. Informs the client that people who undergo total glossectomy (removal of the tongue) can be fitted

with a special maxillofacial prosthesis to allow speech
7. Refers the client to the case manager to assess financial needs

CANCER, OVARIAN

OVERVIEW

- Ovarian cancer is the leading cause of death from female reproductive organ malignancies.
- The most common tumor is the serous adenocarcinoma.
- Tumors grow rapidly, spread quickly, and are often bilateral, with the worst prognosis of all epithelial tumors.
- Cancer spreads by several mechanisms: direct spread to other organs in the pelvis, distal spread through lymphatic drainage, and peritoneal seeding.

COLLABORATIVE MANAGEMENT

- The nurse records the client's
    1. Family history of ovarian cancer
    2. History of breast, bowel, or endometrial cancer
    3. Nullparity
    4. Infertility
    5. History of dysmenorrhea or heavy bleeding
    6. Diet history, including intake of animal fat
- The nurse assesses for
    1. Abdominal pain or swelling
    2. Dyspepsia
    3. Indigestion
    4. Gas and distention
    5. Heavy menstrual flow
    6. Dysfunctional bleeding
    7. Premenstrual tension
    8. Abdominal mass
- Exploratory laparotomy is performed to diagnose and stage ovarian tumors.
- For nursing care, see discussions under Cancer, Cervical, and Cancer, Endometrial.

- The options for treatment depend on the stage of the cancer and include
    1. Chemotherapy: used postoperatively for all stages, although its purpose is usually palliative for stage IV tumors
    2. Intraperitoneal chemotherapy: involves the instillation of chemotherapy agents into the abdominal cavity
    3. Immunotherapy: alters the immunologic response of the ovary and promotes tumor resistance
    4. External radiation therapy: used if the tumor has invaded other organs
    5. Total abdominal hysterectomy and bilateral salpingo-oophorectomy: the surgical procedure for all stages of ovarian cancer
- The nurse
    1. Encourages the client to express feelings about disease
    2. Provides information about ovarian cancer and treatment options
    3. Provides encouragement and support to the client and family

CANCER, PANCREATIC

OVERVIEW

- Pancreatic tumors are highly malignant; they originate in the epithelial cells of the pancreatic ductal system.
- Primary tumors are generally adenocarcinomas and grow in well-differentiated glandular patterns.
- Pancreatic tumors are highly metastatic, with rapid growth and spread to surrounding organs by direct extension and invasion of the lymphatic and vascular systems, lungs, liver, and spleen.

➤ Transcultural Considerations

1. Pancreatic cancer occurs 50% more often in African-Americans than in Caucasians.
2. It is 30% more common in men than women.
3. It occurs twice as frequently in smokers as in nonsmokers.

4. The highest incidence is in people 65 to 79 years of age.

COLLABORATIVE MANAGEMENT
Assessment
- The nurse records the client's
  1. Medical history, including diabetes and pancreatitis
  2. Smoking history
  3. Coffee intake
  4. Employment history to determine exposure to known environmental carcinogens
  5. Skin color if jaundice is present
  6. Ethnic group
  7. Weight loss
- The nurse assesses for
  1. Jaundice (yellow discoloration associated with obstruction) and pruritus (itching)
  2. Clay-colored stool and dark, frothy urine
  3. Enlarged gallbladder and liver
  4. Firm, fixed mass in the left upper abdominal quadrant or epigastric area
  5. Abdominal pain, constant dullness in the right upper quadrant or pain related to eating or activity
  6. Referred back pain
  7. Leg or calf pain with swelling or redness
  8. Weight loss
  9. Anorexia accompanied by early satiety, nausea, flatulence, and vomiting
  10. Dull sound on abdominal percussion indicating ascites
  11. Body image change and fear

Planning and Implementation
Nonsurgical Management
- The nurse provides opioid analgesia with meperidine hydrochloride (Demerol), morphine, or hydromorphone hydrochloride (Dilaudid), as ordered; dependency is not a consideration because of the poor prognosis.
- Chemotherapy has limited success; combining agents such as fluorouracil (5-FU) and carmustine (BCNU) has better results than single-agent chemotherapy. Mitomycin (Mutamycin) and streptozocin (Zanosar) may also be used.

- External radiation therapy to shrink pancreatic tumor cells may provide pain relief but has not increased survival rates.
- Implantation of radon seeds, in combination with systemic or intra-arterial administration of floxuridine (FUDR), has also been used.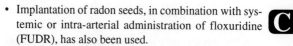

Surgical Management

- Surgical management is the most effective management.
- The classic surgery, or the Whipple procedure, entails extensive surgical manipulation, including resection of the proximal head of the pancreas, the duodenum, a portion of the jejunum, the stomach (partial or total gastrectomy), and the gallbladder, with anastomosis of the pancreatic duct (pancreatojejunostomy), the common bile duct (choledochojejunostomy), and the stomach (gastrojejunostomy) to the jejunum; the spleen may also be removed (splenectomy).
- Palliative measures to relieve obstruction, such as cholecystojejunostomy, may be done as a bypass procedure.
- The nurse provides routine preoperative care.
- The nurse provides intensive postoperative care and monitoring:
  1. Monitors the drainage tubes placed during surgery to remove drainage and secretions from the area and to prevent stress on the anastomosis site
  2. Assesses the tubes and drainage devices for undue stress or kinking; maintains tubes in a dependent position
  3. Monitors drainage for color, consistency, and amount
  4. Observes for fistula formation (drainage of pancreatic fluids are corrosive and irritating to the skin, and internal leakage causes peritonitis)
  5. Places the client in a semi-Fowler's position to reduce stress on the suture line and anastomosis and to optimize lung expansion
  6. Maintains fluid and electrolyte balance
  7. Closely monitors vital signs for decreased blood pressure and increased heart rate, decreased vascular pressures, decreased hemoglobin and hematocrit levels, and electrolyte imbalances
  8. Assesses blood glucose levels for transient hyperglycemia or hypoglycemia due to surgical manipulation of the pancreas

9. Monitors the client for pitting edema of the extremities and dependent edema in the sacrum and back
- Enteral feeding with commercially prepared tube feeding is used while intestinal function is intact.
- A jejunostomy tube is inserted for late stages of pancreatic carcinoma; this method is preferred for lessening reflux and facilitating absorption.
- Hyperalimentation by total parenteral nutrition to optimize nutrition may be used as a single measure or in combination with tube feedings; a Hickman or other type of catheter may be required for long-term use.

Continuing Care

- Many of the care measures are palliative and aimed at providing relief of symptoms.
- Many clients are diagnosed just a few months before death occurs.
- The nurse helps the client identify what needs to be done to prepare for death such as write a will, see family members and friends, make requests for memorial service or funeral known.
- Special home care preparations depend on the client's physical and activity limitations.
- The nurse refers the client to religious leader or support services.
- Regular home care nursing and assistive nursing personnel are scheduled to assist the client and family.
- The nurse provides emotional support to the family and significant others.

CANCER, PROSTATIC

OVERVIEW

- Prostatic cancer is the most common cancer among American men and the second leading cause of deaths due to cancer.
- Although its etiology is unclear, two factors influence its development:
    1. Intact hypothalamic-pituitary-testicular pathway
    2. Advancing age

- Ninety-five percent of prostatic tumors are adenocarcinomas arising from the epithelial cells of the prostate and are usually located in the posterior lobe or outer portion of the gland.
- A prostatic tumor is a slow-growing malignancy with a predictable metastatic pattern to the prostatic and perivesicular lymph nodes, pelvic lymph nodes, bone marrow, and bones of the pelvis, sacrum, and lumbar spine.

→ Transcultural Considerations

1. African-American men experience prostatic cancer twice as frequently as do Caucasians:
   a. They develop it at an earlier age.
   b. The disease is more advanced at the time of diagnosis.
   c. The mortality rate is higher.
2. Hispanic and Asian-American men have a lower incidence of prostatic cancer and a lower mortality rate than do Caucasians.

COLLABORATIVE MANAGEMENT

- Clinical manifestations include
  1. Symptoms related to bladder neck obstruction:
     a. Difficulty in initiating urination
     b. Recurrent bladder infections
     c. Urinary retention
     d. Gross, painless hematuria
  2. Bone pain (advanced disease)
- Prostate cancer screening
  1. Digital rectal examination for a stony hard prostate gland with irregularities or indurations
  2. Prostate-specific antigen (PSA) level as a screening test only
     a. Normal level of PSA is 4ng/mL.
     b. PSA levels are elevated in clients with increased prostatic tissue as a result of various conditions, including cancer of the prostate, benign prostatic hyperplasia, prostatic infarction, and prostatitis.
     c. PSA levels slightly higher in the elderly and African Americans
  3. Biopsy of prostatic tissue
- Management includes

1. Surgical intervention:
   a. Prostatectomy
   b. Prostatectomy with pelvic lymphadenectomy
   c. Radical prostatectomy
   d. Cryosurgical ablation
   e. Bilateral orchiectomy
- Nursing care of the client after a radical prostatectomy includes
   1. Encourage the client to use patient-controlled analgesia (PCA) as needed.
   2. Keep the client on bed rest on the day of surgery. Help the client to get out of bed and ambulate for a short distance by the first postoperative day.
   3. Keep the client NPO, usually until the first or second postoperative day.
   4. Maintain the sequential compression device until the client begins to ambulate. Apply antiembolic stockings until discharge.
   5. Monitor the client for deep vein thrombosis and pulmonary embolus.
   6. Keep an accurate record of intake and output, including Jackson-Pratt or other drainage device.
   7. Teach the client how to care for the urinary catheter because he will be discharged with the catheter in place.
   8. Teach the client how to use a leg bag.
   9. Emphasize the importance of not straining during a bowel movement. Advise the client not to use suppositories or enemas.
   10. Complications of radical prostatectomy include sexual dysfunction and urinary incontinence.
      a. Biofeedback has been used successfully as a noninvasive treatment for urinary incontinence.
      b. An artificial sphincter may be surgically implanted to treat urinary incontinence.
   11. Emphasize the importance of follow-up appointments with health care provider to monitor progress.
- Cryosurgical ablation of the prostate is a minimally invasive procedure used as an alternative to radical prostatectomy.
   1. Advantages of this procedure are minimal blood loss, minimal postoperative pain, decreased risk for postoperative urinary incontinence, a one-to-two day hospital stay, and earlier return to activities such as work.

176

- Interstitial radiation therapy or radioactive seed implantation for localized disease.
- External beam radiation is performed as an alternative curative treatment to surgery for locally contained tumors, as an adjunct to radical prostatectomy, or for palliation of the client's symptoms.
- Androgen deprivation by simple orchiectomy or hormone therapy with estrogens such as diethylstilbestrol (DES) or a gonadotropin-releasing hormone agonist or androgen-blocking agent, such as flutamide.
- Health teaching includes a discussion of quality-of-life issues, including sexuality, body image, and the impact of a cancer diagnosis on life.

CANCER, RENAL

OVERVIEW

- Renal cell carcinoma is also referred to as adenocarcinoma or hypernephroma.
- The healthy functional tissue of the kidney is replaced and displaced by the growth of abnormal, nonfunctional cells.
- Pathophysiologic effects include fever, anemia, erythrocytosis, hypercalcemia, liver dysfunction, and other miscellaneous hormonal effects.
- Complications of renal tumors include metastasis through the blood or lymph to the liver, lungs, and long bones, and other kidney and urinary tract infections.

COLLABORATIVE MANAGEMENT

Assessment

- The nurse assesses the client for
    1. Risk factors, such as smoking or environmental exposures
    2. Weight loss
    3. Changes in urine color
    4. Abdominal or flank pain
    5. Asymmetry or obvious protrusion in the flank area
    6. Hematuria
    7. Renal bruit
    8. Skin pallor

9. Increased pigmentation of the nipples and gyneco-mastia
10. Muscle wasting, weakness, generally poor nutri-tional status
11. Anxiety and fear
12. Red blood cells (RBCs) in the urine
13. Decreased hematocrit and hemoglobin
14. Increased sedimentation rate, adrenocorticotropic hormone, cortisol, and renin
15. Hypercalcemia

Interventions

- Treatment consists of
  1. Chemotherapy
  2. Radical nephrectomy, which may be followed by radiation therapy
- Postoperatively, the nurse
  1. Observes the abdomen for distention due to bleed-ing
  2. Observes for adrenal insufficiency: Large urinary output with subsequent loss of sodium and water leads to hypotension, which is followed by oliguria
  3. Administers intravenous fluids and packed RBCs, as ordered
  4. Monitors intake and output hourly
  5. Weighs the client daily
  6. Monitors vital signs and neurologic signs every 4 hours
  7. Administers pain medication, as ordered: Acute pain control is more effectively achieved when sedatives are used in combination with the opioid analgesic
  8. Administers antibiotics or steroids, as ordered

CANCER, SKIN

OVERVIEW

- Overexposure to sunlight is the major cause of cutane-ous malignancy.
- The most common skin cancers include

1. *Actinic* or *solar keratoses:* premalignant lesions involving the keratinocytes of the epidermis; they are common in chronic sun-damaged skin and may progress to squamous cell carcinoma
2. *Squamous cell carcinomas:* malignant neoplasms of the epidermis characterized by local invasion and potential for metastasis; predisposed by sun exposure and chronic epithelial damage from repeated injury or irritation
3. *Basal cell carcinomas:* lesions that arise in the basal cell layer of the epidermis, resulting primarily from ultraviolet light radiation exposure, genetic predisposition, and chronic irritation
4. *Melanomas:* highly metastatic pigmented malignant lesions originating in the melanin-producing cells of the epidermis

- Risk factors include genetic predisposition and precursor lesions, which resemble unusual moles.

➤ Transcultural Considerations

Skin cancer is highest among light-skinned races and people over 60 years of age.

COLLABORATIVE MANAGEMENT

Assessment

- The nurse records the client's
  1. Risk factors
  2. Age and race
  3. Family history of skin cancer
  4. Past surgical removal of skin growths
  5. Changes in size, color, or sensation of any mole, birthmark, wart, or scar
  6. Sunlight exposure
  7. Exposure to chemical carcinogens
  8. Skin lesions subjected to repeated irritation
- The nurse assesses for
  1. Skin lesions in sun-exposed areas and the entire skin surface
  2. Unusual appearance of moles, warts, birthmarks, and scars
  3. Associated symptoms, such as tenderness and itching

Interventions

- Treatment consists of
    1. *Topical chemotherapy with 5-fluorouracil cream:* for multiple actinic keratoses
    2. *Radiation therapy:* for elderly clients with large, deeply invasive basal cell tumors who are poor surgical risks
    3. *Immunotherapy* is an experimental treatment for clients with melanoma that has metastasized to distant sites
    4. *Cryosurgery* with liquid nitrogen for isolated lesions
    5. Procedures used for small lesions with well-defined borders: *curettage,* to scrape away the cancerous tissue, followed by *electrodesiccation,* which involves placement of an electric probe on the wound surface to destroy the malignant tissue remnants by thermal and electrical energy
    6. *Excision:* for large or poorly defined cancers
    7. *Mohs' surgery:* for basal and squamous cell carcinoma

CANCER, SPINAL CORD

See Tumors, Spinal Cord.

CANCER, STOMACH

OVERVIEW

- Malignant neoplasms found in the stomach develop from the mucous membrane.
- In advanced disease, invasion extends to the muscularis or beyond.
- Most stomach cancers develop in the pylorus and antrum.

- Methods of extension include spread within the gastric wall into the regional lymphatics and direct organ invasion.
- Adenocarcinomas are the most common type, followed by malignant lymphoma.

 Transcultural Considerations

1. Stomach cancer occurs more frequently in men, in African-Americans, and in lower socioeconomic groups.
2. In the United States, the incidence of gastric cancer is highest in the North Central and Northeast regions.

COLLABORATIVE MANAGEMENT
Assessment

- The nurse assesses for *early* symptoms of disease:
    1. Indigestion
    2. Abdominal discomfort
    3. Anorexia
    4. Weight loss
    5. Fatigue
- The nurse assesses for *late* symptoms of disease:
    1. Vomiting
    2. Epigastric mass
    3. Hepatomegaly
    4. Ascites
    5. Enlarged lymph nodes
    6. Blumer's shelf (peritoneal seeding)
    7. Krukenberg's tumor (metastatic ovarian tumor)
    8. Pallor and cachexia
    9. Acanthosis nigricans (axillary rough and pigmented skin)
    10. Recurrent thrombophlebitis
    11. Evidence of tumor on upper gastrointestinal series
    12. Hypoalbuminemia, elevated carcinoembryonic antigen (CEA) level, anemia

Planning and Implementation

- Combination drug chemotherapy including 5-fluorouracil, doxorubicin, and mitomycin C has proved more effective than single-agent chemotherapy.

181

- Radiation therapy is used in conjunction with surgery.
- Surgical management is usually curative in *early* disease and involves distal subtotal gastrectomy by Billroth I or Billroth II procedure (see Ulcers, Peptic), combined with lymph node dissection.
- Pallitative surgical resection in *late* disease may improve the client's quality of life; total gastrectomy is performed for cancer in the upper portion of the stomach. Gastroenterostomy is done for tumors at the gastric outlet.
- The nurse provides routine postoperative care for the client undergoing general anesthesia and provides care of the nasogastric tube. (Also see "Surgical Management" under Ulcers, Peptic.)
- The nurse
    1. Administers nonopioid agents and opioids; opioids may be administered by patient-controlled analgesia pump
    2. Provides and teaches relaxation techniques, cutaneous stimulation, and visual imagery
- Total parenteral nutrition (TPN) may be required immediately after surgery and in the later recovery period if oral intake is poorly tolerated.
- Postoperative oral intake progresses from oral liquids to small, frequent, solid food feedings; milk and dairy products are often eliminated because of lactose intolerance.
- The nurse
    1. Administers antiemetics, as ordered, for nausea relief
    2. Observes the client for signs and symptoms of dumping syndrome during the postoperative period
    3. In collaboration with the dietitian, provides a diet high in protein and fat and low in carbohydrates to prevent dumping syndrome

Continuing Care

- The nurse provides verbal and written postoperative instructions:
    1. Dietary restrictions individualized to the client
    2. Pain management techniques, including medications
    3. Inspection of incision for redness, tenderness, swelling, and drainage

4. Dressing change procedures, if necessary
5. Side effects of chemotherapy or radiation treatments
- The nurse refers the client and family to home health services, hospice services, and appropriate support groups, such as I Can Cope, provided by the American Cancer Society.

CANCER, TESTICULAR

OVERVIEW

- Testicular cancer is the third leading cause of cancer deaths in young men.
- Primary testicular cancers fall into two groups:
    1. *Germinal* tumors arise from the sperm-producing germ cells and include seminoma and non-seminoma tumors (embryonal, teratoma, and choriocarcinoma)
    2. *Nongerminal* tumors arise from other structures in the testicles and include interstitial cell tumors and androblastoma

Transcultural Considerations

Testicular cancer is found most frequently in Caucasians and is rare in African-Americans.

COLLABORATIVE MANAGEMENT

Assessment

- The nurse records the client's
    1. Age and race
    2. History or presence of undescended testes
    3. Family history of testicular cancer
    4. Family situation:
        a. Desire for children
        b. Interest in sperm storage in a sperm bank
- The nurse assesses for
    1. Palpable lymphadenopathy
    2. Abdominal masses
    3. Gynecomastia

4. Psychologic ramifications of the disease
5. Increased alfa-fetoprotein and the beta subunit of human chorionic gonadotropin

Planning and Implementation

✦ NDx: Potential for Metastasis

Nonsurgical Management

- Combination chemotherapy is dramatically effective in treating nonseminomatous testicular cancer, especially cisplatin (Platinol) in combination with other agents.
- External beam radiation therapy may be used.

Surgical Management

- *Unilateral orchiectomy* (removal of the testis) is done for diagnosis and primary surgical management.
- *Radical retroperitoneal lymph node dissection* is used to stage the disease and to reduce tumor volume so that chemotherapy or radiation therapy is more effective.
- The nurse provides preoperative care:
  1. Provides routine preoperative care
  2. Prepares the client for an extensive surgical procedure and a large incision if radical retroperitoneal lymph node dissection is to be performed.
- The nurse provides postoperative care:
  1. Provides routine postoperative care
  2. Assesses the client for any complications of major abdominal surgery
  3. Administers pain medication, as ordered
  4. Monitors the client for complications of immobility

✦ NDx: Risk for Sexual Dysfunction

- Infertility is related to oligospermia and azospermia.
- The nurse provides important client education about reproduction, fertility, and sexuality in the pretreatment stage, including discussion of options.
- Sperm storage for adequate sperm counts prior to undergoing treatment may be suggested.
- Other options include donor insemination, adoption, or not fathering children.

Continuing Care

- The nurse provides postoperative instructions:

1. Notify the physician of chills, fever, increasing tenderness or pain around the incision, drainage, or dehiscence of the incision.
2. Resume normal activities except lifting objects heavier than 20 pounds or stair climbing.
3. Perform monthly testicular self-examination on the remaining testis.
4. Follow instructions for radiation therapy and/or chemotherapy.
5. Follow-up with visits to the physician(s) for at least 3 years.

CANCER, THYROID

OVERVIEW

- There are four types of thyroid cancer:
    1. *Papillary* carcinoma:
        a. This type is a slow-growing tumor found more frequently in women than men.
        b. If it is localized to the thyroid gland, the prognosis is good.
    2. *Follicular* carcinoma:
        a. Follicular carcinoma primarily affects clients older than 50 years of age.
        b. It invades blood vessels and metastasizes to bone and lung tissue.
        c. It can adhere to the trachea, neck muscles, great vessels, and skin, resulting in dysphagia and dyspnea.
        d. The prognosis is fair if metastasis is minimal at the time of diagnosis.
    3. *Medullary* carcinoma:
        a. Medullary carcinoma is more common in those over age 50.
        b. It involves metastasis that occurs via regional lymph nodes and invades surrounding structures.
        c. It may occur as part of multiple endocrine neoplasia type II, a familial endocrine disorder.
        d. Excessive secretion of calcitonin, adrenocorticotropic hormone, prostaglandins, and serotonin may occur.

4. *Anaplastic* carcinoma:
   a. Anaplastic carcinoma is a rapidly growing, extremely aggressive tumor.
   b. It directly invades adjacent structures, causing stridor, hoarseness, and dysphagia.
   c. Its prognosis is poor.

COLLABORATIVE MANAGEMENT

- The treatment of papillary, follicular, and medullary carcinoma includes
  1. Partial or total *thyroidectomy* with a modified radical neck dissection if regional lymph nodes are involved
  2. Postoperative suppressive doses of thyroid hormone for 3 months, followed by a radioactive iodine (RAI) uptake study; if there is RAI uptake, clients are treated with ablative amounts of RAI
  3. A course of chemotherapy if recurrent thyroid cancer does not respond to RAI
- The treatment for anaplastic carcinoma is palliative surgery, radiation, or chemotherapy. For nursing care, see Cancer and Hyperthyroidism.

CANCER, UROTHELIAL

OVERVIEW

- Urothelial cancers are malignancies of the urothelium, which is the lining of transitional cells in the renal pelvis, ureters, urinary bladder, and urethra.
- Most tumors occur in the urinary bladder; consequently, *bladder cancer* is a general term used to describe urothelial cancer.
- The urothelium is described initially in terms of cellular dysplasia.
- The first stages show nonspecific cellular alteration.
- In the second stage of cell growth, there are superficial low- or high-grade, flat or papillary lesions.
- The third stage refers to local invasion of the tissues.
- Stage 4 represents metastasis into the lymphatics or vasculature.

- Effects of tumors include local inflammation, ischemia, hemorrhage, and urinary obstruction.

 Transcultural Considerations

1. Urothelial cancer occurs more frequently in Caucasian men and three times more often in men than in women.
2. People in northern states show a greater frequency of bladder cancer than those living in southern states.

COLLABORATIVE MANAGEMENT

Assessment

- The nurse records the client's
    1. Active and passive exposure to cigarette smoke
    2. Employment history to determine exposure to harmful environmental agents
- The nurse assesses for
    1. Abdominal tenderness or discomfort
    2. Bladder distention
    3. Abdominal asymmetry
    4. Changes in color, frequency, or amount of urine
    5. Painless hematuria
    6. Dysuria
    7. Frequency
    8. Urgency
    9. Anxiety, fear

Planning and Implementation

✦ **NDx:** Risk for Injury

Nonsurgical Management

- The chemotherapy agents used in the treatment of urothelial cancer include MVAC (methotrexate, vinblastine, Adriamycin, and cisplatin) and CMV (cisplatin, methotrexate, and vinblastine).
- Radiation therapy may be performed in combination with chemotherapy.

Surgical Management

- Cystectomy, or surgical removal of the cancerous bladder with urinary diversion, is performed.
- Surgical techniques include

1. *Ureterostomies,* which divert urine directly to the skin through a ureteral skin opening (stoma). After the procedure, the client must wear a pouch (bag) to collect the urine. Types include
   a. Cutaneous ureterostomy
   b. Cutaneous ureteroureterostomy
   c. Bilateral cutaneous ureterostomy
2. *Conduits* collect urine in a portion of the intestine, which is then opened onto the skin surface as a stoma. The client must wear a pouch to collect the urine. Types include
   a. Ileal (Bricker's) conduit
   b. Colon conduit
3. *Sigmoidostomies* divert urine to the large intestine, so no stoma is required. The client excretes urine during bowel movements, and bowel incontinence may occur. Types include
   a. Ureterosigmoidostomy
   b. Ureteroiliosigmoidostomy
4. *Ileal reservoirs* divert urine into a surgically created pouch or pocket that functions a bladder. The stoma is continent, and the client removes urine by regular self-catheterization. One type is the continent internal ileal reservoir (Kock's pouch).

- The nurse provides preoperative care:
  1. Provides routine preoperative care
  2. Provides educational counseling about the urinary diversion and postoperative care requirements
  3. Assists in the selection of the stoma site (with the enterostomal therapist)
  4. Ensures an accurate understanding of self-care practices, methods of pouching, control of urinary drainage, and minimization of odor

- Postoperative care depends on the type and extent of the surgical procedure; the nurse
  1. Provides routine postoperative care
  2. Maintains drainage tubes
  3. Collaborates with the enterostomal therapist to provide wound and skin care and to manage the urinary drainage system
  4. Monitors urinary output and characteristics of the urine
  5. Administers analgesics, antispasmodics, and antibiotics, as ordered

Continuing Care

- The nurse
  1. Provides dietary instructions, including the avoidance of gas-forming foods if urinary diversion is into the gastrointestinal tract
  2. Teaches care of the external pouch, including application, skin care, pouch care, methods of adhesion, and drainage mechanisms
  3. Instructs the client on catheterization techniques following the Kock pouch procedure
  4. Provides educational and psychologic counseling on the impact of urinary diversions on self-image and self-esteem
  5. Refers the client to local, state, and national support groups

CANCER, UTERINE

See Cancer, Endometrial.

CANCER, VAGINAL

OVERVIEW

- Primary vaginal cancer, a rare disease, usually occurs as an extension of cervical, endometrial, or vulvar cancer.
- Most vaginal cancers are squamous cell carcinomas that develop in the upper third of the vagina.
- Adenocarcinomas are associated with intrauterine exposure to diethylstilbestrol as a result of maternal ingestion during pregnancy.
- The spread of vaginal cancer depends on the tumor location; upper vaginal lesions spread in the same manner as cervical cancer, whereas the spread of lower lesions is similar to that of vulvar cancer.
- Early metastasis occurs.

189

- Predisposing factors associated with development of vaginal cancer include
    1. Repeated pregnancies
    2. Sexually transmitted diseases, such as herpesvirus and papillomavirus infection
    3. Prior radiation therapy
- Both nonsurgical and surgical interventions may be used to treat women with vaginal cancer.

COLLABORATIVE MANAGEMENT

Nonsurgical Management

- Laser therapy is performed after iodine staining of the vagina to identify the affected areas.
- Local application of 5-fluorouracil (5-FU) cream to the vagina daily for 1 week is another treatment.
- Intracavitary radiation therapy (IRT) is used alone for treatment of cancer limited to the vaginal wall.
- External radiation therapy is used in combination with IRT for treatment of cancer that extends beyond the vaginal wall.
- Complications of radiation therapy include vaginal stenosis, adhesions, and drainage.
- The nurse
    1. Teaches the client to use a vaginal dilator
    2. Assesses for sexual dysfunction
- Chemotherapy is used for recurrent disease, but there is no effective therapy.

Surgical Management

- Local wide excision is performed for localized lesions.
- Partial or total vaginectomy (removal of part or all of the vagina) is performed for invasive disease.
- The nurse
    1. Informs the client that vaginectomy affects sexual function
    2. Counsels the client on alternative sexual activities
- Radical hysterectomy or pelvic exenteration may also be performed depending on the extent of the cancer.

CANCER, VULVAR

OVERVIEW

- Vulvar cancer is slow growing, stays localized for a long period, and metastasizes late. Over 50% occur in women over 65 years of age.
- Most vulvar cancers are squamous cell carcinomas and develop in the absence of premalignant changes in the epithelium.
- The first change is usually vulvar atypia or mild dysplasia.
- The cancer can spread directly to the urethra, the vagina, and the anus and through the lymphatic system to the inguinal, femoral, and deep iliac pelvic nodes.

COLLABORATIVE MANAGEMENT

Assessment

- The nurse records the client's
  1. Age
  2. Family history of cervical cancer or diabetes
  3. Obesity
  4. Possible sexually transmitted diseases
- The nurse assesses for
  1. Irritation or itching in the perineal area
  2. Bleeding (a late sign)
  3. Multifocal lesions on the labia

Interventions

- Management depends on the extent of the spread.
- Laser therapy is done for premalignant vulvar lesions.
- Chemotherapy, in the form of a topical application of 5-fluorouracil, is used for carcinoma *in situ*.
- External radiation therapy follows surgery for deep pelvic node involvement.
- Surgical interventions include
  1. Local wide *excision* of the lesion
  2. *Simple vulvectomy:* the removal of the vulva, the labia majora, the labia minora, and possibly the clitoris (used less frequently)

191

3. *Skinning vulvectomy:* the removal of the superficial skin of the vulva, without removal of the clitoris, and replacement of the skin with a split-thickness skin graft
4. *Modified radical* or *radical vulvectomy* for invasive cancer: the removal of the entire vulva—skin, labia, clitoris, subcutaneous tissues, and possibly inguinal and femoral node dissection

- The nurse performs specific preoperative procedures:
    1. Shaves the abdomen and perineum
    2. Administers a douche
    3. Administers an enema
    4. Inserts an indwelling urinary catheter
- Postoperatively, the nurse
    1. Maintains patency of drainage tubes
    2. Provides an egg crate mattress or air mattress and a bed cradle to increase the client's comfort
    3. Applies antiembolism stockings or sequential compression devices to prevent thromboembolism and leg edema
    4. Provides wound care and changes dressings over the incision, as ordered
    5. Monitors the client for indications of infection
    6. Encourages the client to eat a diet rich in vitamin C, iron, and protein to promote wound healing
    7. Provides care of the Foley catheter, according to institutional policy
    8. Administers analgesics, as ordered
    9. Explains changes in sexuality that occur as a result of the surgery
    10. Refers the client for counseling, as needed
- Health teaching is focused on
    1. Relief of postoperative discomfort, including medications
    2. Diet instructions, including intake of vitamin C, iron, and protein
    3. Changes in body image and sexual function

CARCINOMA, BASAL CELL

See Cancer, Skin.

CARCINOMA, PANCREATIC

See Cancer, Pancreatic.

CARCINOMA, RENAL CELL

See Cancer, Renal.

CARCINOMA, SQUAMOUS CELL

See Cancer, Skin.

CARDIAC FAILURE

See Heart Failure.

CARDIOMYOPATHY

OVERVIEW

- Cardiomyopathy is a subacute or chronic heart muscle disease of unknown cause; it is not a common disorder.
- Cardiomyopathies are divided into three categories on the basis of abnormalities in structure and function.

1. *Dilated cardiomyopathy* (DCM), the most common type, involves extensive damage to the myofibrils and interference with myocardial metabolism; it is characterized by dilation of both ventricles and impairment of systolic function.
2. Massive ventricular hypertrophy and small ventricular cavities are typical in *hypertrophic cardiomyopathy* (HCM). Left ventricular (LV) hypertrophy leads to a hypocontractile left ventricle with rigid ventricular walls. Obstruction in the LV outflow results in diastolic filling abnormalities. HCM is transmitted as a single-gene, autosomal dominant trait.
3. *Restrictive cardiomyopathy* (RCM), the least common of the three cardiomyopathies, involves restriction of filling of the ventricles. It is caused by endocardial or myocardial disease and produces a clinical picture similar to that with constrictive pericarditis.

- Sudden death may be the first and only manifestation of cardiomyopathy

COLLABORATIVE MANAGEMENT

Assessment

- The nurse assesses for clinical manifestations of *DCM:*
    1. Left ventricular failure
    2. Progressive dyspnea on exertion
    3. Orthopnea
    4. Palpations
    5. Activity intolerance
    6. Right-sided heart failure late in the disease
    7. Atrial fibrillation
- The nurse assesses for clinical manifestations of *HCM:*
    1. Exertional dyspnea (90% of clients)
    2. Angina (75% of clients)
    3. Syncope
    4. Atypical chest pain that occurs at rest, is prolonged, has no relation to exertion, and is not relieved by nitrates
    5. Ventricular dysrhythmias
- The nurse assesses for clinical manifestations of *RCM:*
    1. Exertional dyspnea
    2. Weakness
    3. Exercise intolerance

4. Palpitations
5. Syncope

Interventions

Nonsurgical Management

- Care of the client with DCM or RCM is the same as that for clients with heart failure. (See Heart Failure.)
- The nurse
  1. Administers diuretics, vasodilators, and cardiac glycosides to increase cardiac output
  2. Administers antidysrhythmics to control ventricular dysrhythmias, including tachycardia
  3. Teaches the client to abstain from alcohol because of its cardiac depressant effects
- Management of hypertrophic cardiomyopathy (HCM) is similar to that of myocardial ischemia. (See Coronary Artery Disease.)
- The nurse
  1. Administers beta-adrenergic blocking agents and calcium antagonists, as ordered, to decrease outflow obstruction and heart rate, resulting in less chest pain and dyspnea
  2. Does *not* give vasodilators and cardiac glycosides, which may augment outflow obstruction

Surgical Management

- The type of surgical intervention depends on the type of cardiomyopathy that the client has.
- The most commonly used surgery for HCM is excision of a portion of the hypertrophied ventricular septum.
- *Heart transplantation* is the treatment of choice for clients with severe dilated cardiomyopathy (DCM); a donor heart from a person with a comparable body weight and ABO compatibility is transplanted into a recipient within 6 hours of procurement.
- Criteria for candidates for heart transplantation include
  1. Life expectancy less than 1 year
  2. Age less than 65 years (variable)
  3. New York Heart Association class III or IV (poor functional status)
  4. Normal or only slightly increased pulmonary vascular resistance
  5. Absence of active infection
  6. Stable psychosocial status
  7. No evidence of drug or alcohol abuse

195

- Many clients experience at least one episode of acute rejection of the transplant in the first 3 months after transplantation and then about one rejection episode a year.
- The nurse
    1. Provides postoperative care similar to that provided for clients having open heart surgery (see Coronary Artery Disease, "Surgical Management")
    2. Teaches the client to report signs and symptoms of rejection, such as hypotension, dysrhythmias, weakness, fatigue, and dizziness
    3. Informs the client that the surgeon will perform endomyocardial biopsy at regularly scheduled intervals to detect rejection
    4. Teaches the client the importance of taking immunosuppressants for the duration of his or her life to prevent transplant rejection

CARPAL TUNNEL SYNDROME

OVERVIEW

- Carpal tunnel syndrome (CTS) is a condition in which the median nerve in the wrist is compressed, causing pain and numbness.
- Risk factors include synovitis, hand or wrist trauma from repetitive activities, and congenital or familial problems.
- CTS typically occurs in women between the ages of 30 and 60 years.

COLLABORATIVE MANAGEMENT

Assessment

- The nurse assesses for
    1. Nature, location, and intensity of the pain and numbness
    2. Time of day pain usually occurs
    3. Paresthesia
    4. Positive results for Phalen's test, which produces paresthesia in the median nerve distribution within 60 seconds (the client is asked to relax

the wrist into flexion or place the backs of both hands together and flex both wrists simultaneously)

5. Positive Tinel's sign, which is the same response as for the Phalen's test (elicited by tapping lightly over the area of the median nerve)
6. Weak pinch, clumsiness, and difficulty with fine movements
7. Muscle weakness and wasting
8. Wrist swelling
9. Autonomic changes manifested by skin discoloration, nail changes such as brittleness, and increased or decreased swelling of the hand and wrist
10. Fear that the symptoms are related to a spinal problem or that job or lifestyle changes may have to be made

Interventions

Nonsurgical Management

- The nurse
    1. Administers analgesics such as aspirin and nonsteroidal anti-inflammatory drugs, as ordered
    2. Administers diuretics if edema is present, as ordered
    3. Assists the physician with direct injection of corticosteroids into the carpal tunnel to relieve inflammation
- Wrist immobilization is tried before surgical intervention.

Surgical Management

- Surgery is done to relieve compression on the median nerve; it may be performed as an endoscopic procedure using a laser to free the trapped nerve.
- If CTS is a complication of rheumatoid arthritis, a *synovectomy,* or removal of excess synovium, may resolve the problem.
- The nurse provides routine preoperative care.
- The nurse provides postoperative care:
    1. Checks pressure dressing carefully for drainage and tightness
    2. Elevates the hand and arm for 1 or 2 days
    3. Checks the client's neurovascular status every hour for the first 12 hours
    4. Encourages the client to move all fingers of the affected hand frequently

197

CATARACTS

OVERVIEW

- A cataract is an opacity of the lens that distorts the image projected onto the retina.
- Types of cataracts include
  1. *Age-related:* generally over 65 years of age
  2. *Traumatic:* caused by blunt trauma, penetrating blows, or overexposure to excessive heat, x-rays, or radioactive material
  3. *Toxic:* seen after ingestion of or exposure to certain chemicals, such as extended use of corticosteroids, chlorpromazine, or miotic agents
  4. *Associated:* seen with other diseases, such as diabetes mellitus, hypoparathyroidism, Down's syndrome, and atopic dermatitis
  5. *Complicated:* develops as a result of ocular disorders, such as retinitis pigmentosa, glaucoma, and retinal detachment

🕲 Considerations for Elderly Clients

1. The prevalence of cataracts is 50% in adults aged 65 to 70 years and 70% in adults over 70 years of age.
2. There is an increased incidence of cataract formation in people over age 65 who experience chronic exposure to strong sunlight.

COLLABORATIVE MANAGEMENT

Assessment

- The nurse records the client's
  1. Age
  2. History of trauma
  3. Exposure to radioactive materials or x-rays
  4. Current medical problems, especially systemic diseases, such as diabetes mellitus
  5. Medication history
  6. History of intraocular disease
- The nurse assesses for
  1. Blurred vision

2. Decrease in color vision: Blue, green, and purple appear gray
3. Diplopia
4. Reduced visual acuity progressing to blindness
5. Presence of white pupil (late stage)
6. Anxiety and fear

Planning and Implementation

✦ NDx: Sensory/Perceptual Alterations (Visual)

- Two extraction procedures are commonly performed:
  1. *Extracapsular:* removal of the anterior portion of the capsule
  2. *Intracapsular:* removal of the lens completely within the capsule
- The nurse provides preoperative care:
  1. Provides routine preoperative care and teaching
  2. Allows the client who may be anxious to talk about losing his or her sight
  3. Reviews the procedure for local and retrobulbar anesthesia, which is usually used
  4. Administers preoperative medications, as ordered:
     a. Oral acetazolamide (Diamox) to reduce intraocular pressure
     b. Sympathomimetic drugs, such as phenylephrine (Neo-Synephrine, Spersaphrine◆), to achieve vasoconstriction and mydriasis
     c. Parasympatholytic drops, such as tropicamide (Mydriacyl, Minims Tropcamide◆) or cyclopentolate hydrochloride (Cyclogyl), to induce paralysis and render the ciliary muscles unable to move the lens

🕢 Considerations for Elderly Clients

Because cataract surgery is usually an outpatient procedure and most clients are elderly, adequate preoperative teaching is an essential.

- The nurse provides postoperative care:
  1. Provides routine postoperative care
  2. Administers antibiotics immediately after surgery subconjunctivally, as an antibiotic plus steroid ointment; both are used for several days after surgery
  3. Keeps the client in a semi-Fowler's position or on the unaffected side, as ordered

199

4. Reports drainage on the eye pad to the surgeon
5. Applies cool compresses if the eye itches
6. Administers analgesics, such as acetaminophen, as ordered
7. Restricts the client's coughing, bending at the waist, sneezing, lifting of objects that weigh more than 15 pounds (6.8 kg), and sleeping or lying on the operative side (which increases intraocular pressure)
8. Recommends eyeglasses, sunglasses, or an eye shield during the day and an eye shield at night
9. Observes for and reports complications of surgery, including
   a. Increased intraocular pressure, manifested by severe pain, nausea, and vomiting
   b. Infection
   c. Bleeding into the anterior chamber of the eye, manifested by a change in vision
   d. Secondary membrane or secondary cataract formation, manifested by clouding of the posterior lens
   e. Retinal detachment, manifested when one sees dark spots, an increased number of floaters, or bright flashes of light and when one loses all or part of the visual field

- Rehabilitation options depend on the severity of the problem, the client's age, and the type of surgery:

   1. Eyeglasses (*aphakic spectacles*):
      a. Aphakic spectacles distort images by as much as 25% to 33% and cause vertical lines, such as doorways and lampposts, to look curved.
      b. They cause peripheral vision to be lost.
      c. They cause the two eyes not to function together, resulting in diplopia, if only one eye has been operated on.
      d. Eyeglasses are the least expensive option.
   2. Contact lenses:
      a. Chief advantage of contact lenses over glasses is that image size with the contact lens is only 7% larger than normal size so both eyes function together.
      b. Visual field is not distorted or constricted.
      c. Disadvantages include the necessity for an adequate amount of tears, the manual dexterity required for insertion and removal, and the potential for infection and corneal abrasion.

3. Intraocular lens implant:
   a. Minimal 1% to 3% distortion of the image is produced by the implant.
   b. Return to binocular vision is immediate.
   c. Disadvantages include a higher rate of complications, the possibility of rejection of the lens, and higher cost.

Continuing Care

- The nurse
  1. Discusses the current ability of the client to meet self care needs and activities of daily living
  2. Evaluates how the client's current functional ability will be affected by activity restriction and postoperative needs
  3. Teaches the client required self-care activities, including
     a. Personal care
     b. Shield application
     c. Eyedrop instillation
     d. Activities permitted and restricted
     e. Medications
     f. Monitoring for complications
  4. Informs the client that hair washing is allowed several days after surgery if it can be done with the head tilted back, such as in a hair salon
  5. Advises the client to stand in the shower with the face turned away from the shower head
  6. Advises the client not to drive, operate machinery, and participate in sports until given specific permission to do so
  7. Advises the client that light housekeeping is permitted but vacuuming should be avoided for several weeks
  8. Emphasizes the importance of follow-up visits with the physician(s)

Cellulitis

See Infections, Skin.

CEREBRAL VASCULAR ACCIDENT (BRAIN ATTACK)

OVERVIEW

- Cerebral vascular accident (CVA), commonly referred to as a *stroke* or *brain attack,* is a disruption in the normal blood supply to the brain.
- CVAs may be classified as
  1. Ischemic: caused by the occlusion of a cerebral artery by either a thrombus or embolus:
     a. Types of ischemic CVA include
        (1) *Thrombolic:* commonly associated with the development of atherosclerosis of the blood vessel wall. The artery becomes occluded and blood flow to the area is markedly diminished, causing transient ischemia and then complete ischemia and infarction of brain tissue. Signs and symptoms occur gradually.
        (2) *Embolic:* caused by an embolus or group of emboli that travel to the cerebral arteries through the carotid artery and block the artery, causing ischemia. Sudden and rapid development of focal neurologic deficits occurs. Cerebral hemorrhage may result if the vessel wall is damaged.
     b. Ischemic CVA may be preceded by warning signs, including
        (1) *Transient ischemic attack* (TIA), a transient focal neurological deficit, such as vertigo or blurred vision
        (2) *Reversible ischemic neurologic deficit* (RIND), which lasts longer than a TIA
  2. *Hemorrhagic:* in which the integrity of the vessel wall is interrupted and bleeding occurs into the brain tissue or subarachnoid space. Causes include hypertension, ruptured aneurysm, and arteriovenous malformation (AVM).

a. Aneurysm is an abnormal ballooning or blister on the involved artery, which may become stretched or thinned and rupture.
b. *AVM* is a tangled or spaghetti-like mass of malformed, thin-walled, dilated vessels that form an abnormal communication between the arterial and venous systems.

 Transcultural Considerations

1. CVAs occur more frequently in males than females.
2. African-Americans are affected more frequently than other races, usually because of hypertension.
3. CVAs occur most often in people older than 45 years, with an increased frequency in those over age 65.
4. The number of strokes associated with cocaine abuse has been steadily increasing.

COLLABORATIVE MANAGEMENT

Assessment

- The nurse records the client's
    1. Activity at onset of the CVA
    2. Progression and severity of symptoms, including the presence of a TIA or RIND
    3. Level of consciousness, orientation
    4. Motor status: gait, balance, reading and writing abilities
    5. Sensory status: speech, hearing, vision
    6. Medical history
    7. Social history, with attention toward identifying risk factors, such as smoking, diet, and exercise
    8. Current medications and nonprescribed drugs, especially anticoagulants, aspirin, vasodilators, and illegal drugs
- The nurse assesses for changes in the client's
    1. Level of consciousness, orientation, cognition, memory, judgment, and problem-solving and decision-making abilities
    2. Ability to concentrate and attend to tasks
    3. Motor status (muscle strength, muscle tone, range of motion, proprioception, head and trunk control, balance, gait, coordination, bowel and bladder control)

203

4. Sensory status (response to touch and painful stimuli; ability to distinguish between two tactile stimuli presented simultaneously; ability to read, write, and follow verbal directions; ability to name objects and use them correctly)
5. Speech pattern (rhythm, clarity, aphasia)
6. Visual system (pupil size and reaction to light, visual field deficits [homonymous hemianopsia, bitemporal hemianopsia])
7. Cranial nerve function, especially nerves V, VII, IX, X, and XII
8. Cardiac system (hypertension, dysrhythmias, and murmurs)
9. Body image and self-concept disturbance
10. Coping mechanisms or personality changes
11. Emotional lability
12. Financial status and occupation as a result of hospitalization
- The primary purpose of the intitial CT or MRI is to identify the presence of hemorrhage or a cerebral aneurysm; it will also differentiate stroke from other pathological changes that mimic a stroke.

Planning and Implementation

✦ **NDx:** Altered Tissue Perfusion (Cerebral)

Nonsurgical Management

- The nurse
  1. Performs a neurologic assessment at a minimum of every 2 to 4 hours, checking
     a. Verbal response, orientation
     b. Eye opening, pupil size, and reaction to light
     c. Motor response
  2. Monitors vital signs with neurologic checks:
     a. Asks the physician for acceptable limits for blood pressure
     b. Performs a cardiac assessment
  3. Elevates the head of the bed 30 to 45 degrees
  4. Avoids activities that may increase intracranial pressure:
     a. Positions the client to avoid extreme hip or neck flexion
     b. Avoids clustering nursing procedures
     c. Provides a quiet environment

- Occlusive CVA is treated with anticoagulant therapy (contraindicated in clients with a history of ulcers, uremia, and hepatic failure). Sodium heparin (Hepalean◆) subcutaneously or by continuous intravenous drip is commonly used.
- Thrombolytic therapy was approved for the treatment of acute ischemic strokes in 1996. The stroke should be verified by CT scan.
    1. Tissue plasminogen activator (tPA) or streptokinase is given within 3 hours of the onset of symptoms.
    2. Clients who have bleeding complications or are on anticoagulants are not candidates for this therapy.
    3. Some researchers have found no difference in outcome in clients treated with this therapy than those who were not.
- Anticoagulant therapy and anti-platelet therapy is also controversial and depends on the health care provider's preference.
    1. The nurse obtains a baseline prothrombin time (for oral anticoagulation therapy) and partial thromboplastin time (for heparin [Hepalean◆] therapy) before initiating therapy, 6 to 8 hours after the start of the drug, and every morning thereafter.
        a. International normalized ration (INR) is used to monitor warfarin therapy.
    2. Anticoagulation therapy may cause bleeding. The nurse observes for blood in the urine and stool and easy bruising.
- Enteric-coated or other forms of aspirin (Ancasal◆) or dipyridamole (Persantine) may be used to forestall thrombotic and embolic strokes.
- Other medication used to treat a brain attack include
    1. Phenytoin (Dilantin) may be used to prevent seizures.
    2. Calcium channel blockers (nimodipine; Nimotop) may be administered to treat vasospasm or chronic spasm of the vessel, which inhibits blood flow to the area.
    3. Stool softeners, analgesics for pain, and anti-anxiety drugs may also be ordered.
- The nurse monitors the client for complications:
    1. Hydrocephalus
    2. Vasospasm

3. Rebleeding or rupture of an aneurysm

Surgical Management

- Two surgical procedures may be used.
    1. *Carotid endarterectomy* to remove atherosclerotic plaque
    2. *Extracranial-intracranial bypass* to bypass the occluded area and reestablish blood flow to the affected area
- Surgical procedures to treat AVM include
    1. Injecting an embolic agent such as platinum coils, detachable silicone baloons, liquid acrylic, and polyvinyl alcohol into the carotid artery, which travel to involved vessels, become lodged, and cause the vessels to thrombose
    2. Surgically removing involved vessels
- Surgical procedures to treat *aneurysm* include
    1. Placing a clip or clamp at the base or neck of the aneurysm
    2. Wrapping the aneurysm with muscle, muslin, or plastic coating
- The nursing care for these procedures is similar to that discussed in Tumors, Brain, "Surgical Management."

✦ **NDx:** Impaired Physical Mobility; Self Care Deficit

- The nurse
    1. Performs active and passive range-of-motion exercises at least every 6 hours
    2. Carefully positions the client in proper body alignment
    3. Maintains correct use of splints and braces
    4. Uses antiembolism stockings; frequently positions and mobilizes the client as soon as possible to prevent deep venous thrombosis or pneumonia
    5. Measures thighs and calves daily and checks for positive Homans' sign (indicative of possible deep venous thrombosis)

✦ **NDx:** Sensory/Perceptual Alteration

- The nurse
    1. Uses frequent verbal and tactile cues to help the client perform activities of daily living
    2. Breaks tasks down into small steps when cueing
    3. Approaches the client from the nonaffected side

4. Teaches the client to scan with eyes and turn the head side to side (when visual impairments occur)
5. Places objects within the client's field of vision
6. Places a patch over the affected eye if diplopia is present
7. Removes clutter from the room
8. Orients the client to time, place, and event
9. Provides a structured, repetitious, and consistent routine or schedule
10. Presents information in a clear, simple, concise manner
11. Uses a step-by-step approach
12. Places pictures and other familiar objects in the room

✦ NDx: Impaired Verbal Communication

- The nurse
  1. Gives repetitive, simple directions; breaks each task into simple steps
  2. Faces the client and speaks slowly and distinctly
  3. Allows sufficient time for the client to understand the direction
  4. Uses pictures or a communication board, if necessary
  5. Encourages the client to communicate and positively reinforces this behavior
  6. Repeats the names of objects on a routine basis and teaches the family to do the same

✦ NDx: Impaired Swallowing

- The nurse
  1. Positions the client to facilitate swallowing:
     a. Places the client in a chair or sitting straight up in bed
     b. Positions the client's head and neck slightly forward and flexed
  2. Provides foods that are soft or semisoft and thick fluids (e.g., milkshakes)
  3. Maintains a quiet room with few distractions while the client is eating

✦ NDx: Bowel and Bladder Incontinence

- The nurse
  1. Establishes the cause of the problem and type (bowel or bladder)

2. Determines the client's usual voiding or bowel movement pattern
3. Implements an individualized bladder-training program (see entries on rehabilitation for a thorough discussion):
   a. Uses an intermittent catheterization program if urinary incontinence is due to upper motor lesion
   b. Places the client on a bedpan or commode every 2 hours; encourages fluid intake to 2000 mL/day unless contraindicated
4. Implements an individualized bowel-training program (see entries on rehabilitation for a thorough discussion):
   a. Determines the normal time or routine for bowel elimination
   b. Places the client on a bedpan or commode at the same time each day; uses a suppository or stool softener, if needed
   c. Provides a diet high in bulk or fiber (may require consultation with a dietitian)

Continuing Care

- When possible a case manager should be assigned to help coordinate plans for the client discharged to the home setting
  1. Identifies and suggests corrections of hazards in the home before discharge
  2. Ensures that the client can correctly use all assistive-adaptive devices ordered for home use
  3. Arranges follow-up appointments, as ordered
  4. Provides a detailed plan of care at the time of discharge for clients to be transferred to a rehabilitation center or long-term-care facility (rehabilitation can be a lengthy process; see entries on rehabilitation)
  5. Provides drug information, as needed
  6. Reinforces mobility skills (in collaboration with other therapists):
     a. How to safely climb stairs, transfer from bed to chair, get into and out of a car
     b. How to use adaptive equipment
  7. Provides a variety of publications, availabe from the American Heart Association and National Stroke Association

CEREBROVASCULAR ACCIDENT

See Cerebral Vascular Accident.

CERVICAL CANCER

See Cancer, Cervical.

CERVICAL POLYPS

See Polyps, Cervical.

CHANCROID

- Chancroid is most common in tropical and subtropical countries.
- Recent spread of the causative organism *Haemophilus ducreyi* has made chancroid an important sexually transmitted disease in the United States.
- The incubation period varies from 3 to 10 days.
- A tender papule appears at the site of inoculation.
- The lesion rapidly breaks down to form an irregularly shaped, deep ulcer with purulent discharge that bleeds easily.
- Complications include inguinal adenopathy, balanitis, phimosis, and urethral fistulas.
- Transmission is through contact with the ulcer or with discharge from the infected local lymph glands during sexual intercourse.

- Treatment includes antibiotics, such as erythromycin (E-Mycin, Apo-Erythro◆) for 7 days or a single dose of intramuscular ceftriaxone sodium (Rocephin).
- Health teaching is similar to that for syphilis.

CHF

See Heart Failure.

CHLAMYDIA

See Infections, Chlamydial.

CHLAMYDIAL INFECTIONS

See Infections, Chlamydial.

CHOLECYSTITIS

OVERVIEW

- Cholecystitis is an inflammation of the gallbladder that can occur as an acute or chronic process.
- *Acute* inflammation is usually associated with gallstones (cholelithiasis), although gallstones may not be present.
- *Chronic* cholecystitis results when inefficient bile emptying and gallbladder muscle wall disease contribute to a fibrotic and contracted gallbladder, with decreased motility and deficient absorption.

- *Acalculous* cholecystitis occurs in the absence of gall-stones and is due to bacterial invasion through the lymphatic or vascular systems.
- Complications of cholecystitis include *pancreatitis* and *cholangitis* (inflammation of the common bile duct).
- *Jaundice* (yellow discoloration of body tissues) and *icterus* (yellow discoloration of the sclera) can occur in acute disease but are most commonly seen in the chronic phase of cholecystitis. Jaundice results from increased bilirubin in the body that collects in the skin and sclera. Itching and a burning sensation result.

COLLABORATIVE MANAGEMENT

Assessment

- The nurse records the client's
    1. Height and weight
    2. Sex, age, race, and ethnic group
    3. History of pregnancies, menopause, and use of birth control pills, estrogen, or other hormone supplements
    4. Food preferences, including excess fat and cholesterol intake
    5. Food intolerances and related gastrointestinal (GI) symptoms, including flatulence, dyspepsia (indigestion), eructation (belching), anorexia, nausea, vomiting, and abdominal pain in relation to fatty food intake
    6. Exercise routine or daily activities
    7. Family history of gallbladder disease
- The nurse assesses for
    1. Abdominal pain in the right upper abdominal quadrant of varying intensity, including radiation to the scapula, and asks the client to describe the intensity, duration, precipitating factors, and relief measures
    2. Other GI symptoms, including nausea, vomiting, dyspepsia, flatulence, eructation, and feelings of abdominal heaviness
    3. Guarding, rigidity, and rebound tenderness (Blumberg's sign)
    4. Sausage-shaped mass in the right upper quadrant
    5. Late symptoms seen in chronic cholecystitis, such as jaundice, clay-colored stools, and dark urine
    6. Steatorrhea (fatty stools)

211

7. Elevated temperature with tachycardia and dehydration from fever and vomiting
8. Results of serum liver enzyme and bilirubin tests (may be elevated)
9. Increased white blood cell count
10. Elevated serum and urine amylase levels, if pancreas is affected

Planning and Implementation

Nonsurgical Management

- Food and fluids are withheld during nausea and vomiting episodes; nasogastric decompression is initiated for severe vomiting.
- Clients with chronic cholecystitis are encouraged to consume low-fat meals more frequently and in smaller amounts.
- The nurse administers
  1. Opioid analgesics, as ordered, such as meperidine (Demerol), to relieve pain and reduce spasm
  2. Antispasmodic agents, such as anticholinergics (e.g., dicyclomine hydrochloride [Bentyl, Lomine◆] or propantheline bromide [Pro-Banthine, Propanthel◆]), as ordered, to relax the smooth muscle
  3. Antiemetics, as ordered, to provide relief from nausea and vomiting

Surgical Management

- Cholecystectomy (removal of the gallbladder) is the usual surgical treatment to remove the cause of discomfort. One of two procedures may be performed:
  1. Traditional surgical approach
  2. Laparoscopic laser procedure
- A T tube drain is surgically inserted when the common bile duct is explored to ensure patency of the duct.
- The nurse provides preoperative care for clients having the *traditional* surgical approach:
  1. Stresses the importance of deep breathing, coughing, and turning, as well as early ambulation after surgery
  2. Teaches the use of sustained maximal inspiration (SMI) devices
  3. Teaches how to use a folded blanket or pillow as a splint for the abdomen to prevent jarring during coughing

4. Provides routine preoperative care
- The nurse provides postoperative care:
  1. Administers intravenous (via patient-controlled analgesia) meperidine (Demerol) for pain relief; morphine is not given because it can constrict the sphincter of Oddi and cause biliary ductal spasm
  2. Administers antiemetics, as ordered, for relief of postoperative nausea and vomiting
  3. Ensures that the client receives nothing by mouth (NPO) for 24 to 48 hours
  4. Maintains nasogastric suction
  5. Advances the diet from clear liquids to solid foods, as tolerated by the client
  6. Maintains the client's T tube
     a. Assesses the amount, color, consistency, and odor of drainage
     b. Collects and administers the excess bile output to the client through the nasogastric tube or administers synthetic bile salts, such as dehydrocholic acid (Decholin), as ordered
     c. Reports sudden increases in bile output to the physician
     d. Assesses for foul odor and purulent drainage and reports changes in drainage to the physician
     e. Inspects the skin around the T tube insertion site for signs of inflammation
     f. Keeps the drainage system below the level of the gallbladder
     g. Places the client in a semi-Fowler's position
     h. Avoids irrigation, aspiration, or clamping of the T tube without a physician's order
     i. Assesses the drainage system for pulling, kinking, or tangling of the tubing
     j. Assists the client with early ambulation
     k. Observes the client's stools for brown color
- The laparoscopic laser cholecystectomy is commonly performed by making several small punctures through which the laparoscope is inserted. A laser dissects the gallbladder before removal through a puncture site. This procedure is less invasive and is done on an outpatient (ambulatory) basis.
- No special preoperative care is required for the laparoscopic procedure.
- The nurse provides postoperative care:

1. Teaches the client the importance of early ambulation to absorb the carbon dioxide that is retained in the abdomen.
2. Informs the client that he or she can return to usual activities 3 to 7 days after the procedure.

Continuing Care

- If traditional surgery is performed, the nurse supplies written postoperative instructions:
   1. Inspection of the abdominal incision for redness, tenderness, swelling, and drainage
   2. Dressing change, wound care, and T tube drain care instructions
   3. Pain management, including prescriptions
   4. Signs and symptoms of infection, including when to call the physician (elevated temperature and increased pain)
   5. Activity limitations
- The nurse provides diet therapy instructions based on the client's tolerance of fats, including a low-fat diet and foods to avoid; small, more frequent feedings; and weight reduction, if indicated.

CHOLELITHIASIS

OVERVIEW

- Cholelithiasis (calculous cholecystitis) is a condition in which calculi, or gallstones, lodge in the neck of the gallbladder or in the cystic duct, interfering with or totally obstructing normal bile flow from the gallbladder to the duodenum.
- Vascular congestion results from impeded venous return, with edema and congestion.
- Trapped bile is reabsorbed, acting as a chemical irritant and producing a toxic effect, resulting in tissue sloughing with necrosis and gangrene.
- Contributing factors include supersaturation of bile with cholesterol, excess bile salt losses, decreased gallbladder emptying rates, and changes in bile concentration or bile stasis in the gallbladder.

- There is a familial tendency toward cholelithiasis development. Gallstones are also seen more frequently in clients who are obese, pregnant, on low-calorie or liquid protein diets, or taking drugs such as estrogen and birth control pills. Cholelithiasis is seen in clients with hemolytic bowel disorders, Crohn's disease, and type I diabetes. It can occur after jejunoileal bypass surgery as a treatment for morbid obesity.
- Stones may lie dormant or migrate within the biliary tree, causing obstruction.
- Stones are typically composed of cholesterol, bilirubin, bile salts, calcium, and various proteins; they are designated as cholesterol, mixed, or pigment stones.
- Cholangitis, associated with choledocholithiasis (common bile duct stones), involves infection of the bile ducts.
- Gallstones form in about 10% of the population of the United States.

🕊 Women's Health Considerations

1. Pregnancy worsens gallstone formation and is higher in women who have had multiple births.

➔ Transcultural Considerations

1. Caucasians and Native Americans, particularly the Navajo and Pima tribes, have a higher incidence of gallstones.
2. Cholelithiasis is also prevalent in Asian-Americans and African-Americans.

COLLABORATIVE MANAGEMENT
Assessment

- The nurse records the client's
  1. Height and weight
  2. Sex, age, race, and ethnic group
  3. History of pregnancies, menopause, and use of birth control pills, estrogen, or other hormone supplements
  4. Food preferences, including excess fat and cholesterol intake
  5. Food intolerances and related gastrointestinal (GI) symptoms, including flatulence, dyspepsia, eruc-

tation, anorexia, nausea, vomiting, and abdominal
pain in relation to fatty food intake
6. Exercise routine or daily activities
7. Family or previous history of gallbladder disease
- The nurse assesses for
    1. Abdominal pain, including severity (based on
       whether the stone is stationary or mobile, size and
       location of the stone, degree of obstruction, and
       the presence and extent of inflammation)
    2. Severe pain of biliary colic accompanied by ta-
       chycardia, pallor, diaphoresis, and prostration
    3. Other GI symptoms, including nausea, vomiting,
       dyspepsia, flatulence, eructation, and feelings of
       abdominal heaviness
    4. Guarding, rigidity, and rebound tenderness
    5. Sausage-shaped mass in the right upper abdomi-
       nal quadrant
    6. Jaundice if acute ductal obstruction is present
    7. Increased serum and urinary bilirubin levels if ob-
       struction is present
    8. Absent or low levels of urobilinogen in the feces
    9. Elevated serum and urine amylase levels if the pan-
       creas is involved
    10. Presence of gallstones on x-ray

Planning and Implementation

✦ **NDx:** Pain

Nonsurgical Management

- The nurse
    1. Provides a low-fat diet to prevent further pain of
       biliary colic
    2. Replaces fat-soluble vitamins (A, D, E, and K)
       and bile salts, as ordered, if gallstones cause ob-
       struction, to facilitate digestion and vitamin ab-
       sorption
    3. Withholds food and fluids if nausea and vomiting
       occur
    4. Administers opioid analgesia with meperidine hy-
       drochloride (Demerol), as ordered (not with mor-
       phine, which interferes with biliary flow)
    5. Administers antispasmodic or anticholinergic
       drugs, as ordered, to relax smooth muscles and
       decrease ductal tone and spasm
    6. Administers antiemetics, as ordered, to control
       nausea and vomiting

7. Administers bile acid therapy, as ordered, to dissolve gallstones; chenodeoxycholic acid (chenodiol; Chemix) or ursodiol (Actigall) reduces cholesterol stones by maintaining normal cholesterol solubility in bile

8. Administers cholestyramine (Questran), as ordered, which binds with bile salts in the intestine, removing excess bile salts, and reduces itching (administered in powder form with fruit juices or milk)

- When conservative measures are unsuccessful, extracorporeal shock wave lithotripsy involves the use of a lithotriptor to generate powerful shock waves to shatter gallstones.
- Percutaneous insertion of a transhepatic biliary catheter may be performed to decompress obstructed extrahepatic ducts.

Surgical Management

- Surgical intervention includes
    1. *Cholecystotomy,* an incision into the gallbladder
    2. *Choledocholithotomy,* an incision into the common bile duct to remove stones with common bile duct exploration and T tube placement
    3. *Cholecystectomy,* gallbladder removal for stones confined to the gallbladder
- The nurse provides routine preoperative care and instructions (see Cholecystitis for preoperative instructions).
- The nurse provides postoperative care:
    1. Provides routine postoperative care and instructions and T tube care (see Cholecystitis for postoperative instructions)
    2. Administers hydrocholeretic drugs, such as dehydrocholic acid (Decholin, Cholan, or Neocholin), to increase cholesterol solubility and promote drainage of bile through the T tube drainage system

Continuing Care

- The nurse provides verbal and written postoperative instructions, including
    1. Inspection of abdominal incision for redness, tenderness, swelling, and drainage
    2. Dressing change, wound care, and T tube drain care instructions
    3. Pain management, including prescriptions

4. Signs and symptoms of infection, including when to call the physician (elevated temperature and increase in pain)
   5. Activity limitations
   6. Symptoms of postcholecystectomy syndrome (recurring calculi), including jaundice of skin or sclera, dark urine, light-colored stools, pain, fever, and chills
- Dietary instructions are based on the client's tolerance of fats, including a low-fat diet and foods to avoid; small, more frequent feedings and weight reduction may be indicated.

CHOLESTEATOMA

- A cholesteatoma is a benign growth of squamous cell epithelium, which is most common in clients who have chronic otitis media with a perforated tympanic membrane that fails to heal.
- It appears as a grayish white, shiny mass behind or involving the tympanic membrane and is often described as having a cauliflower-like appearance.
- Clinical management depends on structures that are damaged by the tumor; effects include decreased hearing, chronic otitis media, vertigo, and facial paralysis.
- Treatment includes
   1. Antibiotics if an infection is present
   2. Surgical removal of the tumor:
      a. *Myringoplasty* to repair the tympanic membrane
      b. *Tympanoplasty* to repair or replace the ossicles to improve conductive hearing
      c. *Mastoidectomy* for more extensive growths

CHOREA, HUNTINGTON'S

See Huntington's Chorea.

CHRONIC AIRFLOW LIMITATION

See Airflow Limitation, Chronic.

CHRONIC GLOMERULONEPHRITIS

See Glomerulonephritis, Chronic.

CHRONIC OBSTRUCTIVE PULMONARY DISEASE

See Airflow Limitation, Chronic.

CHRONIC PANCREATITIS

See Pancreatitis, Chronic.

CHRONIC RENAL FAILURE

See Renal Failure, Chronic.

CIRRHOSIS

OVERVIEW

- Cirrhosis is a chronic, progressive liver disease characterized by diffuse fibrotic bands of connective tissue that distort the liver's normal architectural anatomy.
- It is essentially an irreversible reaction to hepatic inflammation and necrosis.
- The four main types of cirrhosis are
    1. *Laennec's cirrhosis* (also known as alcohol-induced, nutritional, or portal cirrhosis):
        a. Alcohol has a direct toxic effect on liver cells, causing liver inflammation (alcoholic hepatitis).
        b. Metabolic changes lead to fatty infiltration of the hepatocytes and scarring between the liver lobules.
        c. The liver becomes enlarged with cellular infiltration by fat, leukocytes, and lymphocytes.
        d. Early scar formation is caused by fibroblast infiltration and collagen formation.
        e. Damage to the hepatic parenchyma progresses, and widespread scar tissue forms with fibrotic infiltration of the liver as a result of cellular necrosis.
    2. *Postnecrotic cirrhosis:*
        a. This occurs after massive liver cell necrosis, resulting as a complication of acute viral hepatitis or after exposure to industrial or chemical hepatotoxins.
        b. Broad bands of scar tissue cause destruction of liver lobules and entire lobes.
    3. *Biliary cirrhosis:*
        a. This develops from chronic biliary obstruction, bile stasis, and inflammation, resulting in severe obstructive jaundice.
        b. Primary biliary cirrhosis results from intrahepatic bile stasis.
        c. Secondary biliary cirrhosis is caused by obstruction of the hepatic or common bile ducts, producing hepatic bile stasis, which causes progressive fibrosis, hepatocellular destruction, and regenerated nodules.

4. *Cardiac cirrhosis:*
   a. This is associated with severe right-sided congestive heart failure; it results in an enlarged, edematous, congested liver.
   b. The liver serves as a reservoir for a large amount of venous blood that the failing heart is unable to pump into circulation.
   c. The liver becomes anoxic, resulting in liver cell necrosis and fibrosis.

- Complications of cirrhosis include
  1. *Portal hypertension*—a persistent increase in pressure within the portal vein developing as a result of increased resistance or obstruction to flow.
  2. *Ascites*—the accumulation of free fluid containing almost pure plasma within the peritoneal cavity. Increased hydrostatic pressure from portal hypertension results in venous congestion of the hepatic capillaries, causing plasma to leak directly from the liver surface and portal vein; other contributing factors include reduced circulating plasma protein and increased hepatic lymphatic formation.
  3. *Bleeding esophageal varices*—fragile, thin-walled, distended esophageal veins that are irritated and rupture. Varices occur most frequently in the lower esophagus and also occur in the proximal esophagus and stomach.
  4. *Coagulation defects*—decreased synthesis of bile fats in the liver that prevent the absorption of fat-soluble vitamins. Without vitamin K, and clotting factors II, VII, IX, and X, the client is susceptible to bleeding.
  5. *Jaundice*—caused by one of two mechanisms:
     a. Hepatocellular jaundice: The liver is unable to metabolize bilirubin.
     b. Intrahepatic obstruction: Edema, fibrosis, or scarring of the hepatic bile duct channels and bile ducts interferes with normal bile and bilirubin excretion.
  6. *Portal systemic encephalopathy* (also known as hepatic encephalopathy and hepatic coma)—end-stage hepatic failure and cirrhosis; manifested by neurologic symptoms, characterized by altered level of consciousness, impaired thinking processes, and neuromuscular disturbances.

7. *Hepatorenal syndrome*—progressive, oliguric renal failure associated with hepatic failure resulting in functionally impaired kidneys; manifested by a sudden decrease in urinary flow and elevated serum urea nitrogen and creatinine levels, with abnormally decreased urine sodium excretion and increased urine osmolarity.

COLLABORATIVE MANAGEMENT

Assessment

- The nurse records the client's
    1. Age, sex, and race
    2. Employment history, including working conditions exposing the client to harmful chemical toxins
    3. History of individual and family alcoholism
    4. Previous medical conditions, including acute viral hepatitis, biliary tract disease, viral infections, recent blood transfusions, and history of heart disease or respiratory disorders
- The nurse assesses for
    1. Generalized weakness
    2. Weight loss
    3. Gastrointestinal (GI) symptoms, including loss of appetite, early morning nausea and vomiting, dyspepsia, flatulence, and changes in bowel habits
    4. Abdominal pain or tenderness
    5. Jaundice of the skin and sclera
    6. Dry skin, rashes
    7. Petechiae or ecchymosis
    8. Palmar erythema
    9. Spider angiomas on the nose, cheeks, upper thorax, and shoulders
    10. Hepatomegaly palpated in the right upper quadrant
    11. Ascites revealed by bulging flanks and dullness on percussion of the abdomen
    12. Protruding umbilicus
    13. Dilated abdominal veins (*caput medusae*)
    14. Presence of blood in vomitus or nasogastric drainage
    15. Fetor hepaticus, the fruity, musty breath odor of chronic liver disease
    16. Amenorrhea or testicular atrophy
    17. Gynecomastia (enlarged breasts)
    18. Impotence

19. Asterixis (liver flap), a coarse tremor characterized by rapid, nonrhythmic extension and flexions in the wrist and fingers
20. Elevated serum liver enzyme and serum bilirubin levels
21. Decreased total serum protein and albumin levels
22. Elevated serum globulin level
23. Prolonged prothrombin time
24. Elevated serum ammonia level
25. Enlarged liver on x-ray

Planning and Implementation

✦ NDx: Fluid Volume Excess

Nonsurgical Management

- The nurse
  1. Provides a low-sodium diet initially, restricting sodium to 500 mg to 2 grams/day
  2. Suggests alternative flavoring additives to foods such as lemon, vinegar, parsley, oregano, and pepper
  3. Collaborates with the dietitian to explain purpose of diet and meal planning
     a. Suggests elimination of table salt, salty foods, canned and frozen vegtables, and salted butter and margin
  4. Restricts fluid intake to 1500 mL/day
  5. Supplements vitamin intake with thiamine, folate, and multivitamin preparations
  6. Administers diuretics to reduce fluid accumulations and to prevent cardiac and respiratory impairment
  7. Monitors intake and output carefully
  8. Weighs the client daily
  9. Measures abdominal girth daily
  10. Monitors electrolyte balance
  11. Administers low-sodium antacids
  12. Assists the physician with paracentesis to remove ascitic fluid
  13. Elevates the head of the bed to minimize shortness of breath

Surgical Management

- A peritoneovenous shunt may be placed, or a surgical bypass shunting procedure, such as a LeVeen or Denver shunt, may be performed for severe ascites. Ascites is drained through a one-way valve into a silicone rubber tube that terminates in the superior vena cava.

- Preoperative care is aimed at optimizing the client's physical state.
- The nurse provides preoperative care:
  1. Administers fresh frozen plasma, as ordered
  2. Administers vitamin K
  3. Ensures that packed red blood cells are available for surgery
  4. Provides routine preoperative care
- The nurse provides postoperative care:
  1. Provides routine postoperative care
  2. Auscultates breath sounds for the presence of crackles, indicating excessive lung fluid
  3. Assesses for fluid volume excess and hemodilution
  4. Administers diuretics for volume excess
  5. Monitors coagulation study results
  6. Performs daily abdominal girth measurements
  7. Records accurate intake and output daily
  8. Weighs the client daily

✦ NDx: Potential for Hemorrhage

- Esophageal bleeding is controlled by:
  1. *Gastric intubation* to lavage the stomach until the fluid returned is clear
  2. *Esophagogastric balloon tamponade* to treat bleeding esophageal varices. The nurse:
     a. Maintains esophagogastric balloon tamponade with a Sengstaken-Blakemore or Minnesota tube to control bleeding varices, as ordered
     b. Assists the physician with tube insertion
     c. Checks balloon pressures and volumes (pressure should be between 20 and 25 mmHg)
     d. Keeps tube taped and secure
     e. Keeps an extra tube and scissors at the bedside
     f. Monitors the client for respiratory distress caused by obstruction from the esophageal balloon; if distress occurs, cuts both balloon ports to allow for rapid balloon deflation and tube removal
  3. Administering blood products (red blood cells and fresh frozen plasma) and intravenous fluids, as ordered

4. Giving vasopressin intra-arterially or intravenously, as ordered, to lower pressures in the portal venous system to decrease bleeding
5. Injection sclerotherapy, which may be performed to sclerose bleeding esophageal varices. The nurse:
   a. Monitors the client's vital signs and assesses the client for chest pain
   b. Administers pain medication as ordered and reports severe pain to the physician
   c. Assesses lung sounds to determine presence of pneumonia, pleural effusion
6. *Endoscopic ligation* procedure uses bands to ligate the bleeding varices and is now considered the treatment of choice by many physicians.
7. *Transjugular intrahepatic portal-systemic shunt* — a nonsurgical procedure whereby the physician implants a shunt, passed through a catheter, between the portal vein and the hepatic vein to reduce portal venous pressure and therefore control the bleeding.
   a. The procedure is painful even though IV conscious sedation is used.
   b. The nurse reinforces the physician's teaching about complications, which are serious and include blood vessel rupture, liver failure, renal failure, myocardial infarction, and death.

Surgical Management

- Surgical management of portal hypertension and esophageal varices are a last-resort intervention associated with high mortality secondary to coagulation abnormalities, infection, poor tolerance to anesthesia, and ascites.
  1. The *portacaval shunt* diverts the portal venous blood flow into the inferior vena cava to decrease portal pressure.
  2. The *splenorenal shunting* procedure involves a splenectomy with anastomosis of the splenic vein with the left renal vein.
  3. In the *mesocaval shunt,* the superior mesenteric vein is anastomosed to the inferior vena cava.
- Preoperative care includes correcting bleeding and clotting deficits by administering fresh frozen plasma and packed red blood cells.
- After surgery the client is admitted to a critical care unit.

225

- The nurse provides postoperative care:
    1. Provides routine postoperative care
    2. Closely monitors the client's hemodynamic status
    3. Maintains mechanical ventilation and the artificial airway
    4. Carefully administers opioid analgesia for pain and sedation, as ordered
    5. Closely monitors urinary output because clients are susceptible to oliguria
    6. Monitors for rebleeding from esophageal varices or from shunting procedure anastomosis sites
    7. Observes for postshunt encephalopathy
    8. Administers total parenteral nutrition (TPN), as ordered
    9. Administers albumin, as ordered
    10. Measures abdominal girth and weight daily; reports significant changes to the physician

---

✦ **NDx:** Risk for Altered Thought Processes

Nonsurgical Management

- The nurse
    1. Assesses for neurologic changes
    2. Limits protein intake in the diet to reduce excess protein breakdown by intestinal bacteria and thus decrease ammonia formation
    3. Collaborates with the dietitian to limit dietary protein to 50 to 60 g/day, although this restriction is being questioned (clients with cirrhosis are malnourished and need *additional* protein and calories)
    4. Initiates TPN, as ordered, if GI bleeding precipitates hepatic encephalopathy
    5. Administers lactulose, as ordered, to promote excretion of fecal ammonia
        a. When given orally, the nurse dilutes it with fruit juice to help the client tolerate the sweet taste
        b. The desired effect of lactulose is 2 to 3 soft stools per day; watery diarrheal stools may signify excessive lactulose administration
    6. Administers neomycin sulfate, as ordered, to act as an intestinal antiseptic
    7. Administers stool softeners, as ordered, to prevent constipation in long-term therapy
    8. Restricts drugs, such as opioids, sedatives, and barbiturates

Continuing Care

- Health teaching is individualized for the client, depending on the cause of the disease.
- The nurse teaches the client and family to

  1. Consume a diet high in calories, protein, and vitamins
  2. Restrict sodium intake if ascites occur
  3. Restrict protein if susceptible to encephalopathy
  4. Take diuretics as prescribed, report symptoms of hypokalemia, and consume foods high in potassium
  5. Take antacids or histamine antagonists, such as ranitidine (Zantac), as ordered, for GI bleeding
  6. Avoid all nonprescription medications
  7. Avoid alcohol (refer to Alcoholics Anonymous if client is an alcoholic)
  8. Keep follow-up visits with the physician(s)

CLUSTER HEADACHE

See Headache, Cluster.

COLITIS, ULCERATIVE

OVERVIEW

- Ulcerative colitis is a chronic inflammatory process of the bowel that results in poor absorption of vital nutrients.
- Classified as an inflammatory bowel disease, it is characterized by diffuse inflammation of the intestinal mucosa, resulting in loss of surface epithelium, causing ulceration and abscess formation.
- Ulcerative colitis typically begins in the rectum and proceeds in a uniform, continuous manner proximally toward the cecum.

- *Acute* ulcerative colitis results in vascular congestion, hemorrhage, edema, and ulceration of the bowel mucosa.
- *Chronic* ulcerative colitis causes muscle hypertrophy, fat deposits, and fibrous tissue, with bowel thickening, shortening, and narrowing.
- Complications of the disease include hemorrhage, abscess formation, bowel obstruction, malabsorption, bowel perforation with peritonitis, fissures, and fistula formation.

 Transcultural Considerations

Ulcerative colitis is two to four times more common among people of Jewish origin and four times more common in Caucasians than in people of other races.

COLLABORATIVE MANAGEMENT
Assessment
- The nurse records the client's
    1. Family history of inflammatory bowel disease
    2. Previous and current therapy for illnesses
    3. Diet history, including usual patterns and intolerances of milk products and greasy, fried, or spicy foods
    4. History of liquid, bloody stools
    5. Anorexia
    6. Fatigue
- The nurse assesses for
    1. The presence or absence of bowel sounds
    2. Increased or localized abdominal tenderness or cramping
    3. Bowel elimination patterns; color, consistency, and character of stools and the presence or absence of blood
    4. The relation between the occurrence of diarrhea and the timing of meals, pain, emotional distress, and activity

Planning and Implementation
✦ **NDx:** Diarrhea

Nonsurgical Management
- Management of ulcerative colitis is aimed at relieving the symptoms and reducing intestinal motility, decreasing inflammation, and promoting intestinal healing.

- The nurse
    1. Administers antidiarrheal drugs, assesses and documents their effectiveness in controlling symptoms, and observes for side effects
    2. Monitors the client for side effects of antimicrobial agents administered to help prevent secondary infection:
        a. Photosensitivity
        b. Agranulocytosis
        c. Aplastic anemia
        d. Nausea and vomiting
        e. Hepatic toxicity
    3. Administers corticosteroids as ordered. For rectal symptoms, topical steroids in the form of retention enemas or suppositories may be used
    4. Administers immunosuppressants as ordered, including azathioprine (Imuran), in combination with steroids; observes for side effects, such as diarrhea, secondary infections, dermatitis, alopecia, and bone marrow depression
    5. Administers salicylate compounds such as mesalamine (Asocol) or Sulfasazine E.C.◆ for its antimicrobial action on the bowel.
- The prescribed diet depends on the severity of the disease and whether surgery is performed. Dietary orders may include
    1. Nothing by mouth for the client with severe symptoms
    2. Total parenteral nutrition (TPN)
    3. Elemental formulas, which are absorbed in the upper bowel, thereby minimizing bowel stimulation
    4. Low-fiber diet
    5. Avoidance of foods such as whole wheat grains, nuts, and raw fruits or vegetables
- The nurse
    1. Encourages the client to avoid smoking, caffeinated beverages, pepper, and alcohol
    2. Collaborates with the dietitian to provide a detailed explanation of prescribed diet therapy
    3. Monitors dietary intake (including calorie count) and output
    4. Restricts the client's activity, promoting comfort and intestinal healing
    5. Ensures that the client has easy access to the bedside commode or bathroom

229

Surgical Management

- The need for surgery is based on the client's response to medical interventions.
- Surgical procedures include
    1. *Total proctocolectomy with permanent ileostomy:* removal of the colon, rectum, and anus with anal closure. The end of the terminal ileum forms the stoma, which is located in the right lower quadrant. Postoperatively, the nurse provides skin and ostomy care.
    2. *Kock ileostomy (pouch)* or *continent ileostomy:* an intra-abdominal pouch or reservoir constructed from the terminal ileum where stool can be stored until the pouch is drained by the nurse or client. The pouch is connected to the stoma with a nipple-like valve constructed from an intussuscepted portion of the ileum; the stoma is flush with the skin.
    3. *Ileoanal reservoir:* a two-stage procedure involving the excision of the rectal mucosa; abdominal colectomy, construction of the reservoir or pouch to the anal canal; and a temporary loop ileostomy. Over 3 to 4 months, the capacity of the reservoir is increased by a series of fluid instillations, after which the loop ileostomy is closed.
- The nurse provides extensive preoperative teaching:
    1. Provides routine preoperative instructions
    2. Provides instructions on care of the ostomy
- The nurse provides routine postoperative care.
- Specific nursing care interventions are determined by the procedure performed, including ostomy or perineal wound care.
- The nurse consults the enterostomal therapist, as needed.

✦ NDx: Pain

- The nurse
    1. Assesses the client for changes in complaints and responses to pain that may indicate disease complications, such as increased inflammation, obstruction, hemorrhage, or peritonitis
    2. Assesses for pain, including its character, pattern of occurrence (such as before or after meals, during the night, or before or after bowel movements), and duration
    3. Administers antidiarrheal drugs, as ordered, to control diarrhea

4. Administers anticholinergics, as ordered, before meals to provide relief of pain caused by cramping
5. Provides measures to relieve irritated skin caused by frequent contact with diarrheal stool:
    a. Cleaning with mild soap and water after each bowel movement
    b. Providing frequent sitz baths
    c. Applying a thin coat of mineral oil, petroleum jelly, vitamin A and D ointment, or other skin protective care product
    d. Applying medicated wipes such as witch hazel or Tucks
6. Assists the client to use other pain relief measures:
    a. Position changes
    b. Stress reduction
    c. Heat applications
    d. Diversional activities
    e. Adequate rest and sleep
7. Involves the client in care planning
8. Provides information and explanations
9. Encourages the client to verbalize feelings and concerns

✦ NDx: Potential for Gastrointestinal Bleeding

- The nurse
    1. Monitors the client for signs and symptoms of internal bleeding
    2. Checks all stools for blood, using both gross and occult examination

Continuing Care

- The nurse teaches the client
    1. Information on the nature of the disease, including acute episodes, remissions, and symptom management
    2. Necessity for caution in situations that promote profuse sweating or fluid loss:
        a. Strenuous physical activities
        b. High environmental temperature
        c. Episodes of diarrhea or vomiting
    3. Where to obtain ostomy supplies, along with the name, size, and manufacturer's order number
    4. Self-care of the ileostomy or Kock pouch, including when to empty the pouch and change the pouch system

5. Activity limitations, including avoidance of heavy lifting
- The nurse refers the client to the United Ostomy Association.

COLORECTAL CANCER

See Cancer, Colorectal.

CONGESTIVE HEART FAILURE

See Heart Failure.

CONJUNCTIVITIS

- Conjunctivitis is an inflammation or infection of the conjunctiva of the eye.
- Types of conjunctivitis and their treatment include
  1. *Allergic* or *inflammatory* conjunctivitis:
     a. Associated with a sensitivity to pollens, animal protein, feathers, certain foods or materials, insect bites, or drugs
     b. Manifested by edema of the conjunctiva, burning and itching sensation, excessive tearing, and engorgement of blood vessels
     c. Treated with instillation of vasoconstrictors and corticosteroid eyedrops; the client is taught how to instill the drops

2. *Infectious* conjunctivitis (bacterial or viral):
    a. Referred to as "pink eye" and easily transmitted; often caused by *Staphylococcus aureus, Haemophilus influenzae,* or *Pseudomonas aeruginosa*
    b. Manifested by blood vessel dilation, mild conjunctival edema, tearing, and watery discharge, which becomes purulent
    c. Treated with broad-spectrum antibiotic ointment until the causative organism is identified, and rest
    d. Health teaching consists of
        (1) Hygienic principles to prevent spread of the infection
        (2) Importance of hand washing before and after instilling eyedrops
        (3) How to instill eyedrops
        (4) Importance of not rubbing the eye or carelessly disposing of tissues

Contusions, Pulmonary

- Pulmonary contusion is characterized by interstitial hemorrhage associated with intra-alveolar hemorrhage, resulting in decreased pulmonary compliance.
- Respiratory failure develops over time after blunt chest trauma from rapid deceleration injuries during motor vehicle accidents.
- Manifestations include
    1. Hypoxemia
    2. Dyspnea
    3. Irritated bronchial mucosa
    4. Increased bronchial secretions
    5. Hemoptysis
    6. Decreased breath sounds, crackles, and wheezes
    7. Hazy opacity in the pulmonary lobes or parenchyma
- Treatment is aimed at maintenance of ventilation and oxygenation; the distressed client requires mechanical

ventilation with positive end-expiratory pressure. The major complication is adult respiratory distress syndrome (ARDS).

COPD

See Airflow Limitation, Chronic.

CORNEAL DISORDERS

OVERVIEW

- There are several types of corneal problems:
    1. *Keratoconus:* degenerative disease that causes generalized thinning and forward protrusion of the cornea
    2. *Dystrophies:* characterized by the abnormal deposition of substances; cause changes in the corneal structure
    3. *Keratitis:* inflammation of the cornea caused by infection or irritation
    4. *Corneal ulcer:* break in the normally intact corneal epithelium, which can provide an entrance for bacteria, viruses, and fungi

COLLABORATIVE MANAGEMENT
Assessment

- The nurse assesses for
    1. Location, quantity, quality, timing, and setting:
        a. Eye pain
        b. Impaired vision
        c. Drainage
        d. Photophobia
    2. Hazy or cloudy-looking cornea

3. Altered corneal light reflex

Interventions

Nonsurgical Management

- The nurse
    1. Administers antibiotics, antifungal agents, and antiviral agents depending on the causative organism
    2. Administers steroids in selected causes of ocular herpes to reduce the inflammatory response in the eye
    3. Times ophthalmic administration of drugs carefully so that if two medications must be administered at the same time, 5 minutes separates their instillation
    4. Uses separate, clearly labeled bottles of medication if the same medication is used for both eyes, one of them infected
    5. Wears gloves if drainage is present
    6. Washes hands before and after administration of medication
    7. Assists the client in using his or her functional vision, suggesting sunglasses, indirect lighting

Surgical Management

- *Keratoplasty,* or corneal transplant, is used to restore vision. One of two procedures is performed:
    1. Lamellar, or partial-thickness, keratoplasty
    2. Penetrating, or full-thickness, keratoplasty
- Tissue for a keratoplasty is obtained from a local eye bank or tissue bank. An eye bank obtains corneal tissue from deceased volunteer donors. If a client is a potential donor, the nurse
    1. Raises the head of the bed 30 degrees
    2. Instills antibiotic eyedrops
    3. Closes the eyes and applies a small ice pack
    4. Contacts the family and physician to discuss possible eye donation
- The nurse provides preoperative care:
    1. Provides routine preoperative care
    2. Recognizes that the client often has short notice that a transplant is available and may be anxious upon arrival at the hospital
    3. Informs the client that regional anesthesia is typically used

235

4. Instructs the client in the importance of lying still during the procedure; if the client is unable to lie still, general anesthesia may be used
5. Assesses the client's eye for signs of infection
6. Inserts an intravenous catheter for fluids and medications, as ordered; a sedative, such as diazepam (Valium, Apo-Diazepam◆) or midazolam (Versed), is usually given

* The nurse provides postoperative care:
  1. Leaves the pressure dressing and eye shield in place until a specific order for removal is written by the surgeon
  2. Notifies the physician of any significant drainage
  3. Observes for and reports complications of surgery:
     a. Bleeding
     b. Infection
     c. Graft rejection
     d. Wound leakage
  4. Instructs the client to lie on the nonoperative side to reduce intraocular pressure

- Graft rejection is possible; vision is reduced and the cornea becomes cloudy; it is treated with frequent applications of topical corticosteroids.
- Severe pain or pain accompanied by nausea is indicative of increased intraocular pressure; the nurse notifies the physician immediately and elevates the head of the bed 30 degrees.
- Prior to discharge, the client is shown how to apply the patch.

CORNEAL DYSTROPHY

See Corneal Disorders.

CORNEAL ULCERS

See Corneal Disorders.

CORONARY ARTERY DISEASE

OVERVIEW

- Coronary artery disease (CAD) affects the three major coronary arteries (right, left anterior descending, and left circumflex), which provide nutrients and blood to the myocardium.
- When blood flow is blocked, ischemia and infarction of the myocardium may occur.
- The most common cause of CAD is atherosclerosis, which is characterized by a fibrous plaque lesion that narrows the vessel lumen or obstructs blood flow (see Atherosclerosis).
- Other causes include increased myocardial oxygen requirements (e.g., exercise or aortic stenosis) and transient reductions in blood flow (e.g., hypotension or coronary artery spasm).
- *Angina pectoris* is a temporary imbalance between the ability of the coronary arteries to supply oxygen and the myocardium's demand for it:
    1. *Stable* angina is chest discomfort that occurs with exertion in a pattern that is familiar to the client and that has not increased in frequency, duration, or intensity of symptoms during the past several months. It is usually associated with a stable atherosclerotic plaque.
    2. *Unstable* angina is chest pain or discomfort that occurs at rest or with minimal exertion. It is characterized by an increase in the number of episodes ("attacks") and the intensity of pain. The pain may last longer than 15 minutes or be poorly relieved by rest or nitroglycerin.

🦠 Women's Health Consideration

- Many women experience atypical angina; described as a choking sensation that occurs with exertion.
- Angina is more likely to be the primary presenting symptom of CAD in women than in men.
- Angina is twice as common as myocardial infarction (MI) in women.

- MI occurs when the myocardial muscle is abruptly and severely deprived of oxygen. Ischemia and necrosis (infarction) of the myocardial tissue result if blood flow is not restored.
- The client's response to an MI depends on which coronary arteries were obstructed and which part of the left ventricular wall was damaged—anterior, lateral, septal, inferior, or posterior:
  1. Clients with obstruction of the left anterior descending artery have anterior or septal MIs, or both. Clients with anterior MIs are most likely to experience left ventricular heart failure and ventricular dysrhythmias.
  2. Clients with obstruction of the circumflex artery have lateral wall MIs and sinus dysrhythmias.
  3. Clients with obstruction of the right coronary artery often have inferior MIs. These clients are likely to experience bradydysrhythmias or atrioventricular conduction defects, especially transient second-degree heart block.
- Women have higher morbidity and mortality rates post MI than men.
- Nonmodifiable risk factors include age, sex, family history, and ethnic background.

 Transcultural Considerations

1. African-Americans do not have significantly higher overall heart disease rates than other groups, but their incidence of diabetes, hypertension, and obesity (risk factors for MI) is higher.
2. Hispanic-Americans have lower death rates from heart disease than non–Hispanic-Americans, but their smoking incidence is higher.
3. Native Americans have a high incidence of diabetes and obesity.

COLLABORATIVE MANAGEMENT
Assessment
- The nurse does not obtain a history until the client is pain free.
- The nurse records
  1. Family history

2. Modifiable risk factors, including eating habits, lifestyle, and physical activity level
- The nurse assesses for clinical manifestations of myocardial infarction:
    1. Chest, epigastric, jaw, back, or arm discomfort (often described as tightness, burning, pressure, or indigestion)
    2. Nausea and vomiting
    3. Diaphoresis
    4. Dizziness
    5. Weakness
    6. Palpitations
    7. Shortness of breath
    8. Diminished or absent pulses
    9. Sinus tachycardia with premature ventricular contractions
    10. Abnormal blood pressure
    11. S_3 gallop
    12. Increased respiratory rate
    13. Crackles or wheezes (if heart failure occurs)
    14. Elevated temperature
    15. Denial (early reaction to chest discomfort)
    16. Fear and anxiety
    17. Elevated serum cardiac enzyme levels:
        a. Creatine kinase (CK-MB isoenzyme)
        b. Lactate dehydrogenase (LDH) (LDH1 isoenzyme rises higher than LDH2 in the presence of an MI)
        c. Elevated white blood cell count
    18. Electrocardiography changes
        a. In angina, ST depression or elevation or T-wave inversion
        b. In MI, ST elevation, T-wave inversion, and an abnormal Q wave
    19. Results of thallium scan, MUGA scan, and cardiac catheterization, if performed

Considerations for Elderly Clients

1. About 25% of older adults who experience MI present complaining primarily of shortness of breath.
2. Many elderly clients do not typically experience chest discomfort but have disorientation or confusion as the primary manifestation.

Planning and Implementation

✦ NDx: Pain

- The nurse administers drug therapy, as ordered:
  1. Nitroglycerin (sublingually), used for angina, to increase collateral blood flow, redistributing blood flow toward the subendocardium; if three repeated doses do not relieve discomfort, the client may be experiencing an MI
  2. Nitroglycerin (IV), administered in a specialized unit to carefully monitor the client's blood pressure; hypotension is a serious side effect of this drug
  3. Morphine sulfate (IV) for clients unresponsive to nitroglycerin
  4. Aspirin 325 mg po (chewed) may be administered immediately
- The nurse
  1. Provides oxygen therapy, as ordered
  2. Places the client in a semi-Fowler position for comfort
  3. Maintains a quiet, calm environment to the extent possible
  4. Administers acetaminophen (Tylenol, Exdol◆), for headaches caused by nitroglycerin, as ordered

✦ NDx: Altered (Cardiopulmonary) Tissue Perfusion

- Thrombolytic agents are given intravenously or by intracoronary route during cardiac catheterization to dissolve thrombi in the coronary arteries and to restore myocardial blood flow. Examples include streptokinase (Kabikinase), tissue plasminogen activator (tPA; Activase), and anisoylated plasminogen-streptokinase activator complex (APSAC; Eminase).
- The nurse
  1. Monitors the client for signs of obvious and occult bleeding, and reports indications of bleeding immediately to the physician (more common in women who receive thrombolytic therapy)
     a. Monitors the client for indications of cerebrovascular bleeding
     b. Observes all IV sites for bleeding
     c. Monitors clotting studies

     d. Observes for signs of internal bleeding (watching hematocrit and hemoglobin)

     e. Test stool, urine, and emesis for occult blood

  2. Monitors for indications that thrombolytic agents were effective, including abrupt cessation of chest pain, sudden onset of ventricular dysrhythmias, and resolution of ST segment depression

  3. Administers intravenous nitroglycerin and heparin, as ordered, after thrombolytic therapy

- The nurse also

  1. Administers one enteric coated aspirin daily or every other day to prevent platelet aggregation at the site of obstruction

  2. Administers beta-adrenergic agents, such as propranolol [Inderal, Apo-Propranolol◆] to clients with MIs; these drugs decrease infarction size, ventricular dysrhythmias, and mortality. The nurse:

     a. Monitors the heart rate

     b. Checks the blood pressure

     c. Checks the client's level of consciousness

     d. Monitors for any chest discomfort

     e. Assess lung sounds for crackles and wheezes

     f. Monitors the client for hypoglycemia, depression, nightmares, and forgetfulness

  3. Administers angiotension-converting enzyme (ACE) inhibitors to prevent ventricular remodeling and the development of heart failure

  4. Administers calcium channel blockers to clients with angina for coronary artery vasodilation and prevention of vasospasm

✦ NDx: Activity Intolerance

- Cardiac rehabilitation is divided into three phases:

  1. Phase 1 begins with acute illness and ends with discharge from the hospital.

  2. Phase 2 begins after discharge and continues through convalescence at home.

  3. Phase 3 involves long-term conditioning.

- The nurse

  1. Promotes rest and assists with activities of daily living

  2. Progresses client mobility gradually, starting with having the client dangle the legs at the side of the bed and proceeding to ambulation

✦ NDx: Ineffective Individual Coping

- The nurse
    1. Assesses the client's coping ability and level of anxiety
    2. Provides simple, repeated explanations of therapies, expectations, and surroundings
    3. During the acute phase of illness, administers anxiolytic drugs, such as alprazolam (Xanax), as ordered
    4. Encourages the client to verbalize frustrations and allows opportunities for client decision-making and control

✦ NDx: Potential for Dysrhythmias in Clients Experiencing an MI

- The nurse
    1. Identifies the dysrhythmia
    2. Assesses the client's hemodynamic status
    3. Evaluates the client for chest discomfort
- Dysrhythmias are treated when they are causing hemodynamic compromise, are increasing myocardial oxygen requirements, or predispose to lethal ventricular dysrhythmias.

✦ NDx: Potential for Heart Failure in Clients Experiencing an MI

- Heart failure is a relatively common complication following MI; the most severe form of heart failure, cardiogenic shock, accounts for most in-hospital deaths following an MI.

Nonsurgical Management

- Decreased cardiac output related to heart failure is a common complication after MI.
- The nurse assesses the client with left ventricular failure and pulmonary edema by aucultating for crackles and identifying their location within the lungs.
- The nurse assesses for
    1. Tachypnea
    2. Frothy sputum
    3. Change in client's orientation or mental status
    4. Urine output below 30 mL/hr
    5. Cold, clammy skin with poor peripheral pulses
    6. Unusual fatigue
    7. Recurrent chest pain

8. Changes in right atrial pressure, pulmonary artery pressure, systolic and diastolic pressures, pulmonary wedge pressure, systemic vascular resistance, cardiac output, and cardiac index

- Classification of post-MI heart failure
   1. Class I often responds well to reduction in preload with IV diuretics.
      a. The nurse monitors hourly the urine output, vital signs, reviews serum potassium levels, and assesses for signs of heart failure.
   2. Class II and Class III may require diuresis and more aggressive medical intervention.
   3. Class IV cardiogenic shock is manifested by tachycardia, hypotension, blood pressure less than 90 or 30 mmHg less than client's baseline.
- The nurse
   1. Administers intravenous morphine, as ordered, which is used to decrease pulmonary congestion and relieve pain
   2. Provides oxygen therapy, as ordered; intubation and mechanical ventilation may be necessary
   3. Uses information from hemodynamic monitoring to titrate drug therapy
   4. Administers diuretics, nitroglycerin, or nitroprusside, as ordered
- Clients who do not respond to drug therapy may require an *intra-aortic balloon pump* (IABP), which is inserted to improve myocardial perfusion, reduce afterload, and facilitate ventricular emptying.
- Immediate reperfusion may be performed on clients with cardiogenic shock. A left-sided cardiac catheterizaton is performed; if the client has a treatable lesion(s), the surgeon performs a percutaneous transluminal coronary angioplasty (PTCA) or the client undergoes a coronary artery bypass graft (CABG).
- The goal of medical management of right-side heart ventricular failure is to improve right ventricular stroke volume.
- The nurse
   1. Administers fluids, as ordered (as much as 200mL/hr), to increase right atrial pressure to 20mmHg
   2. Monitors pulmonary artery wedge pressure (attempting to maintain it below 15–20)
   3. Auscultates the lungs to ensure left-side heart failure not developing

4. Monitors cardiac output to ensure that fluid administration is having desired effect

---

✦ NDx: Potential for Recurrent Chest Discomfort and Extension of Injury

---

- Recurrent chest pain despite medical therapy is a major indicator of surgery.

Surgical Management

- *Percutaneous transluminal coronary angioplasty* (PTCA), an invasive but technically nonsurgical technique, is performed to provide symptom reduction for clients with chest discomfort without a significant risk of complications. PTCA is done by introducing a balloon-tipped catheter into the area of the coronary artery occlusion. When the balloon is inflated, it presses the atherosclerotic plaque against the vessel wall to reduce or eliminate the occlusion.
- Techniques used to ensure patency of the vessel are laser angioplasty, stents, and atherectomy devices.
- The nurse
  1. Monitors vital signs frequently and observes for hypotension
  2. Instructs the client to report the development of chest pain immediately
  3. Monitors cardiac rhythm pattern carefully for the development of dysrhythmias
  4. Monitors circulation to the limb where the catheter was inserted frequently; reports changes immediately to the physician
  5. Maintains immobilization of the affected limb for at least 6 hours
  6. Maintains pressure dressing and sandbag over the insertion site
  7. Elevates head of the bed slowly, per hospital protocol
  8. Instructs the client to
     a. Return to usual activities in 1 to 2 weeks or when instructed by the physician
     b. Avoid heavy lifting for several weeks
     c. Apply manual pressure if there is bleeding from the insertion site and to notify the physician if the bleeding is extensive or if oozing persists for more than 15 minutes
     d. Take long-term nitrates, calcium channel blockers, and aspirin, as prescribed

- *Coronary artery bypass graft* (CABG) surgery is indicated when other treatments have been unsuccessful. This procedure is performed with the client under general anesthesia and undergoing cardiopulmonary bypass (CPB). The graft, either the saphenous vein or internal mammary artery, bypasses the occluded vessel to restore blood supply to the myocardium.
- The nurse provides preoperative care:
    1. If surgery is done as an elective procedure, familiarizes the client and family with the cardiac surgical critical care environment
    2. Teaches the client what to expect during the postoperative period
- The nurse provides immediate postoperative care in a specialized unit:
    1. Maintains mechanical ventilation for 6 to 24 hours
    2. Monitors chest tube drainage system
    3. Monitors pulmonary artery and arterial pressures
    4. Assesses vital signs and cardiac rate and rhythm frequently
    5. Treats symptomatic dysrhythmias according to unit protocols or physician order
    6. Monitors for complications of CABG surgery, including
        a. Fluid and electrolyte imbalances
        b. Hypotension
        c. Hypothermia
        d. Hypertension
        e. Bleeding
        f. Cardiac tamponade
        g. Altered level of consciousness
        h. Pain
- The nurse provides continued postoperative care:
    1. Encourages deep breathing and coughing every 2 hours while splinting incision
    2. Assists the client in slowly resuming activity and ambulation
    3. Monitors for dysrhythmias, especially atrial fibrillation, which occurs on the second or third postoperative day
    4. Assesses for wound or sternal infection (mediastinitis), such as prolonged fever (more than 4 days), reddened sternum, purulent incisional drainage, and elevated white blood cell (WBC) count

5. Observes for indications of postpericardiotomy syndrome: pericardial and pleural pain, pericarditis, friction rub, elevated temperature and WBC count, and dysrhythmias; problem may be self-limiting or may require treatment for pericarditis
- Minimally Invasive Direct Coronary Arterial Bypass (MIDCAB) is indicated for clients with a lesion of the anterior descending artery.
- The nurse
   1. Assesses the client for postoperative chest pain and EKG changes because occulusion of the IMA graft occurs acutely in 10% of clients
   2. Encourages the client to cough and deep breathe (chest tube and thoracotomy incision)
- Transmyocardial Laser Revascularization is an experimental procedure for clients with unstable angina and inoperable coronary artery disease.

Continuing Care

- The client should be assigned to a case manager at the beginning of the hospitalization to provide constant care and assist with the transition to home or long-term care facility.
- Most clients are still recovering from their illness or surgery when discharged from the hospital; home health services may be required.
- The nurse teaches the client and family about
   1. The pathophysiology of angina and MI
   2. Risk factor modification:
      a. Smoking cessation
      b. Dietary changes (decreasing fat intake)
      c. Blood pressure control
      d. Blood glucose control
   3. Gradual increase in physical and sexual activity, according to cardiac rehabilitation protocol
   4. Cardiac medications
   5. Occupational considerations, if any
- The nurse
   1. Provides reassurance and an opportunity for clients to express their fears and concerns
   2. Identifies support systems for the client
   3. Refers the client to the American Heart Association for information
   4. Refers the client for continued cardiac rehabilitation

5. Refers the client who has had CABG surgery to Mended Hearts, a nationwide program that provides education and support to clients and their families

CORPUS LUTEUM CYSTS

See Cysts, Ovarian.

CRF

See Renal Failure, Chronic.

CROHN'S DISEASE

OVERVIEW

- Crohn's disease, or regional enteritis, is an inflammatory disease that occurs anywhere in the gastrointestinal (GI) tract but most often affects the terminal ileum with patchy lesions that extend through all bowel layers.
- This inflammatory bowel disease is similar to ulcerative colitis and is characterized by remissions and exacerbations; its cause is unknown.
- Chronic pathologic changes within the colon and small bowel include thickening of the bowel wall and narrowing of the lumen.
- In advanced disease, the bowel mucosa has nodular swelling, called granulomas, intermingled with deep ulcerations, which contribute to fistula formation.
- Complications of Crohn's disease include malabsorption, fistulas, hemorrhage, abscess formation, bowel obstruction, and cancer (usually after the client has the disease for 15 to 20 years).

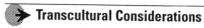

Crohn's disease is most common among those of Jewish descent, Caucasians, and those of middle European origin.

COLLABORATIVE MANAGEMENT
Assessment

- The nurse assesses for
  1. Family history of inflammatory bowel disease
  2. Previous and current therapy for illnesses
  3. Diet history, including usual patterns and intolerance to milk products and greasy, fried, or spicy foods
  4. History of diarrheal stools, anorexia, and fatigue
  5. Right lower quadrant abdominal pain or tenderness or periumbilical pain before and after bowel movements
  6. Diarrhea with steatorrhea (the stool does not usually contain blood)
  7. Weight loss (indicates serious nutritional deficiencies)
  8. Results of barium enema and upper GI series, which show narrowing, ulcerations, strictures, and fistulas consistent with Crohn's disease

Interventions

- The care of the client with Crohn's disease is similar to that for the client with ulcerative colitis (see Colitis, Ulcerative).
- Impaired skin integrity results from fistula formation; the degree of associated problems is related to the location of the fistula, the client's general health status, and the character and amount of fistula drainage.
- The nurse
  1. Replaces fluid loss with oral fluids as well as intravenous fluids or total parenteral nutrition, as ordered
  2. Recognizes that the client requires at least 3000 kcal/day to promote fistula healing
  3. Provides high-calorie, high-protein meals with supplements, in collaboration with the dietitian
  4. Applies a pouch to the fistula to prevent skin irritation and to measure the drainage, in collaboration with the enterostomal therapist

5. Covers the area around the fistula with skin barriers, such as Stomahesive or DuoDerm, and applies a wound drainage system over the fistula, securing it to the protective barriers
6. Cleans adjacent skin and keeps it dry; the wound drainage should *never* be allowed to have direct skin contact without prompt cleaning, because intestinal fluid enzymes are caustic

- About 10% of clients with Crohn's disease require surgery, usually a bowel resection. (See Cancer, Colorectal, "Surgical Management.")

Continuing Care
- See Colitis, Ulcerative, "Continuing Care."

CTS

See Carpal Tunnel Syndrome.

CUSHING'S SYNDROME

See Hypercortisolism (Cushing's Syndrome).

CYSTITIS

OVERVIEW
- Cystitis is an inflammation of the urinary bladder from infectious causes, such as bacteria, viruses, fungi, or parasites, or noninfectious causes, such as chemical exposure or radiation therapy.
- Coliform bacteria, especially *Escherichia coli* normally found in the gastrointestinal tract, account for most cases of bacterial cystitis.

- Other factors that contribute to the development or recurrence of cystitis, or urinary tract infections (UTIs), include
    1. Structural or functional abnormalities of the urinary tract
    2. Use of indwelling urinary catheters
    3. Sexual intercourse, diaphragm use, and pregnancy in women (women are at a higher risk then men)
    4. Prostate disease or structural abnormality of the urinary tract in men

---

𝓔 Considerations for Elderly Clients

1. UTIs occur more often in elderly than in younger adults, with males and females equally affected.
2. Elderly clients are at greater risk of having an overwhelming and generalized infection, called urosepsis, caused by a gram-negative bacteremia.

COLLABORATIVE MANAGEMENT
Assessment

- The nurse records the client's
    1. History of prior UTI
    2. History of renal or urologic problems, such as kidney stones
    3. History of health problems, such as diabetes mellitus
- The nurse assesses for
    1. Pain or discomfort on urination
    2. Urgency to void
    3. Difficulty in initiating urination
    4. Feelings of incomplete bladder emptying
    5. Voiding in small amounts
    6. Increased frequency of voiding
    7. Complete inability to urinate
    8. Changes in urine color, clarity, or odor, presence of white or red blood cellls
    9. Abdominal or back pain
    10. Bladder distention
    11. Urinary meatus inflammation
    12. Prostate gland changes or tenderness
    14. Positive urine culture
    15. Elevated white blood cell count (occasionally)

ⓔ Considerations for Elderly Clients

1. The only symptoms may be as vague as increasing mental confusion, or frequent unexplained falls
2. A sudden onset of incontinence or worsening of incontinence may be an early symptom
3. Fever, tachycardia, tachypnea, and hypotension even without any urinary symptoms may be signs of urosepsis
4. Loss of appetite, nocturia, and dysuria are common symptoms

Planning and Implementation

- The nurse, as ordered
  1. Administers analgesics to promote comfort
  2. Administers urinary antiseptics such as nitrofurantoin (Macrodantin, Nephronex◆) and trimethoprim (Proloprim, Trimpex)
  3. Administers antispasmodics, as ordered, to decrease bladder spasm and promote complete bladder emptying
  4. Administers antibiotics, as ordered, for systemic infection; antibiotics may be given in daily bladder instillations or in oral or parenteral form. In simple, acute bacterial cystitis in healthy, ambulatory clients, a 1- to 3-day course of antibiotic treatment may be adequate. Long term antibiotics may be needed for clients with chronic recurring infections
  5. Ensures the client maintains an adequate caloric intake
  6. Ensures a fluid intake of 2 to 3 L/day
  7. Provides warm sitz baths to relieve local symptoms

ⓦ Women's Health Considerations

- Pregnant women require vigorous interventions when bacteriuria is present because of the tendency of cystitis to evolve into acute pyelonephritis.

Surgical Management

- Surgical interventions for management of cystitis include endourologic procedures with stone manipulation or pulverization for the management of urinary retention if bladder or urethral calculus is the cause.

Continuing Care

- The nurse teaches the client to
    1. Self-administer medications and to complete all of the prescribed medication
    2. Expect changes in color of urine as appropriate
    3. Use appropriate techniques to prevent discomfort with sexual activities and how to prevent postcoital infections
    4. Consume liberal fluid intake of at least 2 to 3 L/day
    5. Clean the perineum properly after urination
    6. Empty the bladder as soon as the urge is felt
    7. Obtain adequate rest, sleep, and nutrition
    8. Avoid known irritants, such as bubble baths, nylon underwear, and scented toilet tissue
    9. Wear cotton underwear
    10. Seek prompt medical care if recurrences are suspected
- The nurse refers the client to the National Kidney Foundation if appropriate.
- The nurse refers clients with interstitial cystitis to the Interstitial Cystitis Foundation.

CYSTOCELE

OVERVIEW

- A cystocele is a protrusion of the bladder through the vaginal wall due to weakened pelvic structures.
- Causes include obesity, advanced age, childbearing, and genetic predisposition.

COLLABORATIVE MANAGEMENT

- The nurse assesses for
    1. Difficulty in emptying the bladder
    2. Urinary frequency and urgency
    3. Urinary tract infections
    4. Stress urinary incontinence
    5. Significant bulging of the anterior vaginal wall during pelvic examination

- Management is conservative with mild symptoms and includes
    1. Use of a pessary for bladder support
    2. Estrogen therapy for the postmenopausal client to prevent atrophy and weakening of vaginal walls
    3. Kegel exercises to strengthen perineal muscles
- Surgical intervention (anterior colporrhaphy or anterior repair) is recommended for severe symptoms. (Care is similar to that for other vaginal surgeries.)
- The nurse teaches the postoperative client
    1. To limit her activities
    2. Not to lift anything heavy
    3. To avoid strenuous exercise
    4. To avoid sexual intercourse for 6 weeks
    5. To notify her physician if she has signs of infection, including fever, persistent pain, and purulent, foul-smelling discharge

CYSTS, BARTHOLIN'S

OVERVIEW

- Bartholin's cysts are one of the most common disorders of the vulva.
- The cysts result from obstruction of a duct; the secretory function of the gland continues, and the fluid fills the obstructed duct.
- The cause of the obstruction may be infection, congenital stenosis or atresia, thickened mucus near the ductal opening, or mechanical trauma.
- Ranging in size from 1 to 10 cm, cysts usually appear unilaterally.

COLLABORATIVE MANAGEMENT

- Assessment for *small cysts* may reveal no symptoms or client complaints of dyspareunia, of inadequate genital lubrication, or of feeling a mass in the perineal area
- Assessment for *large cysts* includes
    1. Constant, localized pain
    2. Difficulty walking or sitting

3. Swelling immediately beneath the skin in the posterior vulva
   4. Brown or sanguineous cyst
- For symptomatic cysts, surgical treatment with incision and drainage may provide temporary relief.
- Marsupialization (the formation of a pouch that serves as a new duct opening) may be performed to prevent recurrence.
- Local comfort measures and prophylactic antibiotics may be provided.
- If the cyst becomes infected, an *abscess* can form, which usually ruptures spontaneously within 72 hours.
- Interventions for abscess include bed rest, analgesics, moist heat, antibiotics, and an incision and drainage.

Cysts, CORPUS LUTEUM

See Cysts, Ovarian.

Cysts, FOLLICULAR

See Cysts, Ovarian.

Cysts, OVARIAN

- There are several types of ovarian cysts:
   1. *Follicular cysts:*
      a. Follicular cysts develop in young menstruating females, are non-neoplastic, and do not grow without hormonal influences.
      b. They develop when a mature follicle fails to rupture or an immature follicle fails to reabsorb follicular fluid.

    c. The cyst is usually small (6 to 8 cm) and may be asymptomatic unless it ruptures, causing acute, severe pelvic pain, which usually resolves with bed rest and administration of mild analgesics.

    d. If the cyst does not rupture, it usually disappears in two or three menstrual cycles without medical intervention.

    e. Oral contraceptives may be prescribed for one or two menstrual cycles to depress ovulation, resulting in cyst shrinkage.

    f. Surgery is recommended only before puberty, after menopause, or when cysts are larger than 8 cm.

    g. Cystectomy (removal of cyst) is recommended instead of oophorectomy (removal of an ovary).

2. *Corpus luteum cysts:*

    a. Corpus luteum cysts occur after ovulation and are often associated with increased secretion of progesterone.

    b. The cysts are small, averaging 4 cm, and are purplish red as a result of hemorrhage within the corpus luteum.

    c. The cysts are associated with delay in the onset of menses and irregular or prolonged flow, and may be accompanied by unilateral, low abdominal, or pelvic pain.

    d. Cyst rupture may cause intraperitoneal hemorrhage.

    e. Corpus luteum cysts may disappear in one or two menstrual cycles or with suppression of ovulation.

    f. The treatment is the same as for follicular cysts.

3. *Theca-lutein cysts:*

    a. Theca-lutein cysts, the least common of the functional ovarian cysts, are associated with hydatidiform mole and develop as a result of prolonged stimulation of the ovaries by excessive amounts of human chorionic gonadotropin (hCG).

    b. The cysts regress spontaneously within 3 months with the removal of the molar pregnancy or source of the excess hCG.

- *Polycystic ovary* (Stein-Leventhal) *syndrome* results when elevated levels of luteinizing hormone cause hyperstimulation of the ovaries; endometrial hyperplasia or carcinoma may result.

1. The typical client is obese, is hirsute, has irregular menses, and may be infertile because of anovulation.
2. The best treatment is administration of oral contraceptives because of lutein production inhibition.

- Bilateral *salpingo-oophorectomy* (removal of both tubes and ovaries) and *hysterectomy* (removal of uterus) are advised for women over 35 who no longer desire childbearing.
- Women desiring fertility can be treated with drugs to stimulate ovulation.

CYSTS, THECA-LUTEIN

See Cysts, Ovarian.

DEGENERATION, MACULAR

- Macular degeneration involves deterioration of the macula.
- It is characterized by sclerosing of the retinal capillaries, decrease in central vision, mild blurring, and distortion of vision.
- Loss of central vision may interfere with the client's ability to read, write, drive, and recognize safety hazards.
- Management is directed toward treating the underlying cause and preventing further deterioration of vision.
- Laser therapy may be used to seal leaking blood vessels.
- The nurse assists the client to identify strategies to cope with the loss of vision and makes referrals to community agencies.

DEGENERATIVE JOINT DISEASE

See Joint Disease, Degenerative.

DEHYDRATION

OVERVIEW

- Dehydration is a state in which a person's fluid intake is not sufficient to meet the needs of the body, resulting in a fluid volume deficit.
- There are three types of dehydration:
  1. *Isotonic* dehydration is the most common type and involves general depletion of isotonic fluids from the extracellular fluid (ECF) compartment (both the plasma and interstitial space). Causes of isotonic dehydration include
     a. Hemorrhage
     b. Vomiting, diarrhea
     c. Profuse salivation
     d. Fistulas, abscesses
     e. Ileostomy, cecostomy
     f. Frequent enemas
     g. Profuse diaphoresis
     h. Burns
     i. Severe wounds
     j. Long-term nothing-by-mouth (NPO) status
     k. Diuretic therapy
     l. Gastrointestinal suction, nasogastric suction
  2. *Hypertonic* dehydration occurs when water loss exceeds electrolyte loss. It is caused by
     a. Hyperventilation
     b. Watery diarrhea
     c. Renal failure
     d. Ketoacidosis
     e. Diabetes insipidus
     f. Excessive fluid replacement (hypertonic)

257

g. Excessive sodium bicarbonate administration
h. Tube feedings, dysphagia
i. Impaired thirst
j. Unconsciousness
k. Fever
l. Impaired motor function
m. Systemic infection
3. *Hypotonic* dehydration, the least common type, occurs when electrolyte loss exceeds water loss. Causes of hypotonic dehydration include
a. Chronic illness
b. Excessive fluid replacement (hypotonic)
c. Renal failure
d. Chronic or severe malnutrition

COLLABORATIVE MANAGEMENT
Assessment

- The nurse records the client's
    1. Medical history
        a. Chronic or recent acute illness
        b. Recent surgery
        c. Medication history
    2. Height and weight: A weight change of 1 pound (0.45 kg) corresponds to a fluid volume change of 475 to 500 mL
    3. Changes in degree of tightness of clothing, rings, and shoes: A sudden decrease in tightness may indicate dehydration; an increase in tightness may reflect a fluid shift to the interstitial space with an accompanying deficit in the vascular space
    4. Urinary output:
        a. Frequency and amount of voidings
        b. Usual fluid intake and intake during the previous 24 hours
        c. Type of fluids ingested
    5. Amount of strenuous physical activity

𝓔 Considerations for Elderly Clients

1. The elderly are prone to develop dehydration in response to relatively small fluid losses.
2. The elderly are more likely to have chronic illnesses or to be taking medications that can lead to fluid and electrolyte imbalances.

- The nurse assesses for
  1. Cardiovascular manifestations:
     a. Increased pulse rate
     b. Thready pulse quality
     c. Decreased blood pressure and pulse pressure
     d. Postural hypotension (orthostatic hypotension)
     e. Flat neck and hand veins in dependent positions
     f. Diminished peripheral pulses

  2. Respiratory manifestations:
     a. Increased respiratory rate
     b. Increased depth of respirations (in presence of cidosis); Kussmaul's respirations
  3. Neuromuscular manifestations:
     a. Decreased central nervous system activity (lethargy to coma)
     b. Fever
  4. Renal manifestations:
     a. Decreased urinary output
     b. Increased specific gravity
  5. Integumentary manifestations:
     a. Dry, scaly skin
     b. Turgor poor, tenting present
     c. Mouth dry and fissured; paste-like coat present
  6. Laboratory values:
     a. Increased blood urea nitrogen and creatinine levels
     b. Changes in hemoglobin and hematocrit (depend on type of dehydration)
     c. Increased urine specific gravity (except in hypotonic dehydration)
  7. Additional manifestation of hypotonic dehydration: skeletal muscle weakness
  8. Additional manifestations of hypertonic dehydration
     a. Hyperactive deep-tendon reflexes
     b. Increased sensation of thirst
     c. Pitting edema

𝓔 Considerations for Elderly Clients

1. Skin turgor for an elderly client is assessed over the sternum, forehead, or abdomen because these areas are the most reliable indicators.
2. Fever in an elderly client may cause severe dehydration; temperature may be as low as 100° to 101° F (38° to 38.6° C).

Planning and Implementation

✦ NDx: Fluid Volume Deficit

- The nurse replaces fluids orally; intravenous fluid replacement may be necessary for severe dehydration.
- Oral rehydration therapy is the most cost-effective way to replace fluids and treat clients with diarrhea; commercial formulas that contain glucose and electrolytes are available.
- The rate of replacement and type of fluids used depend on the degree and type of dehydration and the presence of pre-existing cardiac, pulmonary, or renal problems. Commonly used fluids include
    1. Isotonic fluids, such as 0.9% saline, 5% dextrose in water (D_5W), or Ringer's lactate
    2. Hypotonic fluids, such as 0.45% normal saline
    3. Hypertonic fluids, such as 10% dextrose in water, 5% dextrose in 0.9% saline, 5% dextrose in 0.45% saline, or 5% dextrose in Ringer's lactate
- Protein replacement may be needed in clients who have lost proteins (colloids) from the vascular space.
- The nurse
    1. Administers drug therapy, such as antidiarrheal medications, antiemetics, or antipyretics, as ordered, to ameliorate or correct the underlying cause of the dehydration
    2. Provides oral fluid replacement (any substance that is liquid at body temperature is considered in measuring fluid intake such as gelatin, ice pops, and ice cream)

✦ NDx: Decreased Cardiac Output

- Drug therapy may be needed to increase venous return or improve cardiac contractility.
- Oxygen therapy may be ordered when hemoglobin and hematocrit levels are low.
- The nurse
    1. Monitors the client's vital signs and level of consciousness
    2. Monitors skin color and moisture and urinary output every hour until fluid balance is restored

✦ NDx: Altered Oral Mucous Membrane

- The nurse

1. Provides mouth care every 2 to 4 hours, including brushing and flossing the client's teeth
2. Moistens the client's lips with a petroleum-based lubricant
3. Rinses the client's mouth frequently:
   a. Does not use commercial mouthwashes that contain alcohol or glycerin-containing washes and swabs, because these products tend to dry the oral mucosa further and may increase the discomfort by stinging or burning open fissures in the mucosa
   b. Rinses the client's mouth no more than two or three times per day with dilute hydrogen peroxide
   c. Uses lukewarm saline or tap water rinses
4. Assists the client with oral hygiene before meals or snacks
5. Teaches the client to avoid foods that are highly spiced or hard to chew; bland, soft, cool foods are most easily tolerated

✦ NDx: Potential for Dysrhythmia

- The nurse
   1. Monitors electrolyte levels especially hypercalcemia and hyperkalemia
   2. Assesses the rate, rhythm, and quality of the apical pulse
   3. Assesses the client for fatigue, chest pain, shortness of breath
   4. Places the client on a cardiac monitor and monitors for dysrhythmia

Continuing Care

- The nurse
   1. Teaches the client to determine the electrolyte content of prepared foods and medications by carefully reading labels
   2. Obtains a dietary consult for assistance in providing information on the planning and preparation of palatable meals whenever a specific electrolyte restriction is necessary
   3. Teaches the client about specific food or fluid restriction

4. Reviews the signs and symptoms of the specific imbalance for which the client is at risk, as well as what specific information should be reported immediately to the primary health care provider

DI

See Diabetes Insipidus.

Diabetes insipidus

OVERVIEW

- Diabetes insipidus (DI) is a disorder of water metabolism caused by a deficiency of antidiuretic hormone (ADH), resulting from either a decrease in ADH synthesis or an inability of the kidney to respond appropriately to ADH.
- DI is classified into four types:
    1. *Nephrogenic:* an inherited defect in which the renal tubules do not respond to the actions of ADH, which results in inadequate water absorption by the kidney
    2. *Primary:* results from a defect in the pituitary gland related to familial or idiopathic causes
    3. *Secondary:* results from tumors in the hypothalamic-pituitary region, head trauma, infectious processes, surgical procedures, or metastatic tumors, usually from the lung or breast
    4. *Drug-related:* caused by lithium (Eskalith, Lithobid, Carbolith◆) and demeclocycline (Declomycin), which can interfere with the renal response to ADH

COLLABORATIVE MANAGEMENT
Assessment

- The nurse assesses for

1. History of known etiologic factors, such as recent surgery, head trauma, or medication
2. Excretion of large amounts of dilute urine (more than 4 L in 24 hours)
3. Dehydration
4. Increased or excessive thirst
5. Low urine specific gravity (below 1.005) and urine osmolality (50 to 200 mOsm/kg)
6. Indications of circulatory collapse
7. Neurologic changes

Interventions

- The nurse, as ordered
    1. Administers oral chlorpropamide (Diabinese) or clofibrate (Atromid-S) for partial ADH deficiency
    2. Administers aqueous vasopressin for short-term therapy or when the dosage must be changed frequently
    3. Administers nasal sprays (lypressin, desmopressin)
- The nurse teaches the client
    1. Side effects of nasal sprays, including ulceration of the mucous membranes, allergy, sensation of chest tightness, and inhalation of the spray into the lungs, which precipitates pulmonary problems
    2. What to do if side effects occur or if an upper respiratory infection develops; sustained-action vasopressin (vasopressin tannate in oil) is administered intramuscularly
- The nurse
    1. Monitors strict intake and output
    2. Measures urine specific gravity at least daily
    3. Weighs the client every day
    4. Encourages the client to drink fluids equal to the amount of urinary output; if the client is unable to do so, provides intravenous fluids, as ordered
    5. Monitors the client carefully for indications of dehydration: dry skin, poor skin turgor, dry or cracked mucous membranes
    6. Monitors for signs of circulatory collapse, such as vital sign changes
    7. Provides education on vasopressin preparations for the client who will be discharged
    8. Encourages the client with chronic DI to wear a Medic-Alert bracelet or necklace at all times

DIABETES MELLITUS

OVERVIEW

- Diabetes mellitus is a genetically and clinically heterogeneous group of chronic systemic disorders of various causes, affecting the metabolism of carbohydrates, protein, and fat as a result of insulin deficiency.
- Characterized by fasting hyperglycemia or blood glucose levels above defined limits, polyuria, polydipsia, and polyphagia.
- Insulin, an anabolic hormone made in the beta cells of the islets of Langerhans in the pancreas, plays a key role in allowing body cells to store and utilize carbohydrates, fat, and protein. Insulin also acts as a catalyst to stimulate enzymes and chemicals necessary for cell function and energy production.
- Diabetes is classified according to the cause and presentation of the disease:

  1. *Type I diabetes,* previously referred to as insulin-dependent diabetes mellitus (IDDM) is an autoimmune disorder in which beta-cell destruction of the islets of Langerhans in the pancreas occurs:
     a. Is abrupt in onset
     b. Requires insulin injections to prevent ketosis and sustain health
     c. Affects 10% to 15% of the diabetic population
     d. Occurs primarily in childhood or adolescence but can occur at any age
     e. Causes clients to be thin and underweight
     f. May be caused by a virus that initiates autoimmune destruction of pancreatic beta cells, where insulin is produced

  2. *Type II diabetes,* previously referred to as non–insulin-dependent diabetes mellitus (NIDDM) is not a single disease but the result of many conditions that produce hyperglycemia:
     a. Is generally slow in onset
     b. May require insulin or sulfonylurea therapy to correct hyperglycemia
     c. Is usually ketosis-resistant, but ketosis can occur during severe stress or infection
     d. Affects 85% to 90% of the diabetic population

e. Is usually found in middle-aged and older adults but may occur in younger people

f. Results in obesity in 80% of those affected

g. Has unknown cause, but risk factors include family history of diabetes, obesity, age greater than 40, previously identified impaired glucose intolerance, hypertension or significant hyperlipidemia, and history of gestational diabetes or delivery of babies weighing more than 9 pounds (4.1 kg)

3. *Genetic defects of the beta cells,* formerly referred to as MODY (maturity-onset diabetes of the young), is characterized by impaired insulin secretion with little or no defects in insulin action, and is inherited in an autosomal dominant pattern

4. *Secondary diabetes*
   a. May occur with specific disorders, such as pancreatic disease, endocrine disorders, or genetic disorders associated with glucose intolerance
   b. May be infrequently induced by a chemical agent or drug, such as steroids (steroid-induced diabetes)

5. *Gestational diabetes mellitus* (GDM):
   a. Carbohydrate intolerance is noted during pregnancy and is confirmed by an oral glucose tolerance test.
   b. Clients are at high risk for diabetes after pregnancy.
   c. Children of mothers with GDM are at risk for neonatal mortality, congenital malformation, and large body size; they also have an increased risk of obesity and impaired glucose tolerance later in life.

- Acute complications of diabetes mellitus include
   1. *Diabetic ketoacidosis* (DKA):
      a. DKA occurs in people with type I diabetes and is most often precipitated by concurrent illness, especially infection.
      b. Laboratory diagnosis is based on serum glucose level equal to or greater than 300 mg/dL (16.7 mmol/l), arterial pH less than 7.38, arterial bicarbonate level less than 15 mEq/L, serum sodium less than 137 mEq/L, BUN greater than 20 mg/dL, creatinine greater than 1.5 mg/dL, and ketonemia.

    c. Preceded by polyuria, polydipsia, and polyphagia

    d. Clinical evidence of dehydration and acidosis includes decreased skin turgor, dry mucous membranes, hypotension, tachycardia, tachypnea, Kussmaul's respirations, abdominal pain, nausea, and vomiting. Central nervous system depression results in changes in consciousness varying from lethargy to coma.

2. *Hyperglycemic hyperosmolar nonketotic coma* (HHNC):

    a. HHNC is a hyperosmolar state seen in clients with type II diabetes; it is differentiated from DKA by the absence of significant ketosis and by the presence of a plasma glucose level and osmolality that are higher than average.

    b. Laboratory findings include plasma glucose level above 800 mg/dL and serum osmolality of at least 350 mOsm.

    c. Severe dehydration and electrolyte losses occur, and renal impairment results from decreased renal blood flow.

    d. Occurs almost predominantly in the elderly and almost exclusively in clients with Type II diabetes.

    e. Conditions such as silent myocardial infarction, sepsis, pancreatitis, and stroke and drugs such as glucocorticoids, diuretics, phenytoin sodium, propranolol, and calcium channel blockers may precipitate HHNS.

    f. Elderly clients are more at risk due to age-related changes in thirst perception, loss of taste bud, and poor urine-concentrating abilities that lead to dehydration.

3. *Hypoglycemia:*

    a. Neurogenic symptoms, which result from autonomic nervous system discharge triggered by hypoglycemia, including hunger, diaphoresis, weakness, and nervousness, occur when there is an *abrupt* decrease in the blood glucose level.

    b. Neuroglycopenic symptoms, which result directly from brain glucose deprivation, including headache, confusion, slurred speech, behavioral changes, and coma, occur with a more *gradual* decline in blood glucose level.

🎇 Considerations for Elderly Clients

1. Elderly clients with diabetes are at the greatest risk for dehydration and subsequent HHNC. The onset of HHNC is insidious, and elderly clients typically seek medical attention later and are sicker than younger clients.

2. The classic signs and symptoms of hypoglycemia may not appear in elderly diabetic clients; changes in levels of consciousness may be slow and progress through confusion and bizarre behavior. Coma may come without warning.

- Chronic complications of diabetes can be divided into macrovascular (large vessel) and microvascular (small vessel) problems:
    1. Macrovascular complications:
        a. Cardiovascular disease
        b. Peripheral vascular disease (often leading to amputation)
        c. Cerebrovascular disease
    2. Microvascular complications:
        a. Ocular complications (can lead to blindness): diabetic retinopathy, retinal detachment, macular degeneration, myopia, cataracts, glaucoma
        b. Diabetic neuropathy (damage to peripheral and autonomic nerves)
        c. Diabetic nephropathy (renal failure)

➤ Transcultural Considerations

1. High prevalence rates are found in U.S. African-American women and most U.S. Hispanic groups. Mexican-Americans have a prevalence of type II diabetes approximately 3 times higher than among non-Hispanic whites.
2. Diabetes is found in epidemic proportions in Native American populations; results of a recent study found diabetes rates in the Pima/Maricopa/Papago Indian community in Arizona of 65% for men and 72% for women.
3. In all populations, prevalence of diabetes rises with age.
4. There is a strong correlation between relative weight and the prevalence of type II diabetes.

5. Mexican-Americans, African-Americans, and Native Americans are at a higher risk of developing diabetic end-stage renal disease than are non-Hispanic whites.

COLLABORATIVE MANAGEMENT

Assessment

- The nurse records
  1. Occurrence of a recent illness or extreme stress
  2. Omission of insulin or oral medications if the client is a known diabetic
  3. Change in eating habits
  4. Change in exercise schedule or activity level
  5. Duration of polyuria, polydipsia, polyphagia, weight loss, and loss of energy
  6. History of or concurrent cardiovascular disease, such as dysrhythmias, congestive heart failure, hypertension, or cerebral vascular accident
- The nurse assesses the client for
  1. Elevated blood glucose level
     a. Serum glucose
     b. Oral glucose tolerance test
     c. Capillary blood glucose monitoring
     d. Glycosylated hemoglobin assays
     e. Glycosylated serum proteins and albumin
  2. Positive results for urinary ketones
  3. Abdominal pain, nausea, and vomiting (in DKA)
  4. Dehydration
  5. Numbness and tingling of the hands or feet
  6. Decreased reflexes
  7. Positional blood pressure changes
  8. Symptoms of delayed stomach emptying, such as nausea and distention
  9. Impotence in men
  10. Decreased, weak pulse rate
  11. Calf pain
  12. Visual disturbances
  13. Increased blood urea nitrogen (BUN) and creatinine levels

𝓔 Considerations for Elderly Clients

  1. The classic signs of polyuria and glucosuria may not be seen in the elderly.
  2. An estimated 80% of elderly diabetics are women.

3. Clinical manifestations of diabetes in the elderly include
   a. Fatigue
   b. Lethargy
   c. Recurrent infection
   d. Nocturia
   e. Nonspecific instability of balance
   f. Vulvovaginitis
   g. Pruritus
4. The first manifestation may be peripheral or autonomic neuropathy, renal dysfunction, or eye disorders.

Planning and Implementation

✦ **NDx:** Risk for Injury Related to Hyperglycemia

Nonsurgical Management

- Medication is indicated when a client with type II diabetes cannot achieve blood glucose control with dietary modification, regular exercise, and stress management.

   1. *Sulfonylurea* agents are appropriate only for clients with pancreatic beta cell function. Hypoglycemia is the most serious complication; other side effects include hematologic reactions, allergic skin reactions, and gastrointestinal effects.
   2. *Biguanides:* Metformin (Glucophage), the only biguanide available in the U.S., can cause lactic acidosis in clients with renal insufficiency.
   3. *Alpha-glucosidase inhibitors* such as acarbose (Precose) reduce postprandial hyperglycemia by slowing digestion and absorption of carbohydrate within the intestine. Side effects include abdominal discomfort related to undigested carbohydrate in the intestinal tract.
   4. *Insulin resistance inhibitor* such as troglitazone (Rezulin) lowers blood glucose by improving target cell response to insulin. Frequent side effects include infection, headache, pain, and reversible elevations of liver function tests.

- Insulin therapy is necessary for type I diabetes and moderate-to-severe type II diabetes.

   1. Insulin is available in rapid-, short-, intermediate-, and long-acting forms and may be injected separately or mixed in the same syringe.

2. The nurse teaches the client that insulin type and species, site of injection, and individual response can all affect absorption, onset, degree, and duration of insulin activity and reinforces that changing insulin may affect blood glucose control.
3. Insulin regimens include single daily injections, two-dose protocol, three-dose protocol, four-dose protocol, combination therapy, and intensified insulin regimens.
4. Complications of insulin therapy
   a. Hypoglycemia
   b. Hypertrophic lipodystrophy, a spongy swelling at or around injection sites
   c. Lipoatrophic lipodystrophy, a loss of fat at or distant to the injection site
   d. Dawn phenomenon, a fasting hyperglycemia thought to result from nocturnal release of growth hormone secretion that may cause blood glucose elevations about 5 to 6 AM and is treated by providing more insulin for the overnight period
   e. Somogyi's phenomenon, a morning hyperglycemia due to effective counter-regulatory response to nighttime hypoglycemia, is treated by ensuring adequate dietary intake at bedtime and evaluation of insulin dose and exercise programs
5. Insulin may be administered by
   a. Subcutaneous injection
   b. Continuous subcutaneous infusion of insulin administered by an externally worn pump containing a syringe and reservoir with regular insulin connected to the client by an infusion set
   c. Closed-loop insulin delivery accomplished by the use of an "artificial pancreas" and may be used during surgery, labor and delivery, and dialysis procedures
   d. Implanted insulin pumps implanted into the peritoneal cavity where insulin can be absorbed in a more physiologic manner
   e. Injection devices, whereby the needle is replaced by an ultrathin liquid stream of insulin forced through the skin under high pressure
   f. New technologies include nasal spray administered via nebulizer

- The nurse
    1. Teaches the client about storage, dose preparation, injection procedures, and complications associated with drug therapy
    2. Collaborates with the client, physician, and dietitian to formulate an individualized meal plan for the client
    3. Suggests artificial sweeteners such as saccharin, aspartame, and acesulfame K instead of sugar to enhance dietary compliance
    4. Teaches the client that alcohol should be taken in moderation only if diabetes is well controlled
    5. Explains and reinforces the use of the exchange system in meal planning

---

🖎 Considerations for Elderly Clients

1. A realistic approach to diet therapy is essential for elderly diabetic clients.
2. Attempts to change long-time eating habits may be difficult.
3. Clients who live alone, do their own food preparation, and have physical limitations may have difficulty following the diet recommended by the American Diabetes Association; socioeconomic factors may also affect clients' ability to prepare the proper foods.

- Regular physical exercise is a recommended component of a comprehensive diabetes treatment plan.
- The nurse
    1. Collaborates with the client and rehabilitation specialist to develop an exercise program
    2. Instructs the client to have a complete physical examination before starting an exercise program at home
    3. Instructs the client to wear proper footwear with good traction and cushioning and to examine the feet after exercise
    4. Teaches the client about the risks and complications related to exercise such as prolonged alterations in blood glucose levels, vitreous hemorrhage, or retinal detachment in clients with proliferative retinopathy; increased proteinuria, foot and joint injury in clients with peripheral neuropathy

Surgical Management

1. Pancreas transplant
   a. Whole pancreas transplantation can be performed in one of three situations: pancreas transplant alone in the pre-uremic client, pancreas transplant after successful kidney transplantation, and simultaneous pancreas-kidney transplant
   b. Immunosuppressive therapy is given to prevent rejection of the transplanted pancreas
   c. Complications include venous thrombosis, rejection, and infection
2. Islet cell transplantation has been limited by the technical inability to obtain a sufficient number of islet cells

✦ **NDx:** Risk for Injury (stresses of the surgical experience)

- Surgery is a physical and emotional stressor, making the diabetic client more at risk for intraoperative and postoperative complications.
- The nurse provides preoperative care:
  1. Tells the client, as ordered, to discontinue intake of
     a. Chlorpropamide (Diabinese) 36 hours before surgery
     b. Metformin (Glucophage) 48 hours before surgery
     c. All other oral agents on the day of surgery
  2. Oral agents are restarted only after renal function has been reevaluated and found to be normal
  3. Starts intravenous fluids, as ordered, to maintain hydration
  4. Monitors blood glucose results and administers insulin, as ordered
- Intraoperative IV administration of short-acting insulin in 5% to 10% glucose is recommended for all insulin-treated clients, as well as for drug-treated or diet-treated clients who are undergoing general anesthesia and whose diabetes is poorly controlled.
- The nurse provides postoperative care:
  1. Continues glucose and insulin infusions until the client is stable and able to tolerate oral feedings
  2. Administers short-acting insulin, as ordered, until the client's usual medication regimen can be restarted
  3. Monitors for postoperative complications, including

a. Hyperkalemia
b. Hypoglycemia (may be asymptomatic if the client is well controlled on beta blockers)
c. Impaired wound healing or wound infection
d. Myocardial infarction
e. Renal dysfunction
f. Uncontrolled blood glucose

✦ **NDx:** Risk for Injury Related to Sensory Alterations

- Nonhealing foot wounds cause more inpatient hospital days than any other complication of diabetes.
- Diabetes is associated with more than 51% of the nontraumatic lower limb amputations performed in the United States.
- The nurse
    1. Teaches preventive foot care to the client
        a. Sensory neuropathy, ischemia, and infection are the leading causes of foot disease
    2. Recommends that the client have shoes fitted by an experienced shoe fitter such as a certified podiatrist
        a. Instructs the client to change shoes at midday and in the evening and to wear socks or stockings with shoes
    3. Instructs the client how to care for wounds
    4. Refers the client to a specialist for orthotic devices to eliminate pressure on infected or open wounds of the foot
- Topical application of platelet-derived growth factors may be used to accelerate tissue healing for long-standing foot ulcers.

✦ **NDx:** Risk for Injury Related to Visual Sensory/ Perceptual Alterations

- The nurse
    1. Encourages all clients to have a baseline ophthalmic examination and yearly follow-up examinations
    2. Advises the client to seek a retinal specialist if problems are present
    3. Collaborates with the rehabilitation specialist to recommend strategies to improve the client's visual abilities such as improved lighting, placing dark equipment against a white background, coding objects such as insulin vials with bright colors

or felt tip markers, and large-type books, newspapers, etc.
- Various stages of diabetic retinopathy can be treated with laser therapy or vitrectomy.

✦ NDx: Pain

- The nurse
  1. Administers antidepressants, particularly amitriptyline (Elavil, Levate✦), as ordered, to alleviate peripheral neuropathic pain
  2. Administers 0.075% capsaicin cream (e.g., Zostrix) topically to relieve neuropathic pain, as ordered
  3. Uses other non–drug pain management techniques, as appropriate

✦ NDx: Altered (Renal) Tissue Perfusion

- The nurse
  1. Stresses to the client the importance of maintaining normal blood glucose and blood pressure levels below 130/85 mmHg, and the importance of yearly screening for microalbuminuria
  2. Limits protein and phosphorus, in collaboration with the dietitian, to reduce the progression of renal impairment
  3. Teaches the client about the signs and symptoms of urinary tract infection
  4. Adjusts insulin dosages, as indicated, for clients undergoing dialysis

✦ NDx: Potential Complication: Hypoglycemia

- The nurse
  1. Monitors glucose levels before administering hypoglycemic agents, before meals, at bedtime, and when the client is symptomatic
- Treatment of the client with mild (hungry, irritable, shaky, weak, headache, fully conscious, blood glucose less than 60 mg/dL [3.4 mmol/L]) hypoglycemia who is able to swallow includes one of the following
  1. 2–3 glucose tablets
  2. 4 oz. cup of orange or grape juice
  3. 6 oz. cup of regular soft drink
  4. 8 oz of skim milk
  5. 6 saltines or 3 graham crackers
  6. 6–80 hard candies or 4 cubes of sugar or 2 tsp. of sugar

- Blood glucose should be tested after 15 minutes.
- Treatment of moderate hypoglycemia (cold and clammy skin, pale rapid pulse, rapid shallow respirations, marked changes in mood drowsiness, blood glucose less than 40 mg/dL [2.2 mmol/L]) consists of 15–30 g of rapidly absorbed carbohydrates and taking additional food, such as low fat milk or cheese after 10–15 minutes.
- Severe hypoglycemia (unable to swallow, unconscious or convulsion, blood glucose usually less than 20 mg/dL [1.0 mmol/L]) is treated with glucagon subcutaneously or intramuscularly and 50% dextrose intravenously.
- The nurse
  1. Teaches the client how to prevent the four common causes of hypoglycemia associated with excess insulin, deficient food intake, exercise, and alcohol intake
  2. Encourages the client to wear an identification (Medic-Alert) bracelet

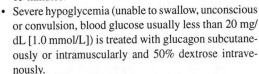

✦ NDx: Potential Complication: Ketoacidosis

- The nurse
  1. Monitors for signs and symptoms of diabetic ketoacidosis (DKA)
  2. Checks the client's blood pressure, pulse, and respirations every 15 minutes until stable
  3. Records urine output, temperature, and mental status every hour
  4. Assesses the client's level of consciousness, hydration status, fluid and electrolyte balance, blood glucose levels every hour until stable then every 4 hours
  5. Gives insulin bolus as indicated followed by a continuous drip
  6. Monitors the client for hypokalemia: muscle weakness, abdominal distention or paralytic ileus, hypotension and weak pulse; prior to administration of potassium ensures that the client's urinary output is at least 30 mL/hour
  7. Instruct the client how to prevent future episodes of DKA by contacting the primary health care provider when the blood glucose is greater than 250 mg/dL, ketonuria is present for more than 24 hours, when unable to take food or fluids, and when illness persists for more than 1–2 days

275

✦ **NDx:** Potential Complication: Hyperglycemic Hyperosmolar Nonketotic Syndrome (HHNS)

- The nurse
  1. Administers IV fluids and insulin as indicated and monitors the client and assesses the client's response to therapy

Continuing Care

- The nurse
  1. In collaboration with the dietitian teaches the client basic survival skills associated with medication, diet, exercise, and complications
  2. Assists the client in purchasing the items needed for the administration of insulin and for glucose monitoring
  3. Provides information about community resources
  4. Teaches the client how to monitor blood sugar level
  5. Teaches the client how to administer medication and prevent hypoglycemia
  6. Helps the client adapt to diabetes, including teaching stress management techniques and identifying coping mechanisms
  7. Refers the client to the American Diabetes Association and its resources
  8. Refers the client to a diabetic educator for the necessary education

DISCOID LUPUS ERYTHEMATOSUS

See Lupus Erythematosus.

DISLOCATION AND SUBLUXATION

- *Dislocation* of a joint occurs when the articulating surfaces are no longer in proximity; a *subluxation* is a partial dislocation.
- These injuries are most often caused by trauma but can be congenital or pathologic, resulting from joint disease such as rheumatoid arthritis.
- Pain, immobility, alteration in the contour of the joint, and rotation and shortening of the extremity are typical manifestations.
- The treatment is a closed manipulation, or reduction, of the joint while the client is anesthetized.
- After reduction, the joint is immobilized by a cast or bandage until healing occurs.
- Clients with recurrent dislocations may require surgical intervention with internal fixation.

DISPLACEMENT, UTERINE

- Uterine displacement is a variation in normal uterine placement resulting from congenital or acquired weakness of pelvic support structures.
- The most common variation is posterior displacement of the uterus, or retroversion, in which the uterus is tilted posteriorly and the cervix rotates anteriorly.
- Other variations include retroflexion, anteversion, and anteflexion.
- Uterine displacement may result in prolapse of the uterus into the vagina.
- Physical findings include
    1. No symptoms
    2. History of backaches
    3. Secondary amenorrhea
    4. Infertility
    5. Dyspareunia (painful intercourse)
    6. Pelvic pressure or heaviness

- Interventions are based on the severity of symptoms and include
  1. Knee-chest positioning
  2. Insertion of a vaginal pessary (a device placed in the vagina to hold the uterus in the correct position)

Dissection, Aortic

OVERVIEW

- Aortic dissection, traditionally referred to as a *dissecting aneurysm,* may be caused by a sudden tear in the aortic intima, opening the way for blood to enter the aortic wall.
- Degeneration of the aortic media and hypertension are contributing factors.
- Aortic dissection is frequently associated with aging and connective tissue disorders, such as Marfan's syndrome.
- Three classes of aortic dissection include
  1. Type I: an intimal tear originates in the ascending (proximal) aorta, with extension into the descending (distal) aorta
  2. Type II: originates in and is limited to the ascending aorta
  3. Type III: arises within the descending thoracic aorta and often progresses distally

COLLABORATIVE MANAGEMENT

Assessment

- The nurse assesses for
  1. Pain that is described as "tearing" or "stabbing" and is located in the anterior chest, back, neck, throat, jaw, or teeth
  2. Diaphoresis
  3. Nausea and vomiting
  4. Faintness and apprehension
  5. Elevated blood pressure
  6. Decreased or absent peripheral pulses
  7. Musical murmur, heard best along the right sternal border

8. Neurologic deficits, such as altered level of consciousness, paraparesis, or cerebral vascular accident

Interventions

- The goals of emergency treatment include the elimination of pain, the reduction of blood pressure, and a decrease in the velocity of left ventricular ejection.
- The nurse
  1. Administers continuous intravenous sodium nitroprusside (Nipride) or trimethaphan (Arfonad), as ordered, to lower blood pressure
  2. Administers intravenous push propranolol (Inderal, Apo-Propranolol◆), as ordered, to decrease left ventricular ejection
- Subsequent treatment is based on the location of the dissection; surgical excision and graft replacement may be necessary.

DIVERTICULA, ESOPHAGEAL

OVERVIEW

- Diverticula are outpouchings anywhere in the esophagus that result in a blind pouch in which ingested foods and liquids are trapped, often to be regurgitated later.
- Clients with esophageal diverticula are at risk for esophageal perforation.

🕲 Considerations for Elderly Clients

The most common form of diverticulum is *Zenker's diverticulum,* which is usually located near the hypopharynx and occurs most often in older adults.

COLLABORATIVE MANAGEMENT
Assessment

- The nurse assesses the client for
  1. Dysphagia
  2. Regurgitation
  3. Feelings of fullness or pressure

4. Halitosis
5. Nocturnal cough
6. Sour taste in the mouth
7. Results of barium swallow

Interventions

- Diet therapy and positioning are the primary interventions for controlling symptoms related to diverticula.
- The nurse
  1. Collaborates with the dietitian to determine the size and frequency of meals as well as the texture and consistency that can best be tolerated by the client
  2. Elevates the head of the bed for sleep
  3. Teaches the client to avoid the recumbent position and vigorous exercising for at least 2 hours after eating
  4. Teaches the client to avoid restrictive clothing and frequent stooping or bending
- Surgical management is aimed at excision of the diverticula.
- The nurse provides postoperative care:
  1. Maintains the client on nothing-by-mouth (NPO) status for several days to promote healing
  2. Does not irrigate the nasogastric tube used for decompression unless specifically ordered by the physician
  3. Maintains hydration and nutrition status through intravenous fluids and tube feedings until oral intake is permitted
  4. Manages the client's postoperative pain
  5. Monitors for bleeding and perforation
  6. Teaches the client to observe for complications at home
  7. Teaches the client the measures that are not conducive to reflux (elevated head of bed, avoidance of recumbent position)

DIVERTICULAR DISEASE

OVERVIEW

- Diverticular disease includes diverticulosis and diverticulitis.
    1. *Diverticulosis* is the presence of several abnormal outpouchings or herniations in the wall of the intestine. These outpouchings, known as diverticula, are caused by significantly high pressures in the lumen of the intestines. They can occur in any part of the intestine but are most common in the sigmoid colon.
    2. *Diverticulitis,* or inflammation of one or more diverticula, results when the diverticulum retains undigested food, which compromises the blood supply to that area and facilitates bacterial invasion of the diverticular sac, which may then perforate. A perforated diverticulum can progress to intra-abdominal perforation with generalized peritonitis.

COLLABORATIVE MANAGEMENT

Assessment

- The nurse records the client's
    1. Report of changes in bowel function, including constipation, diarrhea, and the presence of blood in the stool (diverticulitis)
    2. Recent dietary intake of high-fiber foods, indigestible roughage, or seeds
    3. Known history of diverticulosis
- The nurse assesses for clinical manifestations of diverticulitis:
    1. Abrupt onset of left lower quadrant abdominal pain, which increases with coughing, straining, or lifting, and which may be intermittent
    2. Generalized abdominal pain (peritonitis)
    3. Temperature elevation with tachycardia
    4. Nausea and vomiting
    5. Abdominal distention and tenderness
    6. Palpable, tender abdominal or rectal mass
    7. Blood in the stool (microscopic to larger amounts)
    8. Elevated white blood cell (WBC) count

9. Presence of diverticula on barium enema or upper gastrointestinal tract series (diverticulosis)

Interventions

- Bed rest is recommended in the acute phase of the disease.
- The nurse
    1. Teaches the client to refrain from lifting, straining, coughing, or bending to avoid increased intra-abdominal pressure
    2. Provides clear liquids during the acute phase of the disease
    3. Instructs the client that he or she will be restricted to nothing-by-mouth (NPO) status when experiencing severe symptoms and will receive intravenous fluids; a nasogastric tube is inserted for severe nausea, vomiting, or abdominal distention
    4. Introduces a fiber-containing diet gradually when the inflammation is resolved
    5. Administers oral broad-spectrum antibiotics, as ordered
    6. Administers intravenous antibiotics, as ordered, for severe diverticulitis
    7. Administers pain medication—mild non-opioid drugs, as ordered, for mild cases and opioids for severe cases
    8. Avoids administering laxatives
    9. Administers anticholinergics, as ordered, to reduce intestinal motility

Surgical Management

- Clients with diverticulitis need surgery if one of the following occurs:
    1. Rupture of the diverticulum with subsequent peritonitis
    2. Pelvic abscess
    3. Bowel obstruction
    4. Fistula
    5. Presence of a mass or suspected tumor
    6. Uncontrolled bleeding
- Surgical management includes a colon resection with an end-to-end anastomosis or temporary or permanent colostomy.
- The nurse provides preoperative care:
    1. Reinforces physician teaching about the possible need for a temporary or permanent colostomy

2. Teaches the importance of or provides bowel preparation, consisting of enemas and laxatives (for the client who is *not* in the acute stage of diverticulitis)
3. Administers intravenous fluids, antibiotics, and anti-inflammatory agents, as ordered
4. Maintains NPO status with a nasogastric tube in place for clients having emergency surgery

D

- The nurse provides postoperative care:
  1. Maintains drainage system at the abdominal incision site
  2. Monitors colostomy stoma for color and integrity, if a colostomy was created
  3. Maintains the nasogastric tube for several days until peristalsis returns
  4. Introduces clear liquids slowly, per physician's order
  5. Gives the client an opportunity to express feelings about the colostomy
  6. Provides additional postoperative care as described in Cancer, Colorectal, "Surgical Management"

- The nurse provides written postoperative instructions:
  1. Inspection of the incision for redness, tenderness, swelling, and drainage
  2. Dressing change procedures, if necessary
  3. Avoidance of activities that increase intra-abdominal pressure, including straining at stool, bending, lifting heavy objects, and wearing restrictive clothing
  4. Pain management, including prescriptions

- The nurse teaches the client and family
  1. Signs and symptoms of diverticular disease, including fever, abdominal pain, and bloody stools
  2. To avoid enemas and laxatives other than bulk-forming ones such as psyllium hydrophilic mucilloid (Metamucil)
  3. To follow dietary considerations for diverticulosis:
     a. Eat a diet high in cellulose and hemicellulose, which is found in wheat bran, whole grain breads, and cereals
     b. Eat fruits and vegetables with high-fiber content (unless *diverticulitis* occurs)
     c. Avoid foods containing indigestible roughage or seeds

283

d. Avoid alcohol, which has an irritant effect on the bowel
e. Avoid gas-forming and hot and cold liquids
f. Follow a prescribed weight-reduction plan, if necessary, in collaboration with a dietitian

DIVERTICULITIS

See Diverticular Disease.

DIVERTICULOSIS

See Diverticular Disease.

DJD

See Joint Disease, Degenerative.

DLE

See Lupus Erythematosus.

DUB

See Bleeding, Dysfunctional Uterine.

DUCTAL ECTASIA

See Ectasia, Ductal.

DYSFUNCTIONAL UTERINE BLEEDING

See Bleeding, Dysfunctional Uterine.

DYSTROPHY, CORNEAL

See Corneal Disorders.

DYSTROPHY, MUSCULAR

- Five types of muscular dystrophy are seen in adults:
  1. *Duchenne:*
     a. Sex-linked recessive variety seen only in males
     b. Manifested by symmetric pelvic and shoulder girdle weakness, waddling gait, cardiac involvement, and possible mental retardation
     c. Death from respiratory or cardiac failure usually occurring between ages 10 and 30
  2. *Becker:*
     a. Sex-linked recessive variety also seen exclusively in males
     b. Manifested by wasting of pelvic and shoulder muscles and normal cardiac and mental function; slowly progressive; inability to walk seen 25 years after onset

  c. Normal life span
 3. *Limb-girdle:*
  a. Usually autosomal dominant and seen in either sex
  b. Manifested by upper-extremity and neck muscle weakness and lower-extremity and hip muscle weakness; severe disability within 10 to 20 years
  c. Life span shortened by 10 to 20 years
 4. *Facioscapulohumeral or Landouzy-Dejerine:*
  a. Autosomal dominant and seen in either sex
  b. Manifested by facial and shoulder girdle muscle involvement
  c. Normal life span
 5. *Myotonic:*
  a. Autosomal dominant and seen in either sex
  b. Manifested by muscle atrophy with multiple organ involvement (heart, lungs, smooth muscles, and endocrine system)
  c. Gradual progression if onset in adulthood

- Management and nursing care is supportive. (Also see Rehabilitation, p. 21.)
- An experimental treatment called myoblast transfer therapy (MTT) is being studied and supported by the FDA. It involves injections of healthy muscle cells (myoblasts) taken from a donor and multiplied in a laboratory. The cells are then given to the client with MD where they theoretically fuse with each other and the recipient's unhealthy muscle cells.

EAR INFECTIONS

See Otitis Media.

ECTASIA, DUCTAL

- Ductal ectasia is a benign breast problem in women approaching menopause, caused by dilation and thickening of collecting ducts in the subareolar area.

- The ducts become distended and filled with cellular debris, which initiates an inflammatory response.
- Clinical signs are a hard, tender mass with irregular borders; greenish-brown nipple discharge; enlarged axillary nodes; redness; and edema over the mass.
- Microscopic examination of nipple discharge is performed for atypical or malignant cells.
- The affected area may be excised.
- The nurse
  1. Alleviates anxiety associated with the threat of breast cancer
  2. Supports the client during diagnostic and treatment procedures

Embolism, Pulmonary

OVERVIEW

- Pulmonary embolism occurs when a thrombus that forms in a deep vein detaches and travels to the right side of the heart and then lodges in a branch of the pulmonary artery.
- Physiologic responses include platelet accumulation, triggering the release of potent vasoconstrictors and causing widespread pulmonary vasoconstriction, which impairs ventilation and perfusion.
- Clients prone to pulmonary embolism are those with risk factors for deep venous thrombosis (DVT), including prolonged immobilization, surgery, obesity, pregnancy, congestive heart failure, advanced age, and a history of thromboembolism.

COLLABORATIVE MANAGEMENT

- Nursing interventions are aimed at preventing venous stasis and include range-of-motion exercises, early ambulation, antiembolism or pneumatic compression stockings, and preventing pressure under the popliteal space.

- Subcutaneous heparin injections are given to prevent hypercoagulability.
- The nurse assesses for
  1. Dyspnea accompanied by tachypnea and pleuritic pain exacerbated by inspiration
  2. Dry cough
  3. Blood-tinged sputum
  4. Apprehension; feeling of impending doom
  5. Tachycardia
  6. Crackles
  7. Pleural friction rub
  8. Low-grade fever
  9. Distended neck veins
  10. Cyanosis
  11. S_3 or S_4 heart sound
  12. Positive Homans' sign
  13. Low arterial PCO_2 value
  14. Syncope
  15. Petechiae over chest and axillae
- Interventions include
  1. Oxygen and pulse oximetry
  2. Intubation and mechanical ventilation for severe hypoxemia
  3. Anticoagulation with intravenous heparin (bolus followed by continuous infusion) during the acute phase; warfarin (Coumadin) orally when the heparin drip is discontinued, with prothrombin time and partial thromboplastin time monitored closely
  4. Close monitoring to protect the client from situations that could lead to bleeding
  5. Surgical embolectomy
  6. Insertion of an umbrella filter

EMPYEMA, PULMONARY

OVERVIEW

- Pulmonary empyema is a collection of pus in the pleural space; the fluid is thick, opaque, and foul smelling.

- The most common cause is pulmonary infection, infected pleural effusion or lung abscess, which spreads across the pleura or obstructs lymph nodes and causes a retrograde flood of infected lymph into the pleural space.
- Thoracic surgery and chest trauma are common predisposing conditions in which bacteria are introduced directly into the pleural space.

COLLABORATIVE MANAGEMENT

- Findings on client history include recent febrile illnesses, chest pain, dyspnea, cough, and trauma.
- Physical assessment includes diminished chest wall movement on the affected side, decreased breath sounds, decreased or absent fremitus, a flat percussion note, fever, chills, weight loss, and night sweats.
- Chest x-ray and examination of the pleural fluid by thoracentesis are usually performed to help make the diagnosis.
- Therapy is based on emptying the empyema cavity, re-expanding the lung, and controlling the infection.
- Chest tubes are placed in the inferior parts of the empyema sac to promote drainage and lung expansion, and antibiotics are given.
- An open thoracotomy and lung decortication may be performed for thick pus and marked pleural thickening.

Encephalitis

OVERVIEW

- Encephalitis, an inflammation of the brain parenchyma (brain tissue) and often the meninges, is most often caused by viral agents:
    1. Arboviruses transmitted through the bite of an infected tick or mosquito
    2. Enteroviruses associated with mumps and chickenpox
    3. Herpes simplex virus type I
- Amebas such as *Naegleria* and *Acanthamoeba,* found in warm freshwater, may also be involved.

COLLABORATIVE MANAGEMENT
Assessment

- The nurse assesses the client for
    1. Fever
    2. Nausea and vomiting
    3. Stiff neck
    4. Decreased level of consciousness and mental status
    5. Motor dysfunction
    6. Focal neurologic deficits
    7. Symptoms of increased intracranial pressure
    8. Ocular palsies
    9. Facial weakness
    10. Cerebrospinal fluid analysis
        a. Cell count
        b. Culture
        c. Protein
        d. Glucose
    11. Elevated white blood cell (WBC) count

Interventions

- The treatment for encephalitis is similar to that for meningitis.
- The nurse
    1. Maintains a patent airway
    2. Encourages and assists the client to turn, cough, and deep breathe every 2 hours
    3. Checks vital signs and neurologic signs at least every 2 hours
    4. Elevates the head of the bed 30 to 45 degrees
    5. Administers acyclovir (Zovirax) for herpes encephalitis, as ordered
- Because of permanent neurologic disabilities, the client is usually discharged to a rehabilitation setting or a long-term-care facility.

ENDOCARDITIS, BACTERIAL

See Endocarditis, Infective.

ENDOCARDITIS, INFECTIVE

OVERVIEW

- Infective endocarditis (previously called bacterial endocarditis) is a microbial infection involving the endocardial surface of the heart, including the valves.
- Vegetative lesions form on the endocardium and cardiac valves.
- Infective endocarditis occurs primarily in clients who are intravenous (IV) drug abusers, clients who have had cardiac valve replacements, and clients who have mitral valve prolapse or other structural defects.
- Portals of entry for infecting organisms include
  1. Oral cavity especially if dental procedures have been performed
  2. Skin rashes, lesions, or abscesses
  3. Infections (cutaneous, genitourinary, or gastrointestinal)
  4. Surgery or invasive procedures, including IV line placement

COLLABORATIVE MANAGEMENT

Assessment

- The nurse assesses for
  1. Signs of infection, including high fever, chills, malaise, night sweats, and fatigue
  2. Heart murmurs, usually regurgitant in nature
  3. Right-sided heart failure, evidenced by
     a. Peripheral edema
     b. Weight gain
     c. Anorexia
  4. Left-sided heart failure, evidenced by
     a. Fatigue
     b. Shortness of breath
     c. Crackles
  5. Evidence of arterial embolization, fragments of vegetation, may travel to the spleen, kidneys, gastrointestinal tract, brain, pulmonary circulation, or extremities
  6. Petechiae of the neck, shoulders, wrists, ankles, mucous membranes, or conjunctivae

7. Splinter hemorrhages
8. Osler's nodes (reddish tender lesions with a white center on the pads of the fingers, hands, and toes)
9. Janeway's lesions (nontender hemorrhagic lesions found on the fingers, toes, nose, and earlobes)
10. Splenomegaly and clubbing of the fingers in clients who have had the disease longer than 6 weeks
11. Positive blood culture
12. Low hemoglobin and hematocrit levels

Interventions

- The nurse
  1. Administers IV antibiotic therapy, as ordered
  2. Monitors the client's tolerance to activity
  3. Applies antiembolism stockings
  4. Monitors for signs of embolization, including rapid pulse, dyspnea, new heart murmurs, and signs of heart failure
- Surgical intervention includes removal of the infected valve, removal of congenital shunts, repair of injured valves and chordae tendineae, and abscess drainage.
- Preoperative and postoperative care for the client having surgery involving the valves is similar to that described for clients undergoing a coronary artery bypass grafting or valve replacement (see Coronary Artery Disease).

Continuing Care

- The nurse teaches the client and family
  1. Information on the cause of the disease and its course, medication regimens, practices that help avoid future infections, and signs and symptoms of infection
  2. How to administer IV antibiotic and care for the IV site and ensures that all supplies are available to the client discharged to home
  3. The importance of good personal and oral hygiene such as the use of a soft toothbrush and avoid using irrigation devices and dental floss
  4. The necessity to inform health care providers and dentists of the history of endocarditis, so prophylactic antibiotics are given before treatment

ENDOMETRIAL CANCER

See Cancer, Endometrial.

ENDOMETRIOSIS

OVERVIEW

- Endometriosis is a benign disease of unknown cause characterized by implantation of endometrial tissue outside the uterine cavity.
- The tissue responds to hormonal stimulation and goes through the same cyclic changes.
- Bleeding occurs at the site of implantation, and the blood is trapped in the tissues, causing scarring and adhesions.

COLLABORATIVE MANAGEMENT

Assessment

- The nurse assesses for
    1. Menstrual history
    2. Sexual history
    3. Characteristics of bleeding
    4. Lower abdominal pain occurring before the menstrual flow (the most common symptom)
    5. Rectal pressure
    6. Dyspareunia (painful intercourse)
    7. Painful defecation
    8. Sacral backache
    9. Hypermenorrhea
    10. Infertility

Interventions

- The nurse
    1. Administers mild analgesics or prostaglandin synthetase inhibitors for pain relief, as ordered
    2. Administers hormonal therapy, as ordered:

    a. Pseudopregnancy induced with oral contraceptives and progesterone ingestion

    b. Pseudomenopause or ovarian suppression induced by using danazol (Danocrine, Cyclomen◆), an antigonadotropin testosterone derivative

    c. Reversible medical oophorectomy caused by gonadotropin-releasing hormone (GnRH) agonists

  3. Applies a heating pad to the abdomen or sacrum

  4. Teaches relaxation techniques, yoga, or biofeedback

- Surgical management by removing endometrial implants and adhesions with carbon dioxide laser or hysterectomy may be required.

ENTERITIS, REGIONAL

See Crohn's Disease.

EPIDIDYMITIS

OVERVIEW

- Epididymitis is an infection of the epididymis, which may result from infection of the prostate.
- It occurs as a complication of long-term indwelling catheters, prostatic surgery, and, occasionally, cystoscopic examination.
- *Chlamydia trachomatis* is the major cause of epididymitis in men under the age of 35.

COLLABORATIVE MANAGEMENT

- The nurse assesses for
  1. Pain along the inguinal canal and the vas deferens, leading to pain and swelling in the scrotum and groin
  2. Elevated temperature

3. Pyuria
4. Bacteriuria
5. Chills
- Treatment interventions include
    1. Bed rest with scrotal elevation
    2. Antibiotics
    3. Sexual partner treatment if chlamydial or gonor-rheal in origin
    4. Comfort measures, including ice packs and sitz baths
    5. Orchiectomy (removal of testicle) if abscess develops
    6. Epididymectomy (removal of epididymis from testicle) if condition is recurrent or chronically painful

EPILEPSY

See Seizures.

EPITHELIAL OVARIAN TUMORS

See Tumors, Epithelial Ovarian.

ESOPHAGEAL CANCER

See Tumors, Esophageal.

ESOPHAGEAL DIVERTICULA

See Diverticula, Esophageal.

ESOPHAGEAL TRAUMA

See Trauma, Esophageal.

ESOPHAGEAL TUMORS

See Tumors, Esophageal.

EYE LACERATIONS

See Lacerations, Eye.

FACIAL PARALYSIS

See Paralysis, Facial.

FACIAL TRAUMA

See Trauma, Facial.

FARSIGHTEDNESS

See Refractive Errors.

FATTY LIVER

See Liver, Fatty.

F

FBD

See Breast Disease, Fibrocystic.

FIBROADENOMA, BREAST

- A breast fibroadenoma is the most common breast lump that occurs during the teenage years, although it may occur into the 30s.
- The fibroadenoma is a solid, benign mass of connective tissue unattached to the surrounding breast tissue.
- The lump is characteristically firm, hard but not cystic, easily movable, and clearly delineated from surrounding tissue; it is usually located in the upper outer quadrant of the breast.
- A needle aspiration is performed to establish whether the lump is cystic or solid.
- Solid lumps are usually excised on an outpatient basis by local anesthesia.

Transcultural Considerations

Fibroadenomas are most common in African-American women.

FIBROCYSTIC BREAST DISEASE

See Breast Disease, Fibrocystic.

FIBROMA, OVARIAN

- Ovarian fibromas are the most common benign, solid ovarian neoplasms.
- The fibromas appear as pearly-white tumors of connective tissue origin with low malignancy potential.
- Fibromas range from small nodules to masses weighing more than 50 pounds; the average size is 6 cm.
- The fibromas tend to have a unilateral occurrence and on examination present with slightly irregular contour and are mobile.
- Fibromas larger than 6 cm may be associated with ascites and may cause feelings of pelvic pressure or abdominal enlargement.
- Fibromas often occur after menopause.
- Management is surgical removal of the tumor; oophorectomy (removal of an ovary) may be performed.

FISSURE, ANAL

OVERVIEW

- An anal fissure, or fissure in ano, is an elongated ulcerated laceration between the anal canal and perianal skin.
- Fissures can be primary or secondary, acute or chronic:
    1. *Primary* fissures are idiopathic, with no known cause for their occurrence.

2. *Secondary* fissures are associated with another disorder, such as Crohn's disease, tuberculosis, or perineal trauma, including childbirth. Constipation, diarrhea, and spasm of the anal sphincter are also causes of fissures.

COLLABORATIVE MANAGEMENT

- *Acute* anal fissures are superficial and heal spontaneously with conservative treatment. *Chronic* fissures recur and often warrant surgery.
- Pain during and after defecation is the most common symptom, but bleeding may also occur.
- Diagnosis is made by physical examination.
- Nonsurgical interventions include local, symptomatic relief measures, such as sitz baths, analgesics, and bulk-forming agents.

F

FISTULA, ANAL

- An anal fistula, or fistula in ano, is an abnormal, tract-like communication between the anal canal and the skin outside the anus.
- Most anal fistulas result from anorectal abscesses, but they can be associated with tuberculosis, Crohn's disease, and cancer.
- Symptoms include pruritus, purulent discharge, and tenderness or pain aggravated by bowel movements.
- Because fistulas do not heal spontaneously, surgery (fistulotomy) is necessary.
- Pain relief measures, such as sitz baths, analgesics, and stool softeners, are used to reduce tissue trauma and discomfort.

FISSURE IN ANO

See Fissure, Anal.

FISTULA IN ANO

See Fistula, Anal.

FLAIL CHEST

OVERVIEW

- Flail chest is associated with high-speed motor vehicle accidents; it is associated with a high mortality rate (40%), and is one of the most critical chest injuries.

𝓔 Considerations for Elderly Clients

Flail chest is most common in older clients because their declining agility, vision loss, decreased reaction time and loss of proprioception predisposes them to falls and vehicular accidents.

- Blunt chest trauma results in hemothorax and rib fractures, causing a loose segment of the chest wall to become paradoxical to the expansion and contraction of the rest of the chest wall.
- Paradoxical respiration is the inward movement of the thorax during inspiration with outward movement during expiration; gas exchange and secretion removal are impaired.

COLLABORATIVE MANAGEMENT

- The chest is assessed for paradoxical chest movement, dyspnea, cyanosis, tachycardia, hypotension, pain, and anxiety.
- Interventions include
  1. Humidified oxygen
  2. Pain management
  3. Promotion of lung expansions through deep breathing and positioning
  4. Coughing and tracheal aspiration

300

5. Psychosocial support
6. Intubation with mechanical ventilation with positive end-expiratory pressure for severe flail chest associated with respiratory failure and shock
- The nurse monitors the client's
  1. Arterial blood gases
  2. Vital signs
  3. Fluid and electrolyte balance
  4. Central venous pressure

F

FLU

See Influenza.

FOLIC ACID DEFICIENCY ANEMIA

See Anemia, Folic Acid Deficiency.

FOLLICULAR CYSTS

See Cysts, Ovarian.

FOLLICULITIS

See Infections, Skin.

FOOD POISONING

- Food poisoning is caused by ingestion of infectious organisms in food.
- There are three common types of food poisoning:
  1. *Staphylococcal* food poisoning:
     a. *Staphylococcus* grows in meats and dairy products and can be transmitted by human carriers.
     b. Symptoms of staphylococcal infection include abrupt onset of vomiting, diarrhea, and abdominal cramping, usually 2 to 4 hours after the ingestion of contaminated food.
     c. The diagnosis is made when stool culture yields 100,000 enterotoxin-producing staphylococci.
     d. Treatment includes oral or intravenous (IV) fluids
  2. *Escherichia coli* infection:
     a. Increasingly, *E. coli* is not associated with food poisoning.
     b. Symptoms include vomiting, diarrhea, abdominal cramping, and fever.
     c. Treatment includes IV fluids and antibiotic therapy.
  3. *Botulism:*
     a. Botulism is a severe, life-threatening food poisoning associated with a high mortality rate, most commonly acquired from improperly processed canned foods.
     b. *Clostridium botulinum* enters the bloodstream from the intestines and causes symptoms of diplopia, dysphagia, dysphonia, respiratory muscle paralysis, nausea, vomiting, and diarrhea or constipation.
     c. The diagnosis is made by history and stool culture revealing *C. botulinum.* The serum may be positive for toxins.
     d. Treatment of botulism includes trivalent botulism antitoxin (ABE), stomach lavage, IV fluids, and tracheostomy with mechanical ventilation if respiratory paralysis occurs.
     e. To prevent botulism, cans of food that are punctured, swollen, or have defective seals should be discarded.

- *Salmonellosis* is a bacterial infection that is classified as either a food poisoning or gastroenteritis.
  1. Incubation is 8 to 48 hours after ingestion of contaminated food or drink.
  2. Fever, nausea, vomiting, cramping abdominal pain, and severe diarrhea, which may be bloody, last 3 to 5 days.
  3. Diagnosis is made by stool culture.
  4. Treatment is based on symptoms.
  5. Salmonellosis can be transmitted by the fecal-oral route; therefore, strict hand washing is essential to avoid transmission.

Fracture, Nasal

- A nasal fracture commonly occurs from minor injuries received during falls and sports or from violence or motor vehicle trauma.
- Bone or cartilage displacement can cause airway obstruction and cosmetic deformity.
- Assessment includes deviation of the nose to one side, malaligned bridge, and crepitus and midface ecchymosis.
- Treatment includes
  1. Simple, closed reduction with local anesthesia (the treatment of choice)
  2. Rhinoplasty, or surgical reconstruction, for severe fractures
- Postoperative assessment includes
  1. Checking for edema, bleeding, increased swallowing of blood
  2. Maintaining the client in a semi-Fowler's position
  3. Applying ice to the nose and cool compresses to the eyes and face
- The client is instructed to
  1. Avoid the Valsalva maneuver
  2. Use laxatives or stool softeners
  3. Avoid aspirin and nonsteroidal anti-inflammatory drugs
  4. Take the full antibiotic prescription

FRACTURES

OVERVIEW

- A fracture is a break or disruption in the continuity of a bone.
- Fractures can be classified as complete or incomplete:
    1. *Complete fracture:* The break is across the entire width of the bone such that the bone is divided into two distinct sections.
    2. *Incomplete fracture:* The fracture does not divide the bone into two distinct sections.
- Fractures can also be grouped according to the extent of the soft tissue damage accompanying the fracture:
    1. *Open* or *compound fracture:* The skin surface over the broken bone is disrupted, causing an external wound.
        a. Compound fractures are graded to define the extent of the injury
            (1) Grade I is the least severe injury and skin damage is minimal
            (2) Grade II, an open fracture is accompanied by skin and muscle contusions
            (3) Grade III is the most severe and there is damage to skin, muscle, nerve tissue, and blood vessels; the wound is more than 6–8cm (2.4–3.2 inches) in diameter
    2. *Closed* or *simple fracture:* The break does not extend through the skin.
- Fractures can also be classified based on cause:
    1. *Pathologic* (spontaneous) *fracture:* The break occurs after minimal trauma to a bone that has been weakened by disease.
    2. *Fatigue fracture:* The break results from excessive strain and stress on bone.
- Complications of fractures include
    1. *Acute compartment syndrome* (ACS): ACS is a serious condition in which there is increased pressure within one or more compartments, which causes compromise of circulation to the area; the most common sites are the lower leg and the dorsal and volar compartments of the forearm. Infection, motor weakness, Volkmann's contractures,

and myoglobinuric renal failure can result. Fasciotomy is the surgical treatment.

2. *Shock:* Hypovolemic shock can occur as a result of hemorrhage from severed arteries.

3. *Fat embolism syndrome* (FES): FES is a serious complication in which fat globules are released from the yellow bone marrow into the bloodstream; the emboli migrate to the pulmonary capillary bed, causing confusion (low arterial oxygen), dyspnea, tachycardia, fever, and petechiae.

4. *Thromboembolitic complications:* Deep venous thrombosis is the most common complication of lower extremity surgery or trauma and the most frequently fatal complication of musculoskeletal surgery.

5. *Infection:* Osteomyelitis (bone infection) is most commonly seen in open fractures.

6. *Avascular necrosis* (AVN): AVN, also known as aseptic or ischemic necrosis, is bone death resulting from disruption of blood supply.

7. *Delayed union, nonunion,* and *malunion: Delayed union* is a fracture that has not healed within 6 months of the time of injury; *nonunion* fractures never completely heal; *malunion* is incorrect healing of a fracture.

 Transcultural Considerations

Hip fractures occur less often in African-Americans and men of any race than in Caucasian women.

 Women's Health Considerations

More than 1 million fractures occur annually in the United States secondary to osteoporosis and most occur in middle-aged and elderly women.

COLLABORATIVE MANAGEMENT
Assessment

- The nurse records
    1. Events leading to the fracture and immediate postinjury care
    2. The client's medical history
    3. Current medications, including over-the-counter and illegal drugs, and alcohol use

4. Nutritional history and recreational history
5. Occupation

- The nurse assesses for
    1. Trauma to other body systems (priority assessment)
    2. Change in bone alignment
    3. Shortening or change in bone shape
    4. Neurovascular changes:
        a. Skin color
        b. Skin temperature
        c. Movement (if pain is elicited, stop immediately)
        d. Sensation
        e. Pulses distal to injury
        f. Pain: location, nature, frequency
    5. Changes in skin integrity, such as ecchymosis, subcutaneous emphysema, or swelling
    6. Capillary refill (if an extremity is involved)
    7. Hemorrhage (open fracture)
    8. Muscle spasm
    9. Respiratory compromise

Planning and Implementation

✦ **NDx:** Risk for Peripheral Neurovascular Dysfunction

Nonsurgical Management

- *Closed reduction* involves manipulating the bone ends so that they realign while applying a manual pull, or traction, on the bone.
- *Bandages* and *splints* are used to immobilize areas such as the scapula and clavicle.
- *Casts* are used to hold bone fragments in place after reduction; they allow early mobility, correct and prevent deformity, and reduce pain.
    1. Several cast materials may be used:
        a. *Plaster of Paris* requires application of a well-fitted stockinette and web padding before the application of wet plaster rolls. The cast takes 24 to 72 hours to dry. The client is warned that heat will be felt immediately after the cast is applied. To facilitate drying, the cast is not covered, and the client is turned every 1 to 2 hours. The nurse handles the cast with the palms of the hands to prevent indentations and resulting areas of pressure on skin.

b. *Fiberglass* and *polyester-cotton knit* are lighter weight and take less time to dry.

2. Types of casts:
   a. *Arm cast:* When the client is in bed, a sling is used to elevate the arm above the client's head to reduce edema; when out of bed, the arm is supported by a sling placed around the neck.
   b. *Leg cast:* When the client is in bed, the leg is elevated on several pillows.
   c. A *body cast* encircles the body; a *spica cast* encircles a portion of the trunk and one or two extremities. The client is at risk for skin breakdown, pneumonia or atelectasis, joint contracture, or paralytic ileus. *Cast syndrome,* similar to a claustrophobic reaction, may occur.

3. The nurse provides cast care:
   a. "Petals," or finishes, the cast if the underlying stockinette does not cover the edges of the cast by placing tape over the rough edges (to prevent skin irritation from rough and crumbling edges)
   b. Recognizes that a window may be cut in the cast by the physician so that the wound can be observed and cared for
   c. Ensures that the cast is not too tight by inserting a finger between the cast and the skin; if it is too tight, the physician may cut it to relieve pressure
   d. Recognizes that the physician may bivalve the cast, cutting it lengthwise into two equal pieces; either half can be removed for inspection or provision of care; the two pieces are reunited by an elastic bandage wrap
   e. Encases a long leg or body cast in a protective covering around the perineum to prevent contamination by urine or feces; makes a fracture bedpan available
   f. Monitors the client's neurovascular status frequently
   g. Inspects the cast daily for drainage, cracking, crumbling, alignment, and fit once it is dry
   h. Circles, dates, and monitors areas of drainage on the cast for change; it is not unusual for bloody drainage to seep through the cast from an open fracture site

F

      i. Reports a sudden increase in the amount of drainage or a change in the integrity of the cast to the physician immediately

      j. Cleans a soiled cast with mild detergent and a damp cloth

      k. Does not use lotion or powder on skin around the cast

      l. Teaches the client not to place foreign objects beneath the cast

      m. Smells the cast for foul odor and palpates for hot areas every shift

      n. Has a cast cutter available at all times

4. The nurse observes for and reports complications from casting:
   a. Infection
   b. Circulation impairment
   c. Peripheral nerve damage
   d. Pressure necrosis
   e. Contracture of joint
   f. Degenerative arthritis
   g. Muscle atrophy
   h. Thromboembolism

- Traction is the application of a pulling force to a part of the body to provide reduction, alignment, and rest; it may also decrease muscle spasm and prevent or correct deformity.

  1. Traction types include
     a. *Running,* in which the pulling force is in one direction and the client's body acts as countertraction; moving the bed or body can alter the countertraction force
     b. *Balanced suspension,* which provides the countertraction such that the pulling force of the traction is not altered

  2. Classification of traction includes
     a. *Skin:* A Velcro boot (*Buck's traction*), belt, or halter that is attached to the skin and soft tissues is used; the purpose is to decrease painful muscle spasms, and weight is limited to 5 to 10 pounds.
     b. *Skeletal:* Pins (Steinmann), wires (Kirschner), tongs (Crutchfield), or screws are surgically inserted directly into bone and therefore allow the use of a longer traction time and heavier weights, usually from 15 to 30 pounds (6.8 to 13.6 kg).

     c. *Plaster traction:* A combination of skeletal traction and a plaster cast is used.

     d. *Brace devices:* Braces exert a pull to correct alignment deformities.

3. The nurse provides care for the client in traction:

     a. Maintains correct balance between traction pull and countertraction force

     b. Does not remove weights without a physician's order

     c. Allows the weights to hang freely at all times

     d. Inspects ropes, knots, and pulleys every 8 hours for loosening, fraying, and positioning

     e. Checks the weight for consistency with the physician's order every 8 hours; if not correct, notifies the physician

     f. Notes that if the client complains of severe pain from muscle spasms, the weights may be too heavy or the client may need realignment

     g. Inspects the skin every 8 hours for signs of irritation and inflammation, especially at points of entry of wires, screws, or pins

     h. Performs pin care as required by hospital policy

     i. Performs a neurovascular assessment at least every 8 hours, or more often if clinically indicated

- Large doses of opioid analgesics, anti-inflammatory drugs, and muscle relaxants may be used.
- Mild tranquilizers such as diazepam (Valium) may be given to relax the client and to minimize muscle spasm.
- The nurse
  1. Applies ice or heat
  2. Elevates the involved part, when possible
  3. Provides massage or back rubs
  4. Provides distraction, imagery, or music therapy
  5. Teaches progressive relaxation techniques

🕿 Considerations for Elderly Clients

- The elderly are at risk for problems caused by skin or skeletal traction because of inadequate circulation and sensation.
- Traction of any type is not ideal treatment because it necessitates prolonged immobilization and serious complications such as pneumonia and pulmonary emboli can result.

Surgical Management

- *Open reduction with internal fixation* (ORIF) allows direct visualization of the fracture site and permits early mobilization.
- *External fixation* involves fracture reduction and the insertion of pins into the bone through small percutaneous incisions; the pins are held in place by a large, external metal frame to prevent bone movement.
    1. External fixation allows for early ambulation and exercise while permitting easy access for wound care.
    2. Pin care is performed as required by hospital policy.
    3. The Ilizarov fixator promotes rotation, angulation, shortening, lengthening, and/or widening of bone for congenital anomalies, joint contractures, bone segmental defects, and deformities from malunion or nonunion fractures.
- The nurse provides preoperative care:
    1. Provides routine preoperative care
    2. Recognizes that the client may be placed in traction for a few days before surgery (e.g., fractured hip)
- The nurse provides postoperative care:
    1. Provides routine postoperative care
    2. Monitors neurovascular status at least every hour for the first 24 hours after injury, every 2 hours for the next 12 to 24 hours, and every 4 hours for the next few days
    3. Monitors the complete blood count for signs of anemia resulting from blood loss
    4. Observes for and reports complications such as infection
- Electrical bone stimulation, ultrasound fracture treatment, and bone grafting are methods for treating nonunion.

✦ NDx: Pain

- Musculoskeletal pain is one of the most severe types of pain and may be difficult to manage.
- The nurse
    1. Administers opioid analgesics, anti-inflammatory drugs, and muscle relaxants, as ordered
    2. Observes for effectiveness of drug therapy (an early sign of acute compartment syndrome is the sudden inability of pain medication to relieve pain)

310

3. Uses temporary pain relief measures, such as ice, heat, massage, distraction, imagery, music therapy, and relaxation techniques, as needed

✦ NDx: Risk for Infection

- The nurse
  1. Uses strict aseptic technique for dressing changes, wound irrigations, and pin care
  2. Monitors for signs of infection, such as swelling, drainage, and fever

F

✦ NDx: Impaired Physical Mobility

- The nurse employs measures to prevent complications of immobility
  1. Thromboembolic disease:
     a. Applies thigh-high antiembolism stockings or sequential compression devices (e.g., Venodyne)
     b. Performs active and/or passive range-of-motion exercises and isometric and isotonic exercises
     c. Administers anticoagulation therapy, such as low-dose aspirin, subcutaneous heparin sodium, or warfarin (Coumadin), as ordered
     d. Assesses for the presence of deep venous thrombosis
  2. Respiratory complications:
     a. Encourages the client to turn, cough, and deep breathe every 2 hours and to use an incentive spirometer
     b. Assesses for atelectasis or pneumonia
     c. Assists the client to get out of bed as soon as possible
  3. Skin impairment:
     a. Inspects the skin for signs of redness or irritation, with particular attention to bony prominences
     b. Uses heel or elbow protectors as needed
  4. Alterations in elimination:
     a. Records intake and output, encourages fluids
     b. Provides a diet high in fiber, including raw fruits and vegetables, bran, or prunes
     c. Administers stool softeners and bulk laxatives, as needed
  5. Cerebral dysfunction:
     a. Recognizes that elderly clients may become disoriented

b. Keeps a large clock and calendar in the client's view and asks the family to bring in personal items and pictures

c. Keeps side rails up at all times unless they present an accidental hazard (client consistently crawls over them)

d. Assesses all clients for sensory deprivation

- The nurse collaborates with the physical therapist to promote client mobility.
- *Crutches* require strong upper extremities, balance, and coordination:
    1. To prevent pressure on the axillary nerve, there should be two or three fingerwidths between the axilla and the top of the crutch when the crutch tip is at least 6 inches diagonally in front of the foot.
    2. The crutch is adjusted so that the elbow is flexed no more than 30 degrees.
    3. The most common gait for crutch walking is the three-point gait, which allows no weight-bearing on the affected leg.
- A *walker* is most often used by the elderly client who needs additional support for balance.
- A *cane* is used if minimal support is needed:
    1. The cane is placed on the unaffected side.
    2. The cane should create no more than 30 degrees of flexion of the elbow
    3. Top of cane should be parallel to the greater trochanter of the femur

✦ **NDx:** Altered Nutrition: Less than Body Requirements

- The nurse
    1. Assesses the client's food likes and dislikes
    2. Collaborates with the dietitian to plan meals that are both appealing and nutritional (high protein, high calorie)
    3. Administers supplements of vitamins B and C, as ordered
    4. Teaches the client to increase his or her dietary intake of milk and milk products, because the client is predisposed to hypocalcemia
    5. Encourages consumption of foods high in iron, because anemia may develop; iron supplement may be ordered

Continuing Care

- The nurse
    1. Identifies and suggests corrections for hazards in the home before discharge
    2. Ensures that the client can use all assistive-adaptive devices ordered for home use before discharge
    3. Provides verbal and written instructions for the care of casts, splints, braces, or external fixator
    4. Provides verbal and written instructions on wound care, as needed
    5. Teaches the client and family how to recognize complications such as infection, as well as when and where to contact professional health care should complications arise
    6. Provides a detailed plan of care at the time of discharge for clients to be transferred to a long-term-care or rehabilitation facility, if needed
    7. Emphasizes the importance of follow-up visits with the physician(s) and other therapists

FRACTURES OF SPECIFIC SITES

- *Clavicular:* self-healing. A splint or bandage is used for immobilization.
- *Scapular:* immobilized with a sling and swathe or shoulder immobilizer until healing occurs. Serious internal trauma can occur, including pneumothorax, pulmonary contusions, and fractured ribs.
- *Humeral shaft:* corrected by open reduction and the application of a hanging arm cast or splint. An impacted injury is treated conservatively with a sling. A displaced fracture may require ORIF with pins or a prosthetic device.
- *Olecranon:* treated by closed reduction and application of a cast. Healing may take 2 months, and several additional months may be needed before full use of the elbow returns. For displaced fractures, ORIF is performed, and a splint is worn.

- *Radius* and *ulna:* treated with closed reduction and casting. If displaced, ORIF with intramedullary rods or plates and screws is performed.
- *Wrist* and *hand:* treated with closed reduction and casting.
- *Hip:* classified as *intracapsular* (within the joint capsule) or *extracapsular* (outside the joint capsule). Treatment involves ORIF. Nursing interventions are directed toward management of the following nursing diagnoses:
    1. Risk for Injury related to subluxation or dislocation
    2. Pain related to surgical incision
    3. Risk for Infection related to impaired skin integrity
    4. Impaired Physical Mobility related to hip precautions and surgical pain

---

✐ Considerations for Elderly Clients

1. Hip fractures occur most often in elderly women with osteoporosis
2. As many as 50% of elderly clients who sustain a hip fracture die within one year of injury from medical complications caused by the fracture or by immobility that occurs after the fracture

- *Femur:* seldom immobilized by casting; skeletal traction followed by a cast brace or hip spica cast is used. ORIF may be needed.
- *Patella:* repaired with closed reduction and casting or internal fixation with screws.
- *Tibia* and *fibula:* treated with closed reduction with casting for 8 to 10 weeks; internal fixation and long leg cast for 4 to 6 weeks; or external fixation, used when the fractures cause extensive skin and soft tissue damage.
- *Ankle:* generally spiral, transverse, or oblique breaks that are difficult to treat and present problems in healing. Treatment consists of a combination of closed and open techniques, depending on the severity and extent of the fracture.
- *Foot* or *phalanges:* very painful fractures that are treated with either open or closed techniques.
- *Ribs* and *sternum:* major complication is puncture of the lungs, heart, or arteries by bone fragments or ends.

- *Pelvic:* the second most common cause of death from trauma after head injuries. When a non–weight-bearing part of the pelvis is fractured, treatment involves bed rest. A weight-bearing fracture may require the use of a pelvic sling, skeletal traction, double hip spica cast, or external fixator.

FRACTURES, RIB

- Rib fractures result from direct blunt chest trauma; ribs five through nine are injured most often.
- Rib fractures cause a potential for intrathoracic injury, such as pneumothorax or pulmonary contusion.
- Pain with movement and defensive chest splinting result in impaired ventilation and inadequate clearance of tracheobronchial secretions.
- Clients with preexisting pulmonary disease have an increased risk of pneumonia and atelectasis
- Ribs usually unite spontaneously.
- Pain management is provided to maintain adequate ventilatory status; an intercostal nerve block may be required for severe pain.

FROSTBITE

- Frostbite is a cold injury of the skin; severity depends on temperature, duration of exposure, and tissue hypoxia at exposure.
- Cell death is due to microvascular vasoconstriction, with subsequent interference of blood flow and stasis.
- Continued exposure to cold causes vascular necrosis and gangrene.
- Increased risk factors include age, immobility, alcohol use, vascular disease, and psychiatric disorders.
- Treatment includes rapid and continuous rewarming of the tissue in a warm bath for 15 to 20 minutes or until skin flushing occurs; thawing can be painful.

- Slow thawing or interrupted periods of warmth are avoided because they can contribute to increased cellular damage.
- After thawing, the tissue is exposed so that tissue changes can be monitored.
- Frostbite blisters are left intact.
- Over time, the degree of actual tissue destruction is evident, and local care to eschar is indicated.
- Long-term complications of cold injury include amputation, scarring, depigmentation, and thickened nail plates.

FURUNCLES

See Infections, Skin.

GALLSTONES

See Cholelithiasis.

GASTRIC CARCINOMA

See Cancer, Stomach.

GASTRITIS

OVERVIEW

- Gastritis is defined as the inflammation of the gastric mucosa.

- Mucosal injury occurs and is worsened by histamine release and cholinergic nerve stimulation.
- Hydrochloric acid diffuses into the mucosa and injures small vessels, resulting in edema, hemorrhage, and erosion of the gastric lining.
- Gastritis can be classified as acute or chronic:
    1. *Acute* gastritis, the inflammation of gastric mucosa or submucosa after exposure to local irritants, such as alcohol or aspirin, bacterial endotoxins, ingestion of corrosive substances, or lack of stimulation of normal gastric secretions. It occurs in varying degrees of mucosal necrosis and inflammation, with complete regeneration and healing usually occurring within a few days and complete recovery with no residual damage usually ensuing.
    2. *Chronic* gastritis is a diffuse chronic inflammatory process involving the mucosal lining of the stomach, which usually heals without scarring but can progress to hemorrhage and ulcer formation. It may be caused by chronic local irritation by alcohol, drugs, smoking, radiation, infectious agents (e.g., *Helicobacter pylori*) and environmental agents. Fifty percent of clients with gastric ulcers have associated chronic gastritis.
- The three subtypes of chronic gastritis include
    1. Type A chronic gastritis, which usually involves the body and fundus of the stomach, is autoimmune in cause, and accompanies pernicious anemia.
    2. Type B chronic gastritis usually affects the antrum but may involve the entire stomach. *H. pylori,* a gram-negative microorganism, has been associated with this type.
    3. Atrophic gastritis, in which there is a thickened muscularis with inflammation, occurs in all areas of the stomach, with decreased fundal, parietal, and chief cells (associated with gastric ulcers and cancer).

COLLABORATIVE MANAGEMENT
Assessment
- In acute gastritis the nurse assesses for
    1. General appearance, including facial grimacing, restlessness, or moaning

317

2. Tenderness in the epigastric area, guarding, and distention
3. Increased bowel sounds or visual peristaltic waves
4. Dyspepsia or heartburn, anorexia, nausea, and vomiting
5. Hematemesis

- In *chronic* gastritis, the nurse assesses for
    1. Vague complaints or periodic epigastric distress, which may be relieved by food
    2. Anorexia
    3. Pain that worsens with food, especially spicy or fatty foods
    4. Weight loss

Interventions

- The nurse
    1. Administers H$_2$ antagonists, as ordered, such as cimetidine (Tagamet, Apo-Cimetidine◆), ranitidine (Zantac), famotidine (Pepcid), and nizatidine (Axid), to block gastric acid secretions
    2. Administers antacids as buffering agents and sucralfate (Carafate, Sulcrate◆), as ordered
    3. Administers vitamin B$_{12}$, as ordered, for clients with pernicious anemia
    4. Administers bismuth subsalicylates, metronidazole (Flagyl, Novonidazol◆), tetracycline, or ampicillin (Amcill, Ampicin◆), as ordered, if *Helicobacter pylori* is present
    5. Avoids drugs associated with gastric irritation, including steroids, aspirin, chemotherapeutic agents, and nonsteroidal anti-inflammatory agents
    6. Avoids foods and spices that contribute to distress, including tea, coffee, cola, chocolate, mustard, paprika, cloves, pepper, and Tabasco sauce
    7. Teaches the client to avoid large, heavy meals
    8. Provides a soft, bland diet
    9. Teaches techniques to reduce discomfort, such as progressive relaxation, cutaneous stimulation, guided imagery, and distraction
    10. Teaches the client to stop smoking, if appropriate, and avoid alcohol and caffeine

- Surgery is indicated when conservative measures have failed to control bleeding (see "Surgical Management" under Peptic Ulcer Disease).

GASTROENTERITIS

OVERVIEW

- Gastroenteritis is an inflammation of the mucous membranes of the stomach and intestines, primarily affecting the small bowel.
- The disease may be viral or bacterial in origin, causing an inflammatory response in one of three ways:
    1. Release of enterotoxin, causing local inflammation and diarrhea
    2. Penetration of the organism into the intestine, causing cellular destruction, necrosis, and ulceration (diarrhea occurs with white blood cells or red blood cells)
    3. Attachment of the organism to the mucosal epithelium, destroying cells of the intestinal villi with resultant malabsorption
- *Viral* gastroenteritis can be classified as either epidemic viral gastroenteritis (incubation from 10 to 51 hours and communicable) and rotavirus gastroenteritis (incubation about 48 hours and affecting infants and young children).
- *Bacterial* gastroenteritis can be divided into three general types: (1) *Campylobacter* enteritis, (2) *Escherichia coli* diarrhea, and (3) shigellosis.

COLLABORATIVE MANAGEMENT

Assessment

- The nurse assesses
    1. Onset of diarrhea with accompanying abdominal cramping or pain
    2. Nausea and vomiting
    3. Bloody, mucousy, or watery foul-smelling stool
    4. Fever; temperature may be normal or elevated from 101° to 103° F (38.2° to 39.2° C)
    5. Dehydration exhibited by poor skin turgor, dry mucous membranes, orthostatic blood pressure changes, hypotension, and oliguria
    6. Viral symptoms, such as myalgia, headache, or malaise
    7. Positive result of a stool culture

Interventions

- The nurse replaces fluids, as ordered:
  1. Administers oral rehydration therapy with commercially prepared products, such as Resol
  2. Administers hypotonic intravenous fluids for severe dehydration
  3. Adds potassium supplements to intravenous fluid if the client is hypokalemic
  4. Advises the client to take small volumes of clear liquids with electrolytes (e.g., ginger ale) and then to progress with the diet as tolerated
- The nurse
  1. Provides clear liquid fluids in small amounts as tolerated
  2. Progresses the diet as tolerated, avoiding milk and milk products for 1 week
  3. Avoids intestinal motility suppressants such as antiemetics or anticholinergics for bacterial or viral gastroenteritis
  4. Administers anti-infective agents, as ordered, such as sul-famethoxazole with trimethoprim (Septra, Bactrim) if shigellosis is present
  5. Applies repellent cream, such as zinc oxide, petroleum jelly, Desitin ointment, or Sween products, to protect the skin and anal area
- The nurse teaches the client
  1. To minimize the risk of disease transmission by washing his or her hands after bowel movements
  2. To avoid sharing eating utensils, glasses, and dishes and to maintain strict personal hygiene
  3. To follow written instructions for medication dosage, schedule of administration, and side effects, if ordered
  4. To maintain adequate oral fluid intake
  5. To report returning diarrhea or dizziness to the physician

GASTROESOPHAGEAL REFLUX DISEASE

OVERVIEW

- Esophageal reflux involves the backward flow of gastrointestinal (GI) contents into the esophagus, exposing the esophageal mucosa to the irritating effects of gastric and/or duodenal contents.
- Gastroesophageal reflux disease (GERD) develops when an inflammatory response is initiated.
- The degree of inflammation is related to the acid concentration of the refluxed material, the number of reflux episodes, and the length of time that the esophagus is exposed to the irritant.

COLLABORATIVE MANAGEMENT

Assessment

- The nurse assesses for
  1. Pain location
  2. Heartburn or pyrosis, the primary symptom, described as a burning sensation; severe heartburn may radiate to the neck or jaw or may be referred to the back
  3. Pain aggravated by bending over, straining, or lying in a recumbent position
  4. Pain occurring after each meal and persisting for 20 minutes to 2 hours
  5. Regurgitation not associated with belching or nausea; warm fluid traveling up the throat, resulting in a sour or bitter taste in the mouth
  6. Water brash (reflex salivary hypersecretion)
  7. Dysphagia (difficulty in swallowing)
  8. Chest pain from esophageal spasm
  9. Belching and a feeling of flatulence or bloating after eating
  10. Results of 24-hour pH monitoring, esophageal manometry (motility testing), and scintigraphy (measure of reflux of radioisotope)

Interventions

Nonsurgical Management

- The nurse
    1. Teaches the client to avoid fatty foods, coffee, tea, cola, chocolate, spicy foods, acidic foods, and alcohol because they lower esophageal sphincter (LES) pressure or cause local irritation
    2. Provides four to six small meals a day, in collaboration with the dietitian
    3. Teaches the client to avoid having snacks in the evening or eating 3 hours prior to bedtime
    4. Instructs the client to eat slowly and chew food thoroughly to facilitate digestion and prevent eructation (belching)
    5. Encourages weight reduction if the client is obese
    6. Instructs the client to stop smoking because it decreases LES pressure
    7. Elevates the head of the bed by 8 to 12 inches (3.2 to 4.8 cm) to prevent nighttime reflux
    8. Administers antacids, as ordered, for acid-neutralizing effects
    9. Administers a histamine receptor antagonist, as ordered, such as ranitidine (Zantac), famotidine (Pepcid), or nizatidine (Axid), which reduces gastric acid production, provides symptom improvement, and supports healing of the inflamed esophageal tissue
    10. Administers bethanechol (Urecholine), as ordered, to increase LES and increase the rate of esophageal clearance
    11. Administers metoclopramide (Reglan, Maxeran◆), as ordered, to increase the rate of gastric emptying
    12. Administers proton pump inhibitors as ordererd, such as omeprazole (Prilosec), to reduce gastric acid secretion in clients with severe GERD
    13. Avoids drugs that decrease LES pressure or delay gastric emptying as ordered,, such as anticholinergics, calcium channel blockers, theophylline, and diazepam (Valium, Meval◆)
    14. Cisapride (Propulsid) has been approved for symptomatic treatment of nocturnal heartburn caused by GERD

Surgical Management

- Antireflux surgery is performed only in healthy clients who have not responded to aggressive medical management.
- The three major surgical procedures are *Nissen fundoplication, Belsey's repair,* and *Hill's repair.*
- These procedures involve wrapping and suturing the gastric fundus around the esophagus, which anchors the LES area below the diaphragm and reinforces the high-pressure area.
- The nurse provides routine preoperative care.
- Following wrapping procedures, the nurse provides postoperative care.

    1. Provides routine postoperative care
    2. Avoids repositioning or replacing the nasogastric tube, which was inserted during surgery
    3. Avoids performing endotracheal suctioning on a client with esophageal anastomosis or repair
    4. Assesses the cutaneous suture line for redness, drainage, and other signs of infection
    5. Observes the surgical dressing for bleeding
    6. Cleanses the suture line once each shift with half-strength peroxide, as ordered, and applies antibacterial ointment, as ordered
    7. Elevates the head of the bed 30 degrees at rest and 90 degrees when feeding is instituted
    8. Encourages the client to continue to follow the basic antireflux regime

- Synthetic *Angelchick prosthesis* placement is an alternate surgical procedure. A laparotomy is performed, and a C-shaped silicone prosthesis filled with gel is tied around the distal esophagus, anchoring the LES in the abdomen and reinforcing sphincter pressure.

    1. Prior to the Angelchick procedure, the nurse provides routine preoperative care.
    2. Postoperative care closely parallels that used for the laparotomy procedure.
    3. The nurse additionally
        a. Pays special attention to respiratory care because the surgery is performed close to the diaphragm
        b. Provides adequate analgesia so that the client can cough effectively and clear the airway
        c. Teaches the client that mild dysphagia is common but resolves in time
        d. Encourages the client to eat smaller meals to avoid overdistention of the stomach

GASTROINTESTINAL POLYPS

See Polyps, Gastrointestinal.

GBS

See Guillain-Barré Syndrome.

GENITAL HERPES SIMPLEX

See Herpes Simplex, Genital.

GERD

See Gastroesophageal Reflux Disease.

GLAUCOMA

OVERVIEW
- Glaucoma is a group of ocular diseases characterized by increased ocular pressure.
- Left untreated, glaucoma can result in blindness.
- In most common forms of glaucoma, vision is lost gradually and painlessly, without the person's awareness.

- Types of glaucoma include
  1. Primary, in which the structures that are involved in circulation or reabsorption of the aqueous humor undergo direct pathologic change:
     a. Primary open angle glaucoma (POAG) develops slowly, usually without symptoms.
     b. Angle closure, also known as closed angle, narrow angle, or acute has a sudden onset and is treated as an emergency.
  2. Secondary, which results from ocular diseases that cause a narrowed angle or an increased volume of fluid within the eye

Considerations for Elderly Clients

1. People older than 40 years of age are at higher risk for glaucoma.
2. Incidence of glaucoma is age-related, as high as 10% in people older than 80 years of age.

Transcultural Considerations

Glaucoma is the primary cause of blindness in African Americans.

COLLABORATIVE MANAGEMENT

Assessment

- The nurse assesses for early manifestations of glaucoma:
  1. Increased intraocular pressure
  2. Diminished accommodation
- The nurse assesses for *late* manifestations of glaucoma:
  1. Visual field losses
  2. Decreased visual acuity not correctable with glasses
  3. Appearance of halos around lights
  4. Headache or eye pain (pain is sudden and excruciating in acute glaucoma)
  5. Increased cupping and atrophy of the optic disk
  6. Pale optic disk
  7. Anxiety and fear
  8. Increased tonometry reading

Interventions

Nonsurgical Management

- The nurse administers drug therapy, as ordered:
    1. Miotics to constrict the pupil and contract the ciliary muscle, such as pilocarpine hydrochloride (Pilocar, Isopto Carpine, Spersacarpine♦), carbachol (Isopto Carbachol), and echothiophate iodide (Phospholine Iodide), which may cause blurred vision for 1 to 2 hours after use and adaptation to dark environments may be difficult
    2. Agents to inhibit formation of aqueous humor, which include timolol (Timoptic, Apo-Timoptic♦), and levobunolol (Betagan)
    3. Carbonic anhydrase inhibitors, such as acetazolamide (Acetazolam♦, Diamox) and methazolamide (Neptazane), to reduce production of aqueous humor, with side effects that include numbness and tingling of the hands and feet, nausea, or malaise
    4. Systemic osmotic agents given to clients with acute glaucoma to reduce ocular pressure, including oral glycerin (Osmoglyn) and mannitol (Osmitrol♦)

Surgical Management

- *Laser trabeculoplasty* is performed under local anesthesia for open-angle glaucoma to produce scars in the trabecular meshwork, causing them to tighten and thus increase the outflow of aqueous humor.
- For angle-closure glaucoma, the laser is used to create a hole in the periphery of the iris, which allows aqueous humor to flow from the posterior chamber to the anterior chamber and then into the trabecular meshwork.
- A postoperative ocular steroid ointment may be prescribed following laser surgery.
- Complications of laser surgery are indicated by a headache that is unrelieved by acetaminophen or that is accompanied by nausea, brow pain, or a change in visual acuity.
- Other surgical procedures may be performed if the client's glaucoma fails to respond to pharmacologic or laser management.
- The nurse provides preoperative care:
    1. Provides routine preoperative care
    2. Administers medications to lower intraocular pressure, given topically or intravenously, as ordered
    3. Instills topical antibiotics, as ordered

326

- The nurse provides postoperative care:
    1. Provides routine postoperative care
    2. Provides the antibiotic that is administered subconjunctivally by the ophthalmologist
    3. Adjusts the head of the bed to the position of comfort
    4. Assists the client with ambulating and eating as needed as soon as the effects of anesthesia wear off
    5. Reports any drainage to the physician immediately but does not remove the original dressing unless specific orders are written to do so
    6. Instructs the client not to lie on the operative side
    7. Instructs the client to report symptoms of brow pain, severe eye pain, or nausea
    8. Observes for and teaches the client to report complications of glaucoma surgery:
        a. Increased intraocular pressure, manifested by ocular pain, pain above the eyebrow, and nausea; the client is instructed to avoid bending from the waist, lifting heavy objects, straining while having a bowel movement, coughing, and vomiting
        b. Hypotony—decreased intraocular pressure, which can lead to choroidal hemorrhage, or choroidal detachment, manifested by pain deep in the eye, with a definite onset, diaphoresis, or change in vital signs
        c. Infection
        d. Scar tissue

GLOMERULONEPHRITIS, ACUTE

OVERVIEW

- Acute glomerulonephritis is an inflammatory process of the glomeruli initiated by activation of immunologic responses as a result of infection.
- *Primary* causes from the immune response to pathogens include

1. Group A beta-hemolytic *Streptococcus*
2. Staphylococcal or pneumococcal bacteremia
3. Syphilis
4. Visceral abscesses
5. Bacterial endocarditis
6. Hepatitis B
7. Infectious mononucleosis
8. Measles
9. Mumps
10. Cytomegaloviral infections
11. Parasitic, fungal, or viral infections

- *Secondary* causes related to systemic disease include
    1. Systemic lupus erythematosus
    2. Progressive systemic sclerosis
    3. Thrombocytopenia purpura
    4. Postpartum renal failure
    5. Henoch-Schonlein purpura
    6. Goodpasture's syndrome
    7. Wegener's granulomatosis
    8. Polyarteritis nodosa
    9. Hemolytic-uremic syndrome

COLLABORATIVE MANAGEMENT

Assessment

- The nurse records the client's
    1. History of recent infections, particularly skin and upper respiratory infections
    2. Recent travel
    3. Activities with exposure to viruses, bacteria, fungi, or parasites
    4. Recent illnesses
    5. Recent surgeries or invasive procedures
    6. Known systemic diseases
- The nurse assesses for
    1. Skin lesions or incisions
    2. Edema of the face, eyelids, hands, and peripheral tissue
    3. Hypertension
    4. Changes in patterns of urination
    5. Smoky, reddish-brown, or cola-colored urine
    6. Dysuria
    7. Decreased amount of urine output
    8. Mild to moderate hypertension
    9. Changes in weight

    10. Crackles in lung fields

    11. Fatigue and malaise

    12. Anorexia, nausea, or vomiting

    13. Red blood cells and protein in the urine

- A percutaneous needle biopsy may define the pathologic condition, assist in determining prognosis, and help outline treatment.

Interventions

- Appropriate anti-infectives are given to treat infection such as penicillin, erythromycin, or azithromycin.
- To prevent infection spread, the health care provider may order anti-infective drugs for persons in immediate close contact with the client.
- Sodium and water restriction along with diuretics may be needed for the client with hypertension, circulatory congestions, and edema:

    1. Antihypertensives are given to treat hypertension

    2. The usual fluid allowance is equal to the 24-hour urinary output, plus 500–600 mL for insensible fluid loss

- Potassium and protein intake may be restricted to prevent hyperkalemia and additional uremic manifestations of the elevated BUN.
- Plasmapheresis may also be attempted.
- The nurse

    1. Encourages and promotes a restful environment

    2. Teaches and demonstrates energy conservation techniques

    3. Encourages the client to practice relaxation techniques

- The nurse

    1. Reviews prescribed medication instructions, including purpose, timing, frequency, duration, and side effects

    2. Advises the client to measure weight and blood pressure daily and to notify the health care provider for any sudden changes

    3. Advises the client to exercise each day, as tolerated

    4. Teaches the importance of rest

    5. Instructs the client about peritoneal or vascular access care if short-term dialysis is required to control fluid volume excess or uremic symptoms

G

GLOMERULONEPHRITIS, CHRONIC

OVERVIEW

- Chronic glomerulonephritis, or chronic nephritic syndrome, is the diagnostic name given to known and unknown causes of renal deterioration or renal failure that develop over a period of years.
- The exact pathogenesis is unknown; changes are believed to be due to effects of hypertension, intermittent or recurrent infections and inflammation, and altered metabolism and hemodynamics.
- Kidney tissue atrophies, and the functional mass of nephrons decreases, which alter glomerular filtration.
- Glomerular injury results in proteinuria due to increased permeability of the glomerular basement membrane.
- The process eventually results in end-stage renal disease (ESRD) and uremia, requiring dialysis or transplantation.

COLLABORATIVE MANAGEMENT

Assessment

- The nurse records the client's
    1. Health problems, including systemic disease
    2. Renal or urologic problems
    3. Childhood infectious diseases, such as *Streptococcus*
    4. Recent exposure to infections
    5. Overall assessment of health status
    6. Changes in urinary status, including frequency of voiding and changes in urine color, clarity, and odor
    7. Changes in activity tolerance
    8. Presence of edema
    9. Changes in mental concentration or memory
    10. Proteinuria
    11. Decreased creatinine clearance
    12. Serum electrolyte changes
- The nurse
    1. Inspects the skin for yellow color, ecchymosis, and rashes

2. Inspects for evidence of edema in tissues
3. Measures blood pressure and weight
4. Auscultates the heart for an S_3 sound
5. Auscultates the lungs for the presence of rales or crackles
6. Observes the rate and depth of breathing pattern
7. Inspects neck veins for engorgement
8. Inspects and analyzes urine

Interventions

- Management of chronic glomerulonephritis is similar to conservative management for ESRD.
- Treatment consists of dietary modification, fluid intake sufficient to prevent reduced blood flow volume to the kidneys, and medication therapy to temporarily control the symptoms of uremia.
- Eventually the client requires dialysis or transplantation.

GONORRHEA

OVERVIEW

- Gonorrhea is a sexually transmitted disease (STD) caused by *Neisseria gonorrhoeae,* a gram-negative diplococcus; it continues to be the most reported communicable disease in the United States.
- The disease is transmitted by direct sexual contact and through an infected birth canal to the neonate.
- Initial symptoms occur 3 to 10 days after sexual contact with an infected person, or the client may be asymptomatic.

COLLABORATIVE MANAGEMENT
Assessment

- The nurse assesses for
  1. Male
     a. Dysuria
     b. Penile discharge that is either profuse yellowish-green fluid or clear, scant fluid
     c. Anal itching and irritation

      d. Rectal bleeding

      e. Painful defecation

      f. Pharyngitis

  2. Female

      a. Change in vaginal discharge

      b. Urinary frequency

      c. Dysuria

      d. Anal itching and irritation

      e. Rectal bleeding

      f. Painful defecation

      g. Pharyngitis

- In men, the urethra is the site most commonly affected, but gonorrhea can spread to the prostate, seminal vesicles, and epididymis.
- In women, the cervix and urethra are the most common sites, but upward spread can cause pelvic inflammatory disease, endometritis, salpingitis, and pelvic peritonitis.
- The nurse also assesses for
  1. Sexual history
     a. Types and frequency of sexual activity
     b. Number of sexual contacts
     c. Past history of STD
     d. Potential sites of infection
     e. Sexual preference
  2. Gram's stain smears for gram-negative diplococci (culture provides a definitive diagnosis)

Interventions

- The nurse
  1. Administers ceftriaxone (Rocephin), 250 mg IM in a single dose, plus doxycycline (Vibramycin, Novodoxylin◆), 100 mg orally twice a day, for 1 week, as ordered
  2. Informs the client that sexual partners need to be treated
  3. Informs the client that gonorrheal infections can become systemic and cause
     a. Fever
     b. Chills
     c. Skin lesions
     d. Arthritis
     e. Meningitis and endocarditis (rare)
  4. Teaches the client about
     a. Transmission and treatment

b. Prevention of reinfection
c. Avoidance of sexual activity until the infection is cured
d. Use of condoms if sexually active
e. Need to report the disease
5. Encourages the client to express feelings about having the disease
6. Provides privacy and confidentiality

GOUT

OVERVIEW

- Gout is a systemic disease in which urate crystals deposit in joints and other body tissues.
- Two major types are
    1. *Primary* gout, which results from one of several inborn errors of purine metabolism; uric acid production exceeds the kidney's excretion capability, and sodium urate deposits in synovium and other tissues, resulting in inflammation
    2. *Secondary* gout, which involves excessive uric acid in the blood that is caused by another disease
- Four phases of the disease process include
    1. *Asymptomatic hyperuricemia,* in which there are no symptoms but serum uric acid is elevated
    2. *Acute* gout, which is characterized by excruciating pain and inflammation of one or more small joints, especially the great toe
    3. *Intercritical,* or *intercurrent,* gout, which is asymptomatic, with no abnormalities found on examination (period between acute attacks)
    4. *Chronic* gout, in which repeated episodes of acute gout result in the deposit of urate crystals under the skin and within major organs, especially the renal system

COLLABORATIVE MANAGEMENT
Assessment

- The nurse assesses for

1. A family history of the disease
2. Joint inflammation
3. Excruciating pain in the involved joint(s)
4. Tophi: hard, fairly large, and irregular-shaped deposits in the skin that may break open, with a yellow, gritty substance discharged (seen in chronic gout)
5. Renal stones or dysfunction

Interventions

- The nurse administers drug therapy, as ordered:
  1. For *acute* gout only, colchicine and nonsteroidal anti-inflammatory drugs (NSAIDs) until the inflammation subsides, usually for 4 to 7 days or until severe diarrhea occurs
  2. For *chronic* gout, allopurinol (Zyloprim, Alloprin◆) or probenecid (Benemid), with serum uric acid levels monitored to determine the effectiveness of the drug
- Dietary restrictions are controversial but may include a strict low-purine diet with avoidance of organ meats, shellfish, and oily fish with bones.
- Excessive alcohol intake and fad "starvation'" diets can cause a gout attack.
- The nurse instructs the client to avoid
  1. Aspirin in any form and diuretics
  2. Excessive physical or emotional stress
- The nurse teaches the client
  1. To force fluids
  2. To increase urinary pH by eating alkaline ash foods, such as citrus fruits and juices, milk, and other dairy products

GUILLAIN-BARRÉ SYNDROME

OVERVIEW

- Guillain-Barré syndrome (GBS), also called acute idiopathic polyneuritis, infectious polyneuritis, or

Landry's paralysis, is an acute inflammation and demyelinization of the peripheral nervous system.

- Three stages include
  1. *Initial* period, which begins with the onset of the first definitive symptoms and ends when no further deterioration is noted (usually 1 to 3 weeks)
  2. *Plateau* period, which is a time of little change and lasts several days to 2 weeks
  3. *Recovery* period, which is thought to coincide with remyelination and axonal regeneration and lasts 4 to 6 months
- The cause of GBS remains obscure, although most evidence implicates a cell-mediated immunologic reaction. The client often relates a history of acute illness, trauma, surgery, or immunization 1 to 4 weeks before the onset of neurologic signs and symptoms.
- Three types of GBS include
  1. *Ascending,* the most common clinical pattern, with weakness beginning in the lower extremities and progressing upward to include the trunk and arms; sometimes affecting the cranial nerves and sometimes with respiratory compromise
  2. *Descending,* in which there is weakness of the face or bulbar muscles of the jaw, the sternocleidomastoid muscles, and muscles of the tongue, pharynx, and larynx, and progressing downward to involve the limbs; respiratory compromise can occur quickly
  3. *Miller-Fisher variant,* which consists of a triad of ophthalmoplegia, areflexia, and severe ataxia, with normal motor strength and intact sensory function

G

➡ Transcultural Considerations

1. GBS has worldwide distribution and affects people of all races and ages.
2. Higher rates, however, have been noted in people 45 years old or older, in Caucasians than in African Americans, and in men than in women.

COLLABORATIVE MANAGEMENT
Assessment

- The nurse records the client's
  1. Past medical and surgical history

a. Occurrence of antecedent illness 3 to 4 weeks prior to the onset of GBS
b. Description of symptoms (in chronological order)
- The nurse assesses for
  1. Paresthesia (numbness or tingling)
  2. Pain, resembling that of a charley horse
  3. Cranial nerve dysfunction: facial weakness, dysphagia, diplopia
  4. Difficulty walking
  5. Muscle weakness or flaccid paralysis without muscle wasting in an ascending, distal to proximal, progression
  6. Respiratory compromise or failure: dyspnea, decreased breath sound, decreased tidal volume and/or vital capacity
  7. Bowel and bladder incontinence
  8. Autonomic dysfunction evidenced by labile blood pressure, cardiac dysrhythmias, or tachycardia
  9. Decreased or absent deep-tendon reflexes
  10. Ability to cope with illness
  11. Anxiety, fear, and panic
  12. Anger and depression

Planning and Implementation

✦ **NDx:** Ineffective Breathing Pattern; Ineffective Airway Clearance; Impaired Gas Exchange

- The nurse
  1. Performs a respiratory assessment:
     a. Assesses every 4 hours
     b. Observes for dyspnea, air hunger, or subjective complaints of shortness of breath
     c. Measures vital capacity every 2 to 4 hours
     d. Obtains arterial blood gases as indicated by the client's clinical status
     e. Keeps equipment for intubation and a ventilator available
  2. Performs chest physiotherapy; encourages the client to cough and deep breathe
  3. Changes the client's position frequently

✦ **NDx:** Impaired Physical Mobility

- A grading system is used for muscle testing:
  0: no contraction

1: flicker or trace contraction
2: active movement with gravity eliminated
3: active movement against gravity
4: active movement against gravity and resistance
5: normal power

- The nurse
    1. Applies thigh-high antiembolism stockings
    2. Administers subcutaneous anticoagulant, as ordered
    3. Performs range-of-motion (ROM) exercises
- Plasmapheresis may be performed in which the client's plasma is separated from whole blood, and its abnormal constituents are removed or the plasma is exchanged with normal plasma or a colloidal substitute. It has led to reductions in the length of hospital stay and in the amount of time required before the client resumes walking.
- The nurse monitors vital and neurologic signs routinely throughout the plasmapheresis procedure.
- Complications of plasmapheresis include hypovolemia, hypokalemia, hypocalcemia, temporary circumoral and distal extremity paresthesia, muscle twitching, nausea, and vomiting.
- The nurse
    1. Administers adrenocorticotropic hormone (ACTH), as ordered, to shorten the duration of the disease

✦ NDx: Pain

- The nurse
    1. Assesses the severity and nature of the pain, which is often worse at night and only relieved by opioid analgesics
    2. Uses nondrug pain relief measures, such as repositioning, relaxation techniques, guided imagery, and distractions such as music or visitors

✦ NDx: Impaired Verbal Communication

- The nurse
    1. Assists the client to develop a communication system in collaboration with the speech/language pathologist
    2. Develops a communication board that lists common requests

✦ **NDx:** Powerlessness

- The nurse
    1. Encourages the client to verbalize feelings concerning the illness and its effects
    2. Provides information regarding the disease process
    3. Allows the client to participate in his or her care and make choices as much as possible
    4. Provides encouragement and positive reinforcement
    5. Identifies factors that increase coping abilities through asking the client/family to describe situations that they have successfully coped with in the past
    6. Keeps necessary items (call light, radio, or television control) within the client's reach
    7. Uses the client's own personal items, when feasible

✦ **NDx:** Anxiety; Anticipatory Grieving

- The nurse
    1. Assesses the client/family for verbal and nonverbal behaviors indicative of anxiety, fear, and grieving
    2. Establishes a trusting, therapeutic nurse-client relationship
    3. Encourages the client/family to discuss their fears and concerns
    4. Allows the family to participate in care (if willing and able), such as ROM exercises and massages

✦ **NDx:** Self Care Deficit

- The nurse
    1. Assesses the client's ability to perform activities of daily living; provides assistance based on the level of the client's ability
    2. Monitors response or tolerance of activity
    3. Provides adequate rest periods between activities and therapy sessions
    4. Collaborates with physical, occupational, and speech therapy to identify and obtain needed assistive-adaptive devices

Continuing Care

- The nurse
    1. Provides a detailed plan of care at the time of discharge for clients to be transferred to a long-term-care or rehabilitation facility (rehabilitation may be lengthy)
    2. Assesses the client's and family's knowledge and understanding of the disease
    3. Provides oral and written information:
        a. Techniques to facilitate mobility
        b. Prevention of skin breakdown
        c. ROM exercises
    4. Reinforces the teaching provided by other health care disciplines
    5. Refers the client to local or community agencies for assistance in the home setting
    6. Ensures that adaptive equipment is available
    7. Refers the client to the Guillain-Barré Foundation for information about local resources and educational materials

GYNECOMASTIA

- Gynecomastia is a benign condition of breast enlargement, usually bilateral, in males.
- The condition is caused by proliferation of the glandular tissue, including mammary ducts and ductal stroma.
- Etiologic factors include drugs, aging, and obesity; underlying diseases causing estrogen excess, such as malnutrition, liver disease, or hyperthyroidism; and androgen deficiency states, such as aging or chronic renal failure.
- The client with gynecomastia is evaluated for breast cancer.

HANSEN'S DISEASE

See Leprosy.

HEADACHE, CLUSTER

OVERVIEW

- Cluster headaches are unilateral, oculotemporal, or oculofrontal. They are often described as excruciating, boring, and nonthrobbing; they occur every 8 to 24 hours daily at the same time for 6 to 8 weeks (hence the term cluster).
- The headache, which lasts for approximately 10 to 45 minutes, is accompanied by ipsilateral (same side) tearing of the eye, rhinorrhea or congestion, ptosis, miosis, bradycardia, flushing or pallor of the skin, increased intraocular pressure, and increased skin temperature.

COLLABORATIVE MANAGEMENT
Assessment

- The nurse records
  1. The sequence of events for the headaches
  2. Characteristics of the headaches
  3. Prescribed and nonprescribed drugs used for headache pain
  4. Alcohol intake
  5. Sleep pattern

Interventions

- The nurse
  1. Administers dehydroergotamine (Engomar, Gynergen◆), as ordered, before the onset of the expected attack or immediately at the onset
  2. Administers lidocaine 4% solution intranasal, as ordered, which has been found to decrease the pain associated with cluster headache

3. Administers methysergide (Sansert), prednisone (Deltasone, Winpred◆), or lithium citrate (Cibalith-S), as ordered
4. Instructs the client to wear sunglasses and sit away from the window while the headache is occurring
5. Provides oxygen, as ordered, to reduce cerebral blood flow and to inhibit the activity of the carotid bodies
6. Helps the client identify precipitating factors, such as bursts of anger, excessive physical activity, and excitement
7. Teaches the client the importance of a consistent sleep-wake cycle

Headache, Migraine

OVERVIEW

- A migraine headache is an episodic vascular disorder manifested by headache and often accompanied by nausea, vomiting, anorexia, and sensitivity to light (photophobia).
- Risk factors for migraine headaches include
  1. Premenstrual period
  2. Familial history
  3. Stress (can precipitate an episode)
  4. Contraceptive hormones
  5. Pregnancy
  6. Menopause
- Two forms of migraine headache are migraine *with* aura ("classic migraine") and migraine *without* aura.

Interventions

- For preventive therapy the client may take a
  1. Beta-blocker, such as propranolol (Inderal, Apo-Propranolol◆), an ergot derivative, such as methysergide (Sansert), or an antidepressant, such as amitriptyline (Elavil, Levate◆)
  2. Calcium channel blocker, such as verapamil (Calan) or monoamine oxidase inhibitor (e.g., phenelzine [Nardil]), as ordered

- Drugs used to treat pain after the headache starts include
  1. Ergotamine tartrate (Cafergot)
  2. Nonsteroidal anti-inflammatory drugs such as indomethacin (Indocin, Indocid◆) or naproxen (Naprosyn, Novonaprox◆)
  3. Antiemetics
- The nurse
  1. Teaches the client how to self-administer sumatriptan succinate (Imitrex) subcutaneously, as ordered
  2. Provides a dark, quiet environment
  3. Teaches behavior therapy techniques, such as relaxation or biofeedback
  4. Helps the client determine which factors precipitate episodes, such as certain foods, beverages, odors, or stress

Head and Neck Cancer

See Cancer, Head and Neck.

Head Trauma

See Trauma, Head.

Hearing Loss

OVERVIEW

- Hearing loss, one of the most common physical handicaps in North America, is generally thought of as conductive, sensorineural, or a combination of the two:
  1. *Conductive* hearing loss occurs when sound waves are blocked from coming to the inner-ear nerve fibers because of external-ear or middle-ear disor-

ders, such as an inflammatory process or an obstruction.

2. *Sensorineural* hearing loss is caused by a pathologic process of the inner ear or of the sensory fibers that lead to the cerebral cortex (VIII cranial nerve). Common causes are prolonged exposure to loud noise, ototoxic drugs, aging (presbycusis), metabolic and circulatory disorders, and bacterial or viral infections.

3. *Mixed conductive-sensorineural* hearing loss is a combination of the two.

- The etiology of hearing loss determines the degree to which the hearing loss can be corrected and the amount of normal hearing that will return.

ℰ Considerations for Elderly Clients

1. It is estimated that 30% of adults older than 60 years of age have some degree of hearing loss.
2. The prevalence increases sharply to 90% among elderly clients living in institutions.

COLLABORATIVE MANAGEMENT
Assessment

- The nurse assesses for *early* warning signs of a hearing loss: the client
  1. Frequently asks people to repeat statements
  2. Understands words better in small groups
  3. Strains to hear
  4. Turns the head to favor one ear or leans forward
  5. Complains of ringing in the ears
  6. Fails to respond when not looking in the direction of the sound
  7. Exhibits irritability
  8. Answers questions incorrectly
  9. Raises the volume of television or radio
  10. Avoids large groups
- The nurse also assesses for
  1. Abnormality of the tympanic membrane or ear canal
  2. Client's speaking softly or loudly
  3. Abnormal Rinne test:
     a. Air conduction greater than bone conduction in *conductive* hearing loss

    b. Bone conduction greater than air conduction in *sensorineural* hearing loss

  4. Abnormal Weber test:

    a. Lateralization to the affected ear in *conductive* hearing loss

    b. Lateralization to the unaffected ear in *sensorineural* hearing loss

  5. Client's hearing poorly in a loud environment; high-frequency soft-discriminating consonants are lost first, especially sounds such as *s, sh, f, th,* and *ch*

  6. Social isolation

Planning and Implementation

✦ **NDx:** Sensory/Perceptual Alterations (Auditory)

Nonsurgical Management

- The nurse
  1. Uses the written word if the client is able to see, read, and write
  2. Uses pictures of familiar phrases and objects
  3. Eliminates distracting noises when talking to the client
  4. Ensures that there is adequate lighting in the room, especially if the client can read lips, when appropriate
  5. Does not shout
  6. Keeps his or her hands and other objects away from the mouth when talking to the client
  7. Moves close to the client (positions self in front of the client) and speaks slowly and clearly
  8. Uses lower tones when communicating with a client with a high-frequency hearing loss
  9. Validates with the client the understanding of statements made by asking the client to repeat what was said
  10. Administers antibiotics, analgesics, and antiemetics, as ordered, to treat the underlying cause of the hearing loss
  11. Prevents sudden movements of the client or the client's bed
- Cochlear implant is a new and experimental method to treat a sensorineural hearing loss.
- Hearing with a hearing aid can be much different from normal hearing. The nurse

1. Encourages the client to start using the aid slowly to develop an appreciation for the device
2. Reminds the client that background noises will be amplified as well
3. Reminds the client to remove the hearing aid when he or she is fatigued

Surgical Management

- The type of surgery done depends on the cause of the hearing loss.
- *Tympanoplasty* involves reconstruction of the middle ear:
    1. Type I tympanoplasty is also known as a myringoplasty.
    2. Higher grades of tympanoplasties require more extensive reconstruction.
- The nurse provides preoperative care:
    1. Instills antibiotic drops and irrigates the ear
    2. Instructs the client to avoid people with upper respiratory infections, get adequate rest, and maintain nutrition and hydration
    3. Teaches the importance of deep breathing postoperatively (forceful coughing is avoided)
- The nurse provides postoperative care:
    1. Provides routine postoperative care
    2. Keeps the client flat with the operative ear up for at least 12 hours postoperatively
    3. Monitors ear canal packing and dressing for drainage; changes dressing when needed using sterile technique
    4. Administers prophylactic antibiotics, as ordered
    5. Uses communication techniques for the hearing impaired until the packing is removed
    6. Instructs the client in postoperative care and activity restrictions:
        a. Avoid straining when having a bowel movement.
        b. Do not drink through a straw for 2 to 3 weeks.
        c. Avoid air travel for 2 to 3 weeks.
        d. Avoid coughing excessively for 2 to 3 weeks.
        e. Stay away from people with colds.
        f. Blow the nose gently, one side at a time with mouth open.
        g. Avoid getting the head wet, washing hair, and showering for the first week after surgery.

h. Keep the affected ear dry for 6 weeks by placing a cotton ball coated with petroleum jelly in it; change the cotton ball daily.

i. Avoid rapid head movements, bouncing, and bending over for 3 weeks.

j. Change the dressing on the ear every day or as directed by the physician.

k. Report excessive drainage from the ear immediately to the physician.

- A *partial stapedectomy* or *complete stapedectomy* with a prosthesis is most effective for clients with otosclerosis.

- The nurse provides preoperative care:

    1. Assesses for signs and symptoms of external ear infection

    2. Reviews the expectations from surgery, including an initial increase in hearing loss

    3. Reinforces with the client that complications, such as permanent deafness, prolonged vertigo, infection, and facial nerve damage, are possible

- The nurse provides postoperative care:

    1. Provides routine postoperative care

    2. Reminds the client that hearing is temporarily worse after surgery as a result of ear packing and tissue swelling

    3. Administers antibiotics and analgesics, as ordered

    4. Observes for surgical damage to cranial nerves VII, VIII, and X, including facial weakness, changes in tactile sensation, and changes in taste sensation

    5. Administers antivertiginous drugs, such as meclizine hydrochloride (Antivert, Bonamine◆), and antiemetic drugs, such as droperidol (Inapsine), as ordered, for vertigo, nausea, and vomiting

    6. Assists the client with ambulation during the first 1 to 2 days after surgery, because vertigo is a common complaint

    7. Teaches the client the precautions listed earlier under postoperative care for the client having a tympanoplasty (see No. 6 on the previous page)

✦ NDx: Anxiety

- The nurse

    1. Uses special techniques for communicating with the hearing-impaired client (as listed under the di-

agnosis of Sensory Perceptual Alteration, "Non-surgical Management")
2. Suggests obtaining closed-captioned programming for the television and an amplifier for the telephone
3. Reminds the client to wear a hearing aid, if appropriate
4. Recommends formal lip reading and sign language classes
5. Helps the client identify support systems and resources to make social contact satisfying

Continuing Care

- The nurse
    1. Assists the client and family in identifying potential hazards at home to prevent falls associated with vertigo
    2. Provides verbal and written instructions about how to take medications and when to return for follow-up care
    3. Refers the client to the American Speech-Language-Hearing Association, the National Association of Hearing and Speech Agencies, and Self-Help for Hard-of-Hearing People (Shhh)

Heart Failure

OVERVIEW

- *Heart failure,* also called *cardiac failure* or *pump failure,* is the inability of the heart to pump sufficient blood to meet the demands of the body.
- Heart failure was once called *congestive heart failure (CHF),* but this term is not as accurate because congestion, or fluid, is not always evident.
- Heart failure results in inadequate tissue perfusion and pulmonary and systemic congestion.
- Basic cardiac physiologic mechanisms, such as stroke volume, heart rate, cardiac output, and contractility, are altered in heart failure.
- Compensatory mechanisms to maintain normal cardiac function are

1. Increased sympathetic nervous system response, causing increased heart rate, improved stroke volume (Starling's "law of the heart" states that increased myocardial stretch results in more forceful contraction, increasing stroke volume and cardiac output), and arterial vasoconstriction (which also increases afterload)
2. Sodium and water retention (caused by activation of the renin-angiotensin-aldosterone mechanism when blood flow to the kidney decreases)
3. Myocardial hypertrophy, which provides more muscle mass, resulting in more effective cardiac contractility, and further increasing cardiac output

- Compensatory mechanisms may eventually cause harmful effects on pump function, contributing to increased myocardial oxygen consumption, causing the signs and symptoms of heart failure.
- The classifications of heart failure include
  1. *Systolic versus diastolic dysfunction:*
     a. Systolic dysfunction results when the heart is unable to eject adequate amounts of blood into the circulation, resulting in diminished tissue perfusion.
     b. Diastolic dysfunction represents a relaxation and filling abnormality of the ventricles; an increase in *preload* results in increased volume and pressure in the pulmonary vessels and pulmonary and/or systemic congestion.
  2. *Left versus right ventricular failure:*
     a. Left ventricular (LV) failure, which usually occurs first, is caused by hypertensive disease, coronary artery disease (CAD), or valvular insufficiency, involving the mitral or aortic valves; pulmonary congestion and edema usually signal the onset of LV failure.
     b. Right ventricular (RV) failure is most often caused by LV failure but may result from RV myocardial infarction (MI).
     c. Sustained pulmonary hypertension also develops into RV failure, leading to systemic venous congestion and peripheral edema.
  3. *Low- versus high-cardiac output syndrome:*
     a. Low-output syndrome, the more common type, occurs when the heart fails as a pump, resulting in impaired peripheral circulation and vasoconstriction.

b. High-output syndrome results when cardiac output remains normal or above normal but the metabolic needs of the body are not met; causes include increased metabolic needs as seen in hyperthyroidism, fever, and pregnancy, or it may be triggered by hyperkinetic conditions, such as arteriovenous fistulas or Paget's disease.

4. *Functional status:*
   a. Heart failure may also be categorized by its effect on the client's functional status.
   b. Several scales to assess functional status are used; the New York Heart Association categories are frequently used.

H

Considerations for Elderly Clients

1. Heart failure occurs most commonly in older adults; seventy-five percent of clients with heart failure are older than 60 years of age. It is the most common cause of hospitalization for adults older than 65.

COLLABORATIVE MANAGEMENT

Assessment

- The nurse records the client's
  1. Past medical history:
     a. Hypertension
     b. Angina
     c. MI
     d. Rheumatic heart disease
     e. Valvular disorders
     f. Endocarditis
     g. Pericarditis
  2. Perception of breathing pattern
  3. Fluid volume status; urinary pattern
  4. Response to activity
  5. LV failure complaints:
     a. Change in ability to perform ADLs
     b. Unusual fatigue
     c. Feelings of heaviness in arms and legs
     d. Mental status changes, confusion
     e. Nocturnal cough
     f. Dyspnea; orthopnea
  6. RV failure complaints:
     a. Peripheral edema

b. Weight gain

c. Gastrointestinal problems, such as nausea and anorexia

d. Diuresis at night

e. Shoes fit tighter

f. Indentations develop on their swollen feet from shoes or socks

g. Unable to wear ring because of swollen fingers

7. Nutritional history

- The nurse assesses for

1. Clinical manifestations of LV failure:

   a. Weakness

   b. Fatigue

   c. Dizziness

   d. Confusion

   e. Pulmonary congestion (e.g., breathlessness)

   f. Postural hypotension

   g. Increased heart size by palpating the precordium

   h. Tachycardia

   i. S_3 or S_4 heart sounds

   j. Crackles and wheezes

2. Clinical manifestations of RV failure:

   a. Jugular venous distention

   b. Hepatomegaly

   c. Dependent edema

   d. Ascites

3. Possible kidney function study abnormalities, such as elevated blood urea nitrogen (BUN)

4. Abnormal arterial blood gas (low arterial oxygen)

5. Enlarged heart on x-ray

6. Dysrhythmias, ventricular hypertrophy, myocardial ischemia on electrocardiogram (ECG)

7. Elevated pulmonary artery and pulmonary artery wedge pressures in LV failure

Considerations for the Elderly

1. Clients over 65 who have atrial fibrillation or have evidence of thyroid disease should have thyroxine (T4) and thyroid-stimulating hormone (TSH) levels drawn.

Planning and Implementation

✦ NDx: Decreased Cardiac Output

Nonsurgical Management

- The nurse administers drug therapy as ordered to reduce afterload
    1. Angiotension-converting enzyme (ACE) inhibitiors, a group of arterial vasodilators such as enalapril (Vasotec), moexipril (Univasc) and captopril (Capoten) to reduce arterial resistance, decreasing pulmonary artery wedge pressure and increasing stroke volume and cardiac output:
        a. These drugs may cause a rapid drop in blood pressure especially in those with a systolic blood pressure less than 100, are older than 75, have a serum sodium less than 135, or are volume depleted.

- To reduce preload in clients in heart failure who have congestion with total body sodium and water overload, the nurse
    1. Collaborates with the dietician and client to select foods that meet a sodium-restricted diet and to understand the importance of eliminating table salt or possibly salt used in cooking
    2. Limits the clients with excessive aldosterone secretion who experience thirst to 2 L/day of fluids including IV fluids
    3. Weighs the client every morning before breakfast using the same scale

- When diet and fluid restrictions are not effective the nurse administers medications, as ordered
    1. Diuretics, such as furosemide (Lasix, Furoside✦), torsemide (Demadex), and ethacrynic acid (Edecrin) are most effective for treating fluid volume overload:
        a. Elderly clients receiving loop diuretic are prone to dehydration, especially those with type II diabetes mellitus
        b. Thiazide diuretics may be used in elderly clients with mild volume overload to avoid the excessive diuresis and dehydration that may occur with loop diuretics

- The nurse monitors for and and prevents potassium deficiency from diuretic therapy

1. If the client's potassium is below 40 mEq/L:
   a. Add a potassium sparing diuretic to the regimen
   b. Increase client's intake of potassium-rich foods
   c. Potassium supplement
- The nurse recognizes that clients with renal problems may develop *hyperkalemia*. Renal problems are indicated by a creatinine level greater than 1.8.
- The nurse administers venous vasodilators as ordered for the client in heart failure with persistent dyspnea:
   1. Vasodilators, such as nitrates (nitroglycerin, isosorbide dinitrate), to increase cardiac output by dilating peripheral vascular vessels and reducing impedance or resistance to LV outflow
- The nurse administers medications as ordered to clients in heart failure with sinus rhythm and atrial fibrillation:
   1. Digoxin (Lanoxin) increases contractility, reduces heart rate, slows conduction through the arteriovenous node, and inhibits sympathetic activity while enhancing parasympathetic activity:
      a. Elderly clients particulary those who are hypokalemic are suseptible to digoxin toxicity

✦ NDx: Activity Intolerance

- The nurse
   1. Provides for periods of uninterrupted rest
   2. Assesses the client's response to mild exercise, such as moving from the bed to the chair; checks for changes in blood pressure (BP) and pulse (increase in BP of more than 20 mmHg or pulse rate increase of more than 20 beats per minute)
   3. Assesses for increased fatigue, dyspnea, or chest pain when activity increases

✦ NDx: Potential for Pulmonary Edema

- The nurse
   1. Assesses the client with heart failure for acute *pulmonary edema,* a life-threatening event; clinical manifestations include extreme anxiety; tachycardia; "air hunger"; moist cough productive of frothy, blood-tinged sputum; and cold, clammy, cyanotic skin, crackles in lung bases, disorientation, and confusion
   2. Administers rapid-acting diuretics, such as furosemide, given IV push over 1 to 2 minutes, usu-

ally starting with 40 mg and repeating the dose if needed

3. Provides oxygen, as ordered, and maintains the client in a high-Fowler's position
4. Administers morphine sulfate intravenously, 1 to 2 mg at a time, to reduce venous return (preload)
5. Administers other drugs, as ordered, such as bronchodilators and vasodilators
6. Monitors the client carefully to determine the necessity of intubation and mechanical ventilation

Continuing Care

H

- The nurse
  1. Teaches the client and family that heart failure is a chronic disorder for many clients
  2. Reviews activity restrictions based on the client's functional status
  3. Collaborates with the physical and occupational therapists to plan an individualized cardiac rehabilitation program for the client, including exercises
  4. Assists the client in identifying factors that might precipitate symptoms
  5. Instructs the client to watch for and report to the physician: a weight gain of more than 2 pounds (0.9 kg) per day for 2 successive days, swelling of the ankles and feet, persistent cough, or frequent urination at night
  6. Provides oral and written instructions concerning medications, such as digoxin administration, including the importance of monitoring heart rate and rhythm, and side effects
  7. Reviews the signs and symptoms of hypokalemia for clients on diuretics and provides information on foods high in potassium
  8. Recommends the client restrict dietary sodium and provides written instructions on low-salt diets and identifying food flavorings to use as a substitute for salt, such as lemon, garlic, and herbs
  9. Teaches the client the importance of lifestyle changes, including activity and dietary restrictions
  10. Encourages the client to verbalize fears and concerns
  11. Refers the client to home health services, as needed, and the American Heart Association for information and support groups

HEMOPHILIA

OVERVIEW

- Hemophilia is a group of several hereditary bleeding disorders resulting from deficiencies of specific clotting factors that impair the hemostatic response and the capacity to form a stable fibrin clot.
- *Hemophilia A* (classic hemophilia) is a deficiency of factor VIII and accounts for 80% of all cases.
- *Hemophilia B* (Christmas disease) is a deficiency of factor IX and accounts for 20% of all cases.
- Hemophilia is an X-linked recessive trait; female carriers risk transmitting the gene for hemophilia to half of their daughters (who are then carriers) and to half of their sons (who will have overt hemophilia).
- Abnormal bleeding occurs, which may be mild, moderate, or severe, depending on the degree of factor deficiency in response to any trauma.

COLLABORATIVE MANAGEMENT

- The nurse assesses for
    1. Excessive hemorrhage from minor cuts or abrasions
    2. Joint and muscle hemorrhages (degenerative)
    3. Tendency to bruise easily
    4. Prolonged postoperative hemorrhage
    5. Prolonged partial thromboplastin time, normal bleeding time, and normal prothrombin time
- Management includes administration of factor VIII cryoprecipitate.

HEMORRHOIDS

OVERVIEW

- Hemorrhoids are unnaturally swollen or distended veins in the anorectal region that are common and not significant unless they cause pain or bleeding.

- Increased intra-abdominal pressure causes elevated systemic and portal venous pressure, which is transmitted to the anorectal veins.
- *Internal* hemorrhoids cannot be seen on inspection of the perianal area and lie above the anal sphincter.
- *External* hemorrhoids can be seen on inspection and lie below the anal sphincter.
- *Prolapsed* hemorrhoids can become thrombosed or inflamed, or they can bleed.
- Common causes of repeated increased abdominal pressure are straining at stool, pregnancy, and portal hypertension.

COLLABORATIVE MANAGEMENT

Assessment

- Common symptoms are bleeding, which is characteristically bright red and found on toilet tissue or outside the stool, pain associated with thrombosis, itching, and mucous discharge.
- Diagnosis is made by inspection, digital examination, and proctoscopy, if needed.

Interventions

Nonsurgical Management

- Conservative treatment is aimed at reducing symptoms, including application of cold packs to the anorectal area followed by hot sitz baths; witch hazel soaks and topical anesthetics such as lidocaine (Xylocaine); over-the-counter remedies such as Nupercainal ointment; high-fiber diets and fluids to promote regular bowel movements without straining; and stool softeners.

Surgical Management

- Surgical methods are indicated for recurring symptoms, including sclerotherapy, elastic band ligation, cryosurgery, and hemorrhoidectomy.
- The nurse teaches clients with hemorrhoids
    1. To adhere to a high-fiber, high-fluid diet to promote regular bowel patterns
    2. To utilize the local treatments for symptom relief
- Postoperative care includes
    1. Assisting the client to a side-lying position
    2. Keeping ice packs over the dressing, if ordered, until the packing is removed by the physician

3. Utilizing moist heat (e.g., sitz baths) three to four times a day after the first 12 hours postoperatively:
   a. Vasodilation from the sitz bath redirects blood to the rectal area, which might cause the client to feel faint. This may be prevented by placing an ice bag on the client's head during the sitz bath.
4. Administering stool softeners, such as docusate sodium (Colace), as ordered
5. Administering opioid analgesia postoperatively and prior to the first defecation
6. Monitoring for urinary retention, especially for clients who have undergone hemorrhoidectomy

HEMOTHORAX

- Hemothorax is a common problem following blunt chest trauma or penetrating injuries.
- *Simple hemothorax* is a blood loss of less than 1500 mL into the thoracic cavity; *massive hemothorax* is a blood loss of more than 1500 mL.
- The bleeding is caused by injuries to the lung parenchyma and is associated with rib and sternal fractures.
- Massive intrathoracic bleeding stems from injury to the heart, great vessels, or major systemic arteries.
- Physical assessment findings depend on the size of the hemothorax
    1. Asymptomatic for small hemothorax
    2. Respiratory distress for large hemothorax with diminished breath sounds and a dull percussion note on the affected side
- Interventions are aimed at blood evacuation to normalize pulmonary function and prevent infection and include anterior and posterolateral chest tube insertion.
- The nurse
    1. Monitors the client's vital signs
    2. Monitors for increased blood loss
    3. Measures intake and output
    4. Assesses the client's response to chest tubes. Open thoracotomy may be considered if there is an initial evacuation of 1500–2000 mL of blood or persistent bleeding over 200 mL/hr over 3 hours.

5. Administers intravenous fluids and blood, as ordered
   a. Autotransfusion of blood lost through chest drainage may be considered.

HEPATIC ABSCESSES

See Abscesses, Hepatic.

HEPATITIS

OVERVIEW

- Hepatitis is the widespread inflammation of liver cells, resulting in enlargement of the liver and congestion with inflammatory cells.
- Viral hepatitis is the most prevalent type, caused by one of five common viruses.
  1. *Hepatitis A virus (HAV):*
     a. HAV is spread by the fecal-oral route, by the oral ingestion of fecal contaminants, or by oral-anal sexual activity. It is characterized by a mild course and often goes unrecognized. HAV is the most common type of viral hepatitis.
     b. Sources of infection include contaminated water, shellfish caught in contaminated water, and food contaminated by food handlers infected with the HAV.
     c. The incubation period is usually between 15 and 50 days with an average of 4 weeks.
  2. *Hepatitis B virus (HBV):*
     a. Formerly known as serum hepatitis, HBV is transmitted via the percutaneous and permucosal route by contamination with blood and serous fluids.
     b. Lower concentrations of HBV are also found in semen, vaginal fluid, and saliva.

   c. It is also spread via sexual contact, sharing needles, accidental needlesticks or injuries from sharp instruments, blood transfusion, hemodialysis, acupuncture, tattooing, ear/body piercing, and perinatal.

   d. The clinical course is varied, with an insidious onset and mild symptoms to serious sequelae, such as fulminant hepatitis, chronic active or persistent hepatitis, cirrhosis, or hepatocellular carcinoma.

   e. The incubation period is generally between 45 and 180 days.

   f. Chronic liver disease develops in approximately 5% of clients with acute HBV infection.

3. *Hepatitis C virus (HCV):*

   a. The causative virus is similar to HBV and it is transmitted primarily through blood and blood products and sexual contact.

   b. People at risk are those who had blood transfusions prior to July of 1992, hemodialysis patients, recipients of clotting factors before 1987, infants born to infected women, IV drug abusers, and persons with multiple sex partners.

   c. The incubation period is 14 to 180 days, with the average incubation period being 42–63 days.

   d. Estimated that only 225,000 of the 4.5 million Americans with hepatitis C know they are infected.

   e. Chronic liver disease occurs in 705 of those infected; leading indicator for liver transplant.

   f. Treated with interferon alpha; June, 1998, combination drug of interferon and ribaoirin (Rebetron) was approved.

4. *Delta hepatitis (Hepatitis D virus or HDV):*

   a. Hepatitis D is caused by a defective RNA virus that needs the helper function of HBV. HDV coinfects with HBD and needs its presence for viral replications.

   b. Incubation period is 14–56 days.

   c. In the U.S., Canada, and northern Europe it is most prevalent in people exposed to blood and blood products (drug addicts and hemophiliacs).

5. *Hepatitis E virus (HEV)*

   a. HEV was originally identified by its association with epidemics of hepatitis in the Indian subcontinent, and has since been found in epidemics in Asia, Africa, and Mexico.

    b. In the United States and Canada, HEV has oc-
    curred in people who have visited these endemic
    areas.

    c. HEV is transmitted by the oral-fecal route and
    resembles HAV.

- Toxic and drug-induced hepatitis result from exposure to hepatotoxins such as industrial toxins, alcohol, or medication.
- Hepatitis may occur as a secondary infection during the course of other viral infections, such as cytomegalovirus, Epstein-Barr virus, herpes simplex virus, and varicella zoster virus.
- Fulminant hepatitis is a failure of the liver cells to regenerate, with progression of the necrotic process that is frequently fatal.

- When liver inflammation persists longer than 6 months it is considered chronic hepatitis.

COLLABORATIVE MANAGEMENT
Assessment

- The nurse records the client's
  1. Known exposure to hepatitis
  2. Recent blood transfusions
  3. History of hemodialysis
  4. Sexual preferences
  5. Intravenous drug use
  6. Recent ear piercing
  7. Recent tattooing
  8. Living accommodations, including crowded facilities
  9. Health care employment history
  10. Recent travel to foreign countries
  11. Recent ingestion of shellfish or contaminated water
- The nurse assesses for clinical manifestations of viral hepatitis:
  1. Weakness and fatigue
  2. Loss of appetite
  3. General malaise
  4. Myalgias (muscle pain)
  5. Arthritis-like joint pain
  6. Dull headaches
  7. Irritability
  8. Depression
  9. Nausea and vomiting

10. Liver tenderness in the right upper quadrant
11. Jaundice of the skin, mucous membranes, and sclera
12. Dark urine
13. Clay-colored stools
14. Rashes
15. Fever
16. Elevated serum liver enzymes
17. Elevated total bilirubin (serum and urine)
18. Serologic markers for hepatitis A, B, C, or D

- The clinical manifestations of toxic and drug-induced hepatitis depend on the causative agent.

Interventions

- The nurse
    1. Maintains physical rest alternating with periods of activity to promote liver cell regeneration by reducing the liver's metabolic needs
    2. Promotes emotional and psychologic rest
- A special diet is not required, although increased carbohydrates and calories with moderate fat and protein may be given.
- The nurse
    1. Determines food preferences
    2. Collaborates with the dietitian to provide small, frequent meals
    3. Gives supplemental vitamins, as ordered
    4. Administers antiemetics, such as trimethobenzamide hydrochloride (Tigan, Tegamide) or dimenhydrinate (Dramamine, Travamine◆), as ordered, to relieve nausea
    5. Provides mouth care to stimulate appetite
- Liver transplant may be performed for clients with chronic hepatitis

Continuing Care

- The nurse provides health teaching about
    1. Modes of transmission of hepatitis
    2. Observation of measures to prevent infection transmission
    3. Avoiding alcohol and nonprescription hepatotoxic drugs
    4. Determination of activity tolerance and rest
    5. Eating small, frequent meals of high-carbohydrate and low-fat foods

6. Avoiding sexual activity until hepatitis B surface antigen (HBsAg) testing results are negative

Hernia

OVERVIEW

- A hernia is a weakness in the abdominal muscle wall through which a segment of bowel or other structure protrudes; it results from a defect in the integrity of the muscular wall and increased intra-abdominal pressure.
- Common types of hernias include
  1. *Indirect inguinal* hernias, which occur through the inguinal ring and follow the spermatic cord through the inguinal canal
  2. *Direct inguinal* hernias, which pass through the abdominal wall in an area of muscle weakness
  3. *Femoral* hernias, which occur through the femoral ring as a plug of fat in the femoral canal, which enlarges and pulls the peritoneum and the bladder into the sac
  4. *Umbilical* hernias, which are congenital (infancy) or acquired as a result of increased intra-abdominal pressure, most often in obese people
  5. *Incisional* (ventral) hernias, which occur at the site of a previous surgical incision as a result of inadequate healing, postoperative wound infection, inadequate nutrition, or obesity
- *Reducible* hernias allow the contents of the hernial sac to be reduced or placed back into the abdominal cavity.
- *Irreducible,* or incarcerated, hernias cannot be reduced or placed back into the abdominal cavity.
- *Strangulated* hernias result when the blood supply to the herniated segment of the bowel is cut off by pressure from the hernial ring, causing ischemia and obstruction of the bowel loop; this can lead to bowel necrosis and perforation.

ⓔ Considerations for Elderly Clients

1. The elderly client with a strangulated hernia may not complain of pain but usually has nausea and vomiting.

361

2. Direct inguinal hernias occur more often in the elderly.

COLLABORATIVE MANAGEMENT
Assessment

- The nurse assesses for
  1. Presence of the hernia on abdominal inspection
  2. Presence of bowel sounds (absence may indicate obstruction)
  3. Palpable hernia and its location

Interventions

Nonsurgical Management

- The nurse teaches the client that no attempt should be made to reduce an incarcerated hernia.
- A truss (a pad with firm support) may be used for elderly or debilitated clients who are poor surgical risks.

Surgical Management

- *Herniorrhaphy,* the surgical treatment of choice, involves replacing the contents of the hernial sac into the abdominal cavity and closing the opening.
- *Hernioplasty* may be required to reinforce the weakened muscular wall with mesh, fascia, or wire.
- The nurse provides routine preoperative care.
- The nurse gives the client postoperative instructions:
  1. Avoid coughing
  2. Deep breathe and turn frequently to promote lung expansion
  3. For indirect inguinal hernia repair, wear a scrotal support and apply an ice bag to the scrotum to prevent swelling
  4. Elevate the scrotum with a soft pillow
  5. Encourage early ambulation, if the client is able
  6. Use techniques to stimulate voiding, such as allowing the male client to stand
  7. Ensure an intake of at least 1500 to 2500 mL of fluids per day
- The nurse catheterizes the client every 6 to 8 hours if the client is unable to void.

Continuing Care

- The nurse teaches the client
  1. How to care for the incision

2. To limit activity, including avoiding lifting and straining, for 2 weeks after surgery
3. To inspect the incision for redness, tenderness, swelling, and drainage and report the findings to the physician

HERNIA, HIATAL

OVERVIEW

- Esophageal or diaphragmatic hiatal hernias occur when the lower portion of the esophagus, or a portion of the stomach, or both, move into the thorax through the esophageal hiatus.
- There are two major types of hiatal hernia:
    1. *Sliding* hernias, which occur when the esophagogastric junction and a portion of the fundus of the stomach are displaced through the hiatus into the thorax, with the hernia moving freely and sliding into and out of the thorax when there are changes in position or intra-abdominal pressure increases
    2. *Paraesophageal* or rolling hernias, which occur when the gastroesophageal junction stays below the diaphragm but the fundus and portions of the greater curvature of the stomach roll into the thorax beside the esophagus

COLLABORATIVE MANAGEMENT

Assessment

- The nurse assesses for
    1. General appearance and nutritional status
    2. Heartburn
    3. Regurgitation (esophageal reflux)
    4. Chest pain that may mimic angina
    5. Dysphagia
    6. Belching
    7. Feeling of fullness after eating
    8. Feeling of breathlessness or suffocation
    9. Increased symptoms when in a recumbent position

- Barium swallow study with fluoroscopy is the most specific diagnostic test

Interventions

Nonsurgical Management

- The nurse
    1. Administers antacids and histamine receptor antagonists as ordered, in an attempt to control esophageal reflux and its symptoms
    2. Teaches the client to avoid fatty foods, coffee, tea, cola, chocolate, and alcohol, as well as spicy and acidic foods, such as orange juice
    3. Encourages the client to eat four to six small meals per day
    4. Teaches the client to avoid nighttime snacking to ensure that the stomach is empty
    5. Encourages weight reduction since obesity increases intra-abdominal pressure
    6. Elevates the head of the bed 8 to 12 inches (3.2 to 4.8 cm) to reduce the incidence of esophageal reflux
    7. Instructs the client to avoid lying down several hours after eating; straining or excessive vigorous exercise; or wearing tight, constrictive clothing

Surgical Management

- Elective surgery is indicated when the risk of complications such as aspiration are high and damage from chronic reflux is severe.
- The nurse provides routine preoperative care. In addition, the nurse
    1. Teaches the client to reduce weight and stop smoking, if indicated
    2. Informs the client that he or she will have a nasogastric tube (NG) after surgery
- Surgical approaches for sliding hernias involve reinforcement of the lower esophageal sphincter (LES) to restore sphincter competence and prevent reflux, through some degree of *fundoplication,* or the wrapping of a portion of the stomach fundus around the distal esophagus to anchor it and reinforce the LES.
- The nurse provides postoperative care similar to that for any client with esophageal surgery.
    1. The nurse assesses for complications of surgery, such as temporary dysphagia after oral feeding begins, gas bloat syndrome, atelectasis or pneumonia, and obstruction of the NG tube.

2. The nurse also
    a. Elevates the head of the bed at least 30 degrees
    b. Supports the incisional area during coughing and deep-breathing
    c. Ensures correct placement and patency of the NG tube
    d. Supervises the first oral feedings
    e. Teaches the client to avoid drinking carbonated beverages, eating gas-producing foods (especially high-fat foods), chewing gum, and drinking with a straw
    f. Encourages frequent position changes and ambulation

Continuing Care

- The nurse teaches the client
    1. Activity restriction following hiatal hernia repair, including avoidance of straining and lifting and restriction on climbing stairs
    2. Inspection of the surgical wound daily and reporting the incidence of swelling, redness, tenderness, or discharge to the physician
    3. The importance of reporting fever to the physician
    4. Avoidance of prolonged coughing episodes to prevent dehiscence of the fundoplication
    5. Smoking cessation
    6. Diet restrictions, including modifying the size and timing of meals, avoiding irritating foods or liquids, and reporting recurrence of reflux symptoms to the physician

HERPES SIMPLEX, GENITAL

OVERVIEW

- Genital herpes simplex is a sexually transmitted disease of the herpes simplex virus (HSV).
- The two types of herpes simplex are
    1. *Type 1* HSV, which causes most nongenital lesions, including cold sores
    2. *Type 2* HSV, which causes most genital lesions

- The incubation period is 2 to 20 days, with the average being 1 week.

COLLABORATIVE MANAGEMENT

Assessment

- The nurse assesses for
  1. Tingling sensation on the skin
  2. Appearance of vesicles (blisters) in a characteristic cluster on the penis, scrotum, vulva, perineum, vagina, cervix, and/or perianal region
  3. Headaches
  4. Fever
  5. Generalized malaise
  6. Painful urination
  7. Positive result of a culture
- After lesions heal, the virus remains in a dormant state in the nerve ganglia.
- Periodically, the virus may activate, and episodes of infection recur.
- Activation may be stimulated by factors that include stress, fever, sunburn, menses, and sexual activity.
- Long-term complications of genital herpes include the risks of cervical cancer, neonatal transmission, and HIV infection.

Interventions

- Viral shedding occurs, and the client is infectious.
- Acyclovir, an antiviral drug, partially controls signs and symptoms and accelerates healing. The Centers for Disease Control and Prevention (CDC) recommends 200 mg orally five times a day for·7 to 10 days for the first infection.
- Most recurrent episodes do not benefit from treatment with acyclovir.
- Management is focused on decreasing pain, promoting healing without secondary infection, decreasing viral excretion, and preventing transmission of the infection.
- The nurse
  1. Teaches the client to prevent infection by
     a. Encouraging genital hygiene and keeping the skin clean and dry
     b. Wearing gloves while applying ointments
     c. Avoiding sexual activity when lesions are present

d. Using condoms during all sexual activity
2. Helps clients cope with the diagnosis:
   a. Assesses the client's response to the diagnosis of genital herpes
   b. Is sensitive and supportive during care
   c. Refers the client to support groups, such as HELP

HIATAL HERNIA

See Hernia, Hiatal.

HIV INFECTION

See AIDS.

HODGKIN'S DISEASE

See Hodgkin's Lymphoma.

HODGKIN'S LYMPHOMA

OVERVIEW

- Hodgkin's lymphoma is a cancer originating in a single lymph node or a single chain of nodes. The lymphoid tissues within the node undergo malignant transformation. These nodes contain a specific transformed cell type, the Reed-Sternberg cell, which is a characteristic marker of Hodgkin's lymphoma.

- The initially localized disease first metastasizes to other adjacent lymphoid structures and eventually invades nonlymphoid tissues.
- This malignancy occurs primarily in young adults, although another peak occurs among people older than 50 years of age.
- Factors implicated as causes include viral infections and exposure to alkylating chemical agents.

COLLABORATIVE MANAGEMENT

- The nurse assesses for staging of Hodgkin's disease, which determines treatment:
    1. Stage Ia: confined to a single lymph node region or only one extranodal site
    2. Stage Ib: confined to a single lymph node region or only one extranodal site, and with the client experiencing symptoms of persistent fever, night sweats, and weight loss
    3. Stage IIa: confined to either two or more lymph node regions on the same side or contiguous extranodal sites on the same side of the diaphragm
    4. Stage IIb: confined to either two or more lymph node regions on the same side or contiguous extranodal sites on the same side of the diaphragm, and with the client experiencing systemic symptoms
    5. Stage IIIa: extending to lymph node regions on both sides of the diaphragm
    6. Stage IIIb: extending to lymph node regions on both sides of the diaphragm, and with the client experiencing systemic symptoms
    7. Stage IIIc: extending to lymph node regions on both sides of the diaphragm, with the client experiencing systemic symptoms and involvement of the spleen
    8. Stage IV: with widely disseminated foci of involvement
- The nurse assesses for
    1. Greatly enlarged, painless lymph nodes (usually the earliest manifestation)
    2. Persistent fever
    3. Malaise
    4. Night sweats
    5. Weight loss

- Treatment includes extensive external radiation of involved lymph node regions for stages I and II without mediastinal node involvement; more extensive disease requires radiation coupled with aggressive multiagent chemotherapy.
- The nurse monitors for and teaches the side effects of radiation or drug therapy:
    1. Infection
    2. Bleeding
    3. Anemia
    4. Nausea and vomiting
    5. Skin irritation and breakdown at the site of radiation
    6. Impaired hepatic function
    7. Permanent sterility in men receiving radiation in an inverted Y pattern to the abdominopelvic region along with specific chemotherapeutic agents (Men are given the option of sperm storage in a sperm bank before treatment begins.)

HSV

See Herpes Simplex, Genital.

Huntington's Chorea

OVERVIEW

- Huntington's chorea is a hereditary disorder transmitted as an autosomal dominant trait at the time of conception.
- It is most prevalent in people of western European ancestry.
- The two main symptoms of the disease are progressive mental status changes, leading to dementia, and choreiform movements.
- Other clinical manifestations of Huntington's chorea include poor balance, hesitant or explosive speech,

dysphagia, impaired respirations, and bowel and bladder incontinence. Mental status changes include decreased attention span, poor judgment, memory loss, personality changes, and later, dementia.

COLLABORATIVE MANAGEMENT

- There is no known cure or treatment of the disease.
- The only way to prevent transmission of the gene is for those affected to refrain from having children.
- Genetic testing is an option for people at risk of Huntington's chorea to see if they have the gene on chromosome 4; results of the test are, however, subject to error.
- Management of the disease is symptomatic.
- Nursing interventions are directed toward treating nursing diagnoses:
    1. Impaired physical mobility
    2. Altered nutrition: less than body requirements
    3. Total incontinence
    4. Total self-care deficit
    5. Body image disturbance and altered role performance
    6. High risk for injury
    7. Ineffective airway clearance, ineffective breathing pattern, and impaired gas exchange
- As the symptoms progress, the client's status deteriorates, and death occurs from complications of immobility, such as pneumonia or sepsis.

HYDROCELE

OVERVIEW

- A hydrocele is a cystic mass, usually filled with straw-colored fluid, that forms around the testes.
- A hydrocele is the result of a disorder in the lymphatic drainage of the scrotum, causing a swelling of the tunica vaginalis, which surrounds the testes.

COLLABORATIVE MANAGEMENT

- A hydrocele may be aspirated via needle and syringe or surgically removed.

- The nurse provides postoperative care:
    1. Informs the client that if an incision drain is present, there is usually some serosanguineous drainage for the first 24 to 48 hours after surgery
    2. Teaches the client the importance of wearing a scrotal support to keep the scrotal dressing in place and keep the scrotum elevated to prevent edema
    3. Assesses the client for pain and infection
    4. Reassures the client that swelling will subside over several weeks

HYDRONEPHROSIS, HYDROURETER, AND URETHRAL STRICTURE

OVERVIEW

- Several disorders are associated with obstruction of the outflow of urine.
- In *hydronephrosis,* the kidney becomes enlarged as urine accumulates in the renal pelvis and the calyces; obstruction within the pelvis or ureteropelvic junction results in renal pelvic distention, and extensive damage to the vasculature and renal tubules can result.
- *Hydroureter* is the obstruction of the ureter at the point of the iliac vessel crossing or the ureterovesical entry; dilation of the ureter occurs at the point proximal to the obstruction as urine accumulates.
- A *urethral stricture* is the most distal point of obstruction, with bladder distention occurring before hydroureter and hydronephrosis.
- *Urinary tract obstruction* results in direct pressure buildup on the tissue, causing structural damage.
- Within the nephron, the tubular filtrate pressure increases as drainage through the collecting system is impaired, resulting in decreased glomerular filtration and renal failure.
- Causes of hydronephrosis and hydroureter include tumors, stones, trauma, congenital structural defects, and retroperitoneal fibrosis; pregnancy may cause ureteral dilation.

- Urethral stricture occurs from chronic inflammation.

COLLABORATIVE MANAGEMENT

- The nurse records the client's
    1. History of known renal or urologic disorders
    2. Childhood urinary tract problems
    3. Pattern of urination, including amount and frequency
    4. Description of urine, including color, clarity, and odor
    5. Report of symptoms, including flank and/or abdominal pain, chills, fever, and malaise
- The nurse assesses for
    1. Flank asymmetry and pain
    2. Abdominal tenderness or pain
    3. Bladder distention
    4. Urine leakage with abdominal pressure
    5. Bacteria or white blood cells in the urine if infection is present
    6. Enlarged ureter or kidney on x-ray and intravenous pyelography
- Urinary retention and potential for infection are primary problems.
- Treatment measures are aimed at correcting the cause of obstruction.
- Failure to treat the cause of urinary obstruction may result in renal failure.

HYDROURETER

See Hydronephrosis, Hydroureter, and Urethral Stricture.

HYPERALDOSTERONISM

OVERVIEW

- Hyperaldosteronism is defined as an increased secretion of aldosterone by the adrenal glands, resulting in a state of mineralocorticoid excess.

- Primary hyperaldosteronism (Conn's syndrome), due to excessive secretion of aldosterone, is usually caused by the presence of an adenoma.
- Secondary hyperaldosteronism, the continuous excessive secretion of aldosterone resulting from higher levels of angiotensin II, is usually caused by poor renal perfusion, mechanical obstruction of the renal vessels, or the use of thiazide diuretics.
- Hyperaldosteronism is manifested by hypernatremia, hypokalemia, metabolic alkalosis, peripheral edema, hypertension, hypokalemia, hypernatremia.

🐾 Women's Health Considerations

H

1. Hyperaldosteronism occurs three times more frequently in women than in men.

COLLABORATIVE MANAGEMENT

- *Adrenalectomy* is the surgery of choice in most cases, either unilateral or bilateral
- The nurse
  1. Provides a low-sodium diet preoperatively as ordered but no restrictions postoperatively
  2. Prior to surgery or if surgery is inadvisable, administers as ordered Aldactone A, Sincomen (mli), a potassium-sparing diuretic and aldosterone antagonist, to promote fluid balance
  3. Administers temporary glucocorticoid replacement as ordered if a unilateral adrenalectomy is performed or permanent replacement if a bilateral adrenalectomy is performed
  4. Instructs the client about side effects of spironolactone:
     a. Hyperkalemia (in the client with impaired renal function or excessive potassium intake)
     b. Hyponatremia
     c. Gynecomastia
     d. Diarrhea
     e. Urticaria, rash
     f. Inability to maintain an erection, hirsutism, and amenorrhea
  5. Administers potassium supplements, if needed

HYPERCALCEMIA

OVERVIEW

- Hypercalcemia is a serum calcium level exceeding 10 mg/dL or 2.5 mmol/L.
- Small increases in serum calcium can have severe effects on body function.
- Common causes of hypercalcemia include
    1. Increased absorption of calcium:
        a. Excessive oral intake of calcium
        b. Excessive oral intake of vitamin D
    2. Decreased excretion of calcium:
        a. Renal failure
        b. Use of thiazide diuretics
    3. Increased bone resorption of calcium:
        a. Hyperparathyroidism
        b. Malignancy:
            (1) Direct invasion (cancers of breast, lung, prostate, and osteoclastic bone and multiple myeloma)
            (2) Indirect resorption (liver cancer, small cell lung cancer, cancer of the adrenal gland)
        c. Hyperthyroidism
        d. Immobility
        e. Use of glucocorticoids
    4. Hemoconcentration
        a. Dehydration
        b. Use of lithium
        c. Adrenal insufficiency

COLLABORATIVE MANAGEMENT

Assessment

- The nurse assesses for
    1. Cardiovascular manifestations, the most serious and life-threatening changes:
        a. Increased heart rate
        b. Increased blood pressure
        c. Bounding, full peripheral pulses
        d. Electrocardiogram (ECG) abnormalities (severe or prolonged hypercalcemia):
            (1) Shortened ST segment (resulting from a shortened QT interval)

(2) Widened T wave
   e. Potentiation of digitalis-associated toxicities
   f. Decreased clotting time
   g. Late phase:
      (1) Bradycardia
      (2) Cardiac arrest, sinus arrest
2. Neuromuscular manifestations:
   a. Disorientation, lethargy, coma
   b. Profound muscle weakness
   c. Diminished or absent deep-tendon reflexes
3. Gastrointestinal manifestations:
   a. Decreased motility
   b. Hypoactive bowel sounds
   c. Anorexia, nausea
   d. Abdominal distention
   e. Constipation

4. Respiratory manifestations (ineffective respiratory movement related to profound skeletal muscle weakness)
5. Renal manifestations:
   a. Increased urinary output
   b. Dehydration
   c. Formation of renal calculi
6. Psychosocial changes:
   a. Behavioral changes
   b. Mood changes
   c. Impaired short- and long-term memory
   d. Disordered thought processes

Collaborative Management

- The nurse administers drug therapy, as ordered
   1. Immediately stops all intravenous (IV) infusions and oral medications containing calcium
   2. Discontinues oral drugs containing calcium or vitamin D
   3. Stops thiazide diuretics; furosemide (Lasix, Furoside♦) may be administered to increase the excretion of calcium
   4. May administer:
      a. IV normal saline for fluid balance replacement
      b. Calcium chelators or binders
      c. Mithramycin (Mithracin)
      d. Penicillamine (Cupramine, Pendramine♦)
   5. May administer drugs that inhibit calcium resorption from the bone:
      a. Phosphorus

375

b. Calcitonin (Calcimar)

c. Biphosphonates (Etidronate)

d. Prostaglandin synthesis inhibitors (aspirin, non-steroidal anti-inflammatory drugs)

- Peritoneal dialysis, hemodialysis, and/or blood ultra-filtration may be used to treat the client with life-threatening hypercalcemia.
- The nurse institutes continuous cardiac monitoring:

  1. Compares recent ECG tracings with the client's baseline tracings or tracings obtained when the client's serum calcium was normal
  2. Examines the ECG for changes in T waves and the QT interval, as well as for changes in rate and rhythm

Hypercortisolism (Cushing's Syndrome)

OVERVIEW

- Hypercortisolism, or Cushing's syndrome, results from the production of excess amounts of glucocorticoids, causing widespread abnormalities.
- The disorder may be caused by bilateral adrenal hyperplasia secondary to a pituitary or nonendocrine tumor that produces excess adrenocorticotropic hormone (ACTH) or the use of exogenous glucocorticoids or ACTH in the therapy of clinical entities such as organ transplantation, as an adjunct to chemotherapy, or in the treatment of neurologic or cardiothoracic disease.

COLLABORATIVE MANAGEMENT

Assessment

- The nurse records the client's

  1. Change in activity or sleep pattern
  2. Past medical history:
     a. Steroid or alcohol abuse
     b. Frequency of infections
     c. Easy bruising
- The nurse assesses for

1. Fatigue
2. Muscle weakness
3. Bone pain and history of fractures
4. Characteristic physical changes:
   a. Buffalo hump
   b. Centripetal obesity
   c. Supraclavicular fat pads
   d. Round or moon face
   e. Large trunk
   f. Thin arms and legs
   g. Generalized muscle wasting and weakness
5. Characteristic skin changes:
   a. Bruises
   b. Thin, translucent skin
   c. Wounds that have not healed properly
   d. Reddish-purple striae on the abdomen and upper thighs
   e. Fine coating of hair over the face and body
   f. Acne
6. Hypertension
7. Emotional lability, irritability, confusion, or depression
8. Increased plasma cortisol level
9. Increased urinary 17-ketosteroids and 17-hydroxycorticosteroids

Planning and Implementation

Nonsurgical Management

- The nurse administers drug therapy, as ordered:
   1. Mitotane (Lysodren) for inoperable adrenal tumors
   2. Aminoglutethimide (Elipten, Cytadren) and metyrapone to decrease cortisol production
   3. Metyrapone in combination with mitotane to decrease cortisol production
- Radiation therapy is not always effective and may destroy normal tissue.

Surgical Management

- Transsphenoidal removal of the microadenoma is performed if hyperfunction is caused by increased pituitary secretion of ACTH.
- A *hypophysectomy* (surgical removal of the pituitary gland) may be indicated if the microadenoma cannot be located.
- *Adrenalectomy* is indicated if the etiologic agent is an adrenal adenoma or carcinoma.

- The nurse provides preoperative care:
    1. Monitors electrolyte balance
    2. Ensures a high-calorie, high-protein diet
    3. Administers glucocorticoid preparations as ordered
    4. Monitors for and reports hyperglycemia
- The nurse provides postoperative care:
    1. Provides routine postoperative care according to the critical care unit guidelines, including hemodynamic monitoring per protocol
    2. Monitors for signs and symptoms of cardiovascular collapse and shock
    3. Carefully measures intake and output
    4. Weighs the client daily
    5. Monitors serum electrolytes daily
    6. Administers glucocorticoids if necessary
    7. Identifies the need for and provides pain management
    8. Assesses the skin frequently to detect reddened areas, excoriation, breakdown, and edema
    9. Observes venipuncture sites for excessive bleeding
    10. Turns the client frequently (at least every 2 hours)
    11. Pads bony prominences
- The nurse instructs the client
    1. To use a soft toothbrush
    2. To use an electric razor for shaving
    3. To keep the skin clean and dry
    4. To use moisturizing skin lotion
    5. About safety issues and dietary needs:
        a. To consume a high-calorie diet, including milk, cheese, yogurt, and green leafy and root vegetables
        b. To avoid caffeine and alcohol
        c. To keep rooms free of hazardous objects
        d. To use ambulatory aids correctly, if necessary
- The nurse administers medications to minimize gastric irritation such as antacids and histamine blockers.
- The nurse teaches the client and family
    1. Compliance with medication regime and its side effects
    2. Importance of wearing a Medic-Alert bracelet
- Hypercortisolism results in demineralization of bone and may lead to osteoporosis and fracture.

HYPERKALEMIA

OVERVIEW

- Hyperkalemia is a serum potassium level exceeding 5.1 mEq/L.
- The consequences can be life threatening, and the imbalance is generally not seen in people with normally functioning kidneys.
- Causes include
  1. Excessive potassium intake:
     a. Potassium-containing foods or medications
     b. Salt substitutes
     c. Potassium chloride (KCl) administration
     d. Rapid infusion of potassium-containing intravenous (IV) solution
  2. Decreased potassium excretion, which may be seen in Addison's disease and renal failure
  3. Movement of potassium from intracellular fluid to extracellular fluid:
     a. Tissue damage
     b. Acidosis
     c. Hyperuricemia
     d. Hypercatabolism

COLLABORATIVE MANAGEMENT

- The nurse records the client's
  1. Age (decreased renal function occurs in the elderly)
  2. Past medical and surgical history
  3. Medication use, particularly diuretics containing potassium
  4. Urinary output and frequency
  5. Diet history, including the use of salt substitutes and methods of preparing food
- The nurse assesses for
  1. Cardiovascular manifestations (the most common cause of death):
     a. Irregular heart rate, usually slow and weak
     b. Decreased blood pressure
     c. Electrocardiogram (ECG) abnormalities:
        (1) Tall T waves

H

379

          (2) Widened QRS complexes

          (3) Prolonged PR intervals

          (4) Flat P waves

     d. Ectopic beats

     e. Late changes: dysrhythmias, ventricular fibrillation, complete heart block, ventricular standstill

  2. Neuromuscular manifestations:

     a. Early phase or mild hyperkalemia:

          (1) Muscle twitches, cramps

          (2) Paresthesia

     b. Late phase or severe:

          (1) Profound weakness

          (2) Ascending flaccid paralysis in distal to proximal direction involving arms or legs

  3. Gastrointestinal manifestations

     a. Increased motility

     b. Hyperactive bowel sounds

     c. Diarrhea

  4. Respiratory manifestations (profound weakness of skeletal muscles causes respiratory failure in late stage of hyperkalemia)

  5. Laboratory values:

     a. Increased blood urea nitrogen and serum creatinine levels (when renal failure occurs)

     b. Decreased blood pH (acidemia)

- The nurse

  1. Immediately stops infusions of IVs containing potassium; leaves the IV line open

  2. Administers IVs containing substantial amounts of glucose and insulin, as ordered

  3. Withholds oral potassium supplements

  4. Maintains a potassium-restricted diet

  5. Gives sodium bicarbonate, as ordered, if hyperkalemia is accompanied by or caused by metabolic acidosis

  6. Monitors the client closely for hypokalemia or hypoglycemia

  7. Administers oral or rectal cation exchange resins such as sodium polystyrene sulfonate (Kayexalate) as ordered

  8. Administers potassium-excreting diuretics as ordered, such as furosemide (Lasix, Furoside◆)

  9. Compares ECG tracings to baseline (notes changes in rate, rhythm, and waveform)

- Dialysis may be necessary when potassium levels reach lethal levels.
- The nurse reviews diet therapy with the client and family, as needed:
  1. Foods to avoid including salt substitute
  2. Permissible foods
  3. How to examine medication and food package labels to determine potassium content
- The nurse instructs the client and family to report signs and symptoms of hyperkalemia.

HYPERMAGNESEMIA

- Hypermagnesemia is a serum magnesium level exceeding 2.6 mg/dL.
- Common causes of hypermagnesemia include
  1. Excessive ingestion of antacids with a high concentration of magnesium
  2. Renal insufficiency
- Clinical manifestations include
  1. Bradycardia (can lead to cardiac arrest)
  2. Peripheral vasodilation
  3. Hypotension
  4. Electrocardiogram changes:
     a. Prolonged PR interval
     b. Widened QRS complex
  5. Drowsy and lethargic, progressing to coma
  6. Diminished or absent deep-tendon reflexes
  7. Respiratory insufficiency
- Interventions for hypermagnesemia include
  1. Discontinue oral and parenteral magnesium
  2. Intravenous fluids (without magnesium)
  3. Loop diuretics, such as furosemide (Lasix, Furoside◆)
  4 Calcium for severe cardiac manifestations
  5. Dietary restrictions of meat, nuts, legumes, fish, vegetables, and whole-grain cereal products

Hypernatremia

OVERVIEW

- Hypernatremia is a serum sodium level above 145 mEq/L. Common causes include
    1. Decreased sodium excretion:
        a. Hyperaldosteronism
        b. Renal failure
        c. Corticosteroids
        d. Cushing's syndrome
    2. Increased sodium intake:
        a. Excessive oral sodium ingestion
        b. Excessive administration of sodium-containing intravenous (IV) fluids
    3. Decreased water intake, nothing by mouth
    4. Increased water loss:
        a. Increased rate of metabolism
        b. Fever
        c. Hyperventilation
        d. Infection
        e. Excessive diaphoresis
        f. Watery diarrhea
        g. Dehydration

COLLABORATIVE MANAGEMENT

- The nurse assesses for
    1. Central nervous system:
        a. Hypernatremia with normovolemia or hypovolemia (agitation, short attention span, confusion, seizures)
        b. Hypernatremia with hypervolemia (lethargy, stupor, coma)
        c. Mild or early manifestations:
            (1) Spontaneous muscle twitches
            (2) Irregular contractions
        d. Severe or late manifestations:
            (1) Skeletal muscle weakness
            (2) Deep-tendon reflexes diminished or absent
    2. Cardiovascular manifestations:
        a. Decreased myocardial contractility
        b. Diminished cardiac output

   c. Heart rate and blood pressure responsive to vascular volume
3. Respiratory manifestations or problems associated with pulmonary edema when hypernatremia is accompanied by hypervolemia)
4. Renal manifestations:
   a. Decreased urinary output
   b. Increased specific gravity
5. Integumentary manifestations:
   a. Dry, flaky skin
   b. Presence or absence of edema related to accompanying fluid volume changes
6. Psychosocial manifestations (agitation or manic behavior)

Interventions

- The nurse restores fluid balance when caused by fluid loss:
  1. IV infusions of D_5W
  2. IV infusion of isotonic sodium chloride solutions if hypernatremia is caused by fluid and sodium loss
- The nurse administers diuretics, generally loop diuretics, if the condition is caused by inadequate renal excretion of sodium:
  1. Furosemide (Lasix, Furoside◆)
  2. Bumetanide (Bumex)
- The nurse assesses the client frequently for symptoms that indicate excessive loss of fluids, sodium, or potassium.
- Dietary restriction of sodium is prescribed.
- Fluid restriction may be needed.

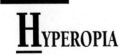

Hyperopia

See Refractive Errors.

HYPERPARATHYROIDISM

OVERVIEW

- Hyperparathyroidism results in increased levels of parathyroid hormone (PTH), which acts directly on the kidney. The result is increased tubular resorption of calcium and phosphate excretion, which contributes to hypercalcemia and hypophosphatemia.
- Primary hyperparathyroidism results when one or more hyperfunctioning glands is unresponsive to the normal feedback of serum calcium, usually caused by a benign, autonomous adenoma in *one* parathyroid gland.
- Secondary hyperparathyroidism is a response to the hypocalcemia in chronic renal disease and in vitamin D deficiency, which results in hyperplasia of the glands.

COLLABORATIVE MANAGEMENT

Assessment

- The nurse inquires about the client's symptoms:
    1. Bone fractures
    2. Recent weight loss
    3. Arthritis
    4. Psychological distress
    5. History of radiation treatment to the head or neck
- The nurse assesses for
    1. Gastrointestinal disturbances, such as anorexia, nausea, vomiting, and constipation
    2. Renal calculi and nephrocalcinosis (deposits of calcium in the soft tissue of the kidney)
    3. Hypergastrinemia (elevated serum gastrin levels)
    4. Fatigue and lethargy
    5. Results of radiographic tests that indicate bone demineralization, bone lesions such as cysts or fractures

Interventions

Nonsurgical Management

- Hydration (usually with intravenous normal saline) and the administration of furosemide (Lasix, Uritol◆, Furoside◆) are used to reduce serum calcium levels.

- The nurse
  1. Records strict intake and output measurements
  2. Observes for changes in blood pressure, rate or rhythm of pulses, and increasing confusion, lethargy, or irritation
  3. Assesses the need for cardiac monitoring
  4. Monitors for congestive heart failure secondary to fluid overload
  5. Monitors serum calcium levels frequently
  6. Instructs the client to report any nausea, vomiting, palpitations, tingling sensations, or numbness
  7. Administers drug therapy, as ordered:
     a. Phosphates to inhibit bone resorption and interfere with calcium absorption (used only when calcium levels must be lowered rapidly)
     b. Calcitonin to decrease skeletal calcium release and increase the renal clearance of calcium (must be given in conjunction with glucocorticoids)
     c. Mithramycin, a cytotoxic antibiotic, the most effective agent to lower calcium levels (monitor closely for thrombocytopenia and renal and hepatic toxicity)

Surgical Management

- The surgery of choice is the removal of the parathyroid glands (*parathyroidectomy*).
- Partial or total parathyroidectomy may be performed, depending on the cause of the hyperparathyroidism.
- The nurse provides preoperative care:
  1. Stabilizes calcium levels per the physician's order
  2. Monitors bleeding times and coagulation studies
  3. Monitors complete blood count
  4. Provides routine preoperative care
  5. Explains postoperative care, including pain control, deep breathing and coughing, and neck support technique to elevate the head
- The nurse provides postoperative care:
  1. Monitors serum calcium levels every 4 hours
  2. Monitors vital signs frequently per protocol
  3. Checks neck dressing for abnormal amounts of drainage or bleeding
  4. Observes for respiratory distress caused by hemorrhage or tissue swelling

5. Has emergency equipment such as a tracheostomy tray, oxygen, and suction at the bedside
6. Monitors for signs of hypocalcemia, such as tingling and twitching of the extremities and face
7. Checks for Trousseau's and Chvostek's signs
8. Administers calcium and vitamin D, as ordered

HYPERPHOSPHATEMIA

- Hyperphosphatemia is a serum phosphate level greater than 4.5 mg/dL.
- Elevations of phosphate are well tolerated.
- Problems are associated with hypocalcemia induced as a result of the increase in serum phosphorus levels.
- Common causes include
    1. Renal insufficiency
    2. Aggressive treatment of cancer (tumor lysis syndrome)
    3. Increased intake of phosphorus
    4. Hypoparathyroidism
- Interventions for hyperphosphatemia include management of the underlying hypocalcemia.

HYPERPITUITARISM

OVERVIEW

- Hyperpituitarism is a pathologic state that occurs as a result of a hormone-secreting adenoma (pituitary tumor) or hyperplasia.
- Common secretory tumors include the prolactinoma (lactotrophic [PRL] secreting tumor), causing decreased reproductive functioning, and the somatotrophic-producing adenoma (growth hormone [GH]), causing gigantism or acromegaly:
    1. *Gigantism,* characterized by rapid proportional growth in the length of all bones

2. *Acromegaly,* characterized by increased skeletal thickness, hypertrophy of the skin, and enlargement of visceral organs

- Hypersecretion of adrenocorticotropic hormone results in overstimulation of the adrenal cortex and may lead to the development of Cushing's disease.

COLLABORATIVE MANAGEMENT
Assessment

- The nurse records the client's
  1. Age, sex, and family history
  2. Complaints of change in hat, glove, ring, or shoe size
  3. Visual difficulties
  4. Sexual history and functioning:
     a. Female clients:
        (1) Amenorrhea
        (2) Irregular menses
        (3) Difficulty becoming pregnant
        (4) Decreased libido
        (5) Painful intercourse
     b. Male clients:
        (1) Decreased libido
        (2) Impotence
- The nurse assesses for
  1. Changes in facial features:
     a. Increase in lip and nose size
     b. Prominent supraorbital ridge
  2. Enlarging head, hand, and foot size
  3. Prominent jaw
  4. Dysphagia, difficulty chewing, and/or dentures that do not fit
  5. Arthritic changes causing pain and decreased mobility
  6. Arrowhead or tufted characteristics on x-ray films and a thickened appearance of the distal phalanges
  7. Increased perspiration and oil secretion on the client's skin
  8. Increased metabolism and strength (initially with acromegaly and gigantism)
  9. Lethargy and weakness (in later stages of gigantism and acromegaly)
  10. Visual changes

11. Organomegaly (cardiac or hepatic)
12. Hypertension
13. Deepening of the voice because of hypertrophy of the larynx
14. Hyperprolactinemia (observed with hypogonadism and galactorrhea)
15. Changes in body image
16. Depression and emotional distress
17. Increased adrenocorticotropic hormone (ACTH) or GH

Planning and Implementation

✦ **NDx:** Body Image Disturbance

Nonsurgical Management

- The nurse
  1. Encourages the client to verbalize concerns and fears related to his or her altered physical appearance
  2. Helps the client to identify his or her strengths and positive characteristics
  3. Administers bromocriptine mesylate (Parlodel), as ordered, to treat hyperprolactinemia or acromegaly by reducing GH levels and decreasing tumor size
  4. Instructs the client regarding drug side effects, which include postural hypotension, gastric irritation, nausea, headaches, abdominal cramps, and constipation
  5. Teaches the client to take the drug with meals or a snack
  6. Instructs the client to stop the drug immediately if she becomes pregnant
- Proton beam or alpha particle radiation therapy is usually effective but slow. Side effects include hypopituitarism, optic nerve damage, oculomotor dysfunction, and/or visual field defects.

Surgical Management

- Surgical removal of the tumor or pituitary gland (*hypophysectomy*) is performed, usually via the transsphenoidal approach:
  1. The client is placed in a semisitting position, and an initial incision is made at the inner aspect of the upper lip.
  2. The sella turcica is entered through the sphenoid sinus, and the gland or tumor is removed.

3. A muscle graft is taken, often from the anterior thigh, to pack the dura and prevent leakage of cerebrospinal fluid (CSF).
4. Nasal packing is inserted, and a dressing is applied under the nose to prevent the packing from dislodging ("moustache" dressing or "drip" pad).

- The nurse
  1. Provides routine preoperative care
  2. Explains to the client that nasal packing will remain in place for 2 to 3 days, which necessitates mouth breathing
  3. Explains that toothbrushing, coughing, sneezing, nose blowing, and bending must be avoided postoperatively
  4. Provides routine postoperative care:
     a. Monitors for changes in neurologic status
     b. Carefully measures intake and output
     c. Observes and reports signs of diabetes insipidus, such as low urine specific gravity and polyuria
     d. Instructs the client to report postnasal drip
     e. Records the amount and color of nasal drainage (clear drainage is tested for glucose, whose presence indicates that the fluid is CSF)
     f. Elevates the head of the bed at all times
     g. Reports severe persistent headache to the physician immediately (may indicate that CSF has leaked into the sinus area)
     h. Observes the client for indications of meningitis, such as headache, fever, and nuchal rigidity
     i. Instructs client *not* to cough because it increases intracranial pressure and may lead to a CSF leak
     j. Performs frequent mouth and lip care because the client has to breathe through his or her mouth
     k. Administers glucocorticoid and thyroid hormones if the entire pituitary gland is removed

- A transfrontal craniotomy is performed if the tumor is inaccessible through the transsphenoidal route.

✦ NDx: Sexual Dysfunction

- The nurse
  1. Identifies the specific problem(s) and encourages the client to discuss any effect that sexual dysfunction has had on the relationship with his or her sexual partner

2. Instructs the client that medication may be helpful
3. Informs the client that sexual dysfunction may occur after a hypophysectomy

Continuing Care

- The nurse identifies the need for adaptive-assistive equipment in the home.
- The nurse teaches the client
  1. To avoid bending over to pick things up or tie shoes
  2. To avoid straining during a bowel movement
  3. To rinse the mouth and use dental floss until brushing of teeth can be resumed after the incision has healed
  4. To expect a decreased sense of smell for 3 to 4 months
  5. To take hormones, as prescribed

Hypertension

OVERVIEW

- Hypertension is defined as systolic blood pressure greater than or equal to 140 mmHg and/or diastolic blood pressure greater than or equal to 90 mmHg, occurring in a client on at least three separate occasions.
- Hypertension is the major risk factor for coronary, cerebral, renal, and peripheral vascular disease.
- Systemic arterial pressure is a product of cardiac output and total peripheral resistance.
- Four control systems play a major role in maintaining blood pressure: arterial baroreceptors, body fluid volume, renin-angiotensin system, and vascular autoregulation.
- These are two major classifications of hypertension:
  1. *Essential,* or primary with no known cause
  2. *Secondary,* from known causes, such as estrogen-containing oral contraceptives, renal vascular and renal parenchymal disease, dysfunction of adrenal medulla or adrenal cortex, coarctation of the aorta, neurogenic disorders such as brain tumors and encephalitis, and psychiatric disorders

- Sustained blood pressure elevation in clients with essential hypertension results in damage to blood vessels in vital organs, causing myocardial infarctions, cerebrovascular accidents (strokes), peripheral vascular disease, or renal failure.
- *Malignant* hypertension is a severe type of hypertension that progresses rapidly and leads to renal failure, left ventricular failure, and stroke unless intervention occurs promptly.

Transcultural Considerations

1. The incidence of hypertension among African Americans is greater than that for Caucasians in the United States.
2. Hypertension is more prevalent in people of all races living in the southeast region of the United States.

Women's Health Considerations

1. Afican-American men have a higher incidence of hypertension than Caucasian men or women, and Hispanic or African-American women.

COLLABORATIVE MANAGEMENT
Assessment

- The nurse records the client's
  1. Age
  2. Race or ethnic origin
  3. Family history of hypertension
  4. Alcohol intake
  5. Smoking history
  6. Exercise habits
  7. Past and present history of renal or cardiovascular disease
  8. Medication use (prescribed and over-the-counter)
- The nurse assesses for
  1. Symptoms of hypertension (although most clients have no obvious symptoms):
     a. Headache
     b. Edema
     c. Nocturia
     d. Lethargy

e. Nosebleeds

f. Vision changes

2. Blood pressure readings in both arms
3. Blood pressure readings in supine and erect positions
4. Peripheral pulse rate, rhythm, and force
5. Bruits over the carotid and abdominal arteries
6. Psychosocial stressors
7. Retinal changes on funduscopic examination
8. Physical findings related to *secondary* hypertension:

   a. Abdominal bruits

   b. Tachycardia, sweating, and pallor

   c. Decreased or absent femoral pulses

Planning and Implementation

✦ NDx: Knowledge Deficit

- The nurse

  1. Advises the client to avoid adding table salt to food, cooking with salt, adding seasonings that contain sodium, and limit eating canned, frozen, and other processed foods
  2. Teaches the client to use salt substitutes, as ordered
  3. Advises the client to lose weight, in collaboration with the dietitian
  4. Advises the client to restrict alcohol intake and smoking
  5. In collaboration with the dietitian, develops a plan to reduce saturated fat and cholesterol in the diet
  6. Assists the client to develop a regular exercise program
  7. Teaches or refers the client to stress management programs
  8. Administers drug therapy, as ordered:

     a. *Diuretics* are particularly effective for African Americans and for clients with asthma, chronic airway limitation, chronic renal disease, and selected clients with congestive heart failure:

        (1) *Thiazide* diuretics prevent sodium and water reabsorption in the kidney's distal tubules, while promoting potassium excretion (e.g., hydrochlorothiazide [HydroDIURIL, Urozide◆]).

(2) *Loop* diuretics depress sodium reabsorption in the ascending loop of Henle and promote potassium excretion (e.g., furosemide [Lasix, Furoside◆]).

(3) *Potassium-sparing* diuretics act on the kidney's distal tubule to inhibit reabsorption of sodium in exchange for potassium ions, thus retaining potassium (e.g., spironolactone [Aldactone, Novospiroton◆]).

b. *Beta-blocking* agents lower blood pressure by blocking beta receptors in the heart and peripheral vessels, reducing cardiac rate and output (e.g., propranolol [Inderal, Apo-Propranolol◆, Novopranol◆, Metoprolol]).

c. *Calcium channel blockers* lower blood pressure by interfering with transmembrane influx of calcium ions, resulting in vasoconstriction (e.g., nifedipine [Procardia]).

d. *Angiotensin-converting-enzyme* (ACE) *inhibitors* convert angiotensin I to angiotensin II (e.g., captopril [Capoten]); these drugs are most effective in young Caucasian adults and are not as effective in African-American clients.

e. *Adrenergic inhibitors* stimulate alpha receptors in the brain to lower blood pressure, which inhibits the sympathetic nervous system vasomotor center and sympathetic outflow (e.g., clonidine hydrochloride [Catapres]).

f. *Vasodilators* relax vascular smooth muscle tone, reducing peripheral resistance (e.g., minoxidil [Loniten]).

• A stepped-care approach to treat hypertension has been recommended. As a result, a variety of drug options and protocols are used by physicians.

ℰ Considerations for Elderly Clients

1. ACE inhibitors are not as effective in older clients.

2. The elderly client is at the highest risk for postural hypotension from ACE inhibitors because of the cardiovascular changes associated with aging.

♦ **NDx:** Risk for Ineffective Management of Therapeutic Regimen

- The nurse
  1. Instructs the client that pharmacologic treatment for essential hypertension usually requires lifetime medication control
  2. Explains the side effects of hypertension
  3. Identifies potential reasons for noncompliance, such as the client's assumption that hypertension is under control when symptoms are gone, adverse side effects, and cost factors

Continuing Care

- The nurse provides educational information for hypertension control:
  1. Salt restriction
  2. Weight maintenance or reduction
  3. Stress reduction
  4. Alcohol restriction
  5. Exercise program
- The nurse gives oral and written information on medication therapy:
  1. Indications
  2. Dosage
  3. Times of administration
  4. Side effects
  5. Drug interactions
  6. Importance of renewing prescriptions
  7. Reporting side effects to the physician
- The nurse instructs the client in the technique of blood pressure monitoring for use at home.
- The nurse teaches the client to record blood pressure readings in a log book or diary.
- The nurse emphasizes the importance of follow-up visits with the physician(s).
- The nurse refers the client to the American Heart Association for information and support.

HYPERTHYROIDISM

OVERVIEW

- Hyperthyroidism occurs as a result of excessive thyroid hormone secretion.
- The most common cause is Graves' disease (toxic diffuse goiter); women between 20 and 40 years of age are most often affected.
- Thyrotoxicosis refers to the signs and symptoms that appear when body tissues are stimulated by increased thyroid hormones.
- Hyperthyroidism produces a state of hypermetabolism with increased sympathetic nervous system activity; it may be transient or permanent.
- *Thyroid storm* is a life-threatening event:
    1. The nurse assesses for signs and symptoms triggered by a major stressor, such as trauma or infection:
        a. Fever
        b. Tachycardia or systolic hypertension
        c. Gastrointestinal symptoms: nausea, vomiting, and diarrhea
        d. Agitation, tremors, and anxiety
        e. Restlessness, confusion, or psychosis
        f. Seizures
    2. The nurse provides interventions, as ordered:
        a. Maintains a patent airway and adequate ventilation
        b. Administers antithyroid drugs, such as propylthiouracil (PTU) and methimazole (Tapazole), as ordered
        c. Administers sodium iodide solution
        d. Administers propranolol (Inderal, Apo-Propranolol◆) if life-threatening dysrhythmias are present
        e. Administers glucocorticoids, as ordered, to prevent release of thyroid hormone
        f. Provides comfort measures, including a cooling blanket
        g. Monitors vital signs frequently
        h. Administers nonsalicylate antipyretics, as ordered, to reduce fever

i. Monitors continually for cardiac dysrhythmias

COLLABORATIVE MANAGEMENT

Assessment

- The nurse records the client's
  1. Age and sex
  2. Usual weight (the client may report weight loss and increased appetite)
  3. Heat intolerance or diaphoresis
  4. Palpitations or chest pain
  5. Changes in breathing pattern (dyspnea with or without excretion may occur)
  6. Changes in vision: blurring, double vision, or eyes tiring easily
  7. Changes in ability to perform activities of daily living (ADL): fatigue, weakness, insomnia
  8. Changes in menses (amenorrhea, decreased menstrual flow)
  9. Increased libido
  10. Previous medical history
      a. Thyroid surgery
      b. Radiation therapy to the neck (some clients may be resistant to radiation therapy)
      c. Past or current medications, noting the use of thyroid hormones or antithyroid drugs
- The nurse assesses for
  1. Two types of ophthalmopathy
     a. Eyelid retraction and eyelid lag
     b. Globe lag
  2. Exophthalmos (seen in Graves' disease)
     a. Impaired vision
     b. Problems with focusing
     c. Possible corneal ulcerations and infections
     d. Excessive tearing
     e. Photophobia
  3. Mass or general enlargement of the thyroid gland
  4. Fine, soft, silky hair and smooth, moist skin
  5. Proximal muscle weakness
  6. Hyperactive deep tendon reflexes or tremors
  7. Restlessness and irritability
  8. Fatigue
  9. Increased serum triiodothyronine (T_3) and serum thyronine (T_4)
  10. Increased radioactive iodine (RAI) uptake on thyroid scan

11. Electrocardiogram (ECG) changes: tachycardia, atrial fibrillation, and alterations in P and T wave-forms

Planning and Implementation

Nonsurgical Management

- The nurse
    1. Monitors vital signs at least every 4 hours
    2. Instructs the client to report palpitations, dyspnea, vertigo, and/or chest pain immediately
    3. Provides a quiet, restful environment
    4. Administers drug therapy, as ordered
        a. Antithyroid drugs, such as propylthiouracil (PTU) and methimazole (Tapazole)
        b. Iodide preparations
        c. Lithium carbonate
        d. Beta-adrenergic blocking agents, such as propranolol

- The nurse teaches the client about radioactive iodine therapy:
    1. ^{131}I is taken orally (one dose usually on an outpatient basis)
    2. Radiation precautions are generally not required.
    3. Relief of symptoms usually does not occur for 6 to 8 weeks
    4. Hypothyroidism may occur as a complication

Surgical Management

- All (total thyroidectomy) or part of the thyroid gland (subtotal thyroidectomy) may be removed.
- The nurse provides preoperative care:
    1. Provides routine preoperative care
    2. Administers antithyroid drugs and iodine preparations, as ordered, to place the client in a euthyroid state and to decrease the size and vascularity of the gland
    3. Monitors cardiac status
    4. Monitors nutritional status
- The nurse provides postoperative care:
    1. Provides routine postoperative care
    2. Places sandbags or pillows to support the client's head and neck
    3. Maintains the client in a semi-Fowler's position
    4. Administers pain medication as ordered
    5. Provides humidification

6. Encourages the client to turn, cough, and deep breathe every 1 to 2 hours
7. Inspects the neck dressing for drainage (a moderate amount of drainage is expected if a drain is left in place)
8. Keeps equipment for a tracheostomy at the bedside
9. Keeps calcium gluconate or calcium chloride at the bedside for emergency use
10. Administers fluids, as ordered
11. Applies an ice bag to the neck to reduce swelling
12. Observes for complications:
    a. Hemorrhage
    b. Respiratory distress
    c. Hypocalcemia and tetany, caused by parathyroid gland injury
       (1) Tingling around the mouth or of the toes and fingers
       (2) Muscular twitching
       (3) Positive Chvostek's and Trousseau's signs
    d. Damage to laryngeal nerves (hoarseness and a weak voice)
- The infiltrative ophthalmopathy of Graves' disease is not influenced by medical therapy.
- The nurse
   1. For mild symptoms
      a. Elevates the head of the bed at night
      b. Applies eye lubricant or artificial tears
   2. For severe symptoms
      a. Tapes the eyes closed
      b. Administers short-term steroids, as ordered
      c. Administers diuretics, as ordered
- In extreme cases, surgical intervention (orbital decompression) may be necessary.

Continuing Care

- The nurse teaches the client
   1. Pertinent drug information, including side effects
   2. The necessity to report any temperature elevation, sore throat, or symptoms of infection
   3. The signs and symptoms of hyperthyroidism or hypothyroidism
   4. Inspection of the incision for redness, tenderness, drainage, and swelling
   5. The importance of follow-up visits with the physician(s)

- Home health services may be necessary for the client who has difficulty with ADL.

HYPOCALCEMIA

OVERVIEW

- Hypocalcemia is a serum calcium level below 8.6 mg/dL or 2.15 mmol/L.
- Small changes in serum calcium levels have major effects on body function.
- Hypocalcemia is usually not a primary disease or condition but a result of other diseases or conditions.
- Common causes of hypocalcemia include
  1. Inhibition of calcium absorption from the gastrointestinal (GI) tract:
     a. Inadequate oral intake of calcium
     b. Lactose intolerance
     c. Malabsorption syndromes:
        (1) Celiac sprue
        (2) Crohn's disease
     d. Inadequate intake of vitamin D
  2. Increased calcium excretion:
     a. Renal failure (polyuric phase)
     b. Diarrhea
     c. Steatorrhea
     d. Wound drainage (especially GI)
  3. Conditions that decrease the ionized fraction of calcium:
     a. Alkalosis
     b. Calcium chelators or binders:
        (1) Citrate
        (2) Mithramycin (Mithracin)
        (3) Penicillamine (Cupramine, Pendramine◆)
        (4) Cellulose sodium phosphate (Calcibind)
     c. Acute pancreatitis
     d. Hyperphosphatemia
     e. Immobility
  4. Endocrine disturbances
     a. Removal or destruction of the parathyroid glands:
        (1) Thyroidectomy
        (2) Radiation to the thyroid

      (3) Strangulation
      (4) Neck injuries

 Transcultural Considerations

1. African Americans with a lactose intolerance may have difficulty obtaining adequate calcium intake; milk and other dairy products are rich in calcium and vitamin D but contain lactose.

 Women's Health Considerations

1. Postmenopausal women are susceptible to hypocalcemia, which may be related to reduced weight-bearing activities and a decrease in estrogen levels.

 Considerations for Elderly Clients

1. The elderly client is more likely to be taking medications that affect fluid and electrolyte balance.
2. The elderly client may have an inadequate calcium intake related to economic conditions or general problems with obtaining, preparing, or eating food.

COLLABORATIVE MANAGEMENT

Assessment

- The nurse assesses for
    1. Neuromuscular manifestations (the most common):
        a. Anxiety, irritability, psychosis
        b. Paresthesia followed by numbness
        c. Irritable skeletal muscles—twitches, cramps, tetany, seizures
        d. Hyperactive deep-tendon reflexes
        e. Positive Trousseau's sign:
            (1) Testing is accomplished by placing a blood pressure cuff around the upper arm, inflating the cuff to greater than systolic pressure, and keeping it there for 1 to 4 minutes.
            (2) The hand and fingers spasm in palmar flexion.
            (3) Spasms continue for 20 to 30 seconds after the cuff has been released.

f. Positive Chvostek's sign (tapping on the face just below and anterior to the ear—over the facial nerve—triggers facial twitching that includes one side of the mouth, nose, and cheek)
2. Cardiovascular manifestations:
   a. Decreased heart rate
   b. Decreased myocardial contractility
   c. Diminished peripheral pulses
   d. Hypotension
   e. Electrocardiogram abnormalities:
      (1) Prolonged ST interval
      (2) Prolonged QT interval
   f. Congestive heart failure (especially with severe or prolonged hypocalcemia, or in clients taking calcium channel blocking agents)
3. GI manifestations:
   a. Increased gastric motility
   b. Hyperactive bowel sounds
   c. Abdominal cramping
   d. Diarrhea

Interventions

- The nurse administers drug therapy, as ordered
   1. Oral supplements of calcium carbonate, calcium citrate, calcium gluconate, or calcium lactate used for mild hypocalcemia:
      a. Use with thiazide diuretics can increase risk for hypercalcemia
      b. Do not give phenytoin within 3 hours of calcium administration
   2. Parenteral calcium for severe hypocalcemia of calcium acetate, calcium chloride, or calcium gluconate:
      a. Give slowly, not to exceede 27 g/min: warm before administration.
      b. Monitor cardiovascular status; ideally the client should be on a cardiac monitor.
      c. Potential for hypercalcemia and hypomagnesemia.
      d. Assess the infusion site for infiltration.
      e. Vitamin D enhances the intestinal absorption of calcium.
      f. Aluminum hydroxide, magnesium chloride, and/or magnesium sulfate increases calcium levels.

- The nurse provides diet therapy:
  1. High-calcium, low-phosphorus diet for mild cases and those with chronic pathologic conditions that put them at risk for hypocalcemia
  2. Foods high in calcium:
     a. Low-fat yogurt
     b. Skim and whole milk
     c. Raw collard greens
     d. Rhubarb
     e. Cheddar and American cheese
     f. Tofu
     g. Broccoli
- The nurse
  1. Administers drugs, as ordered, to decrease the degree of nerve and muscle responsiveness and overstimulation:
     a. Methocarbamol (Robaxin)
     b. Orphenadrine (Banflex, Flexoject, Myolin)
     c. Carisoprodol (Soma, Vanadom)
     d. Magnesium sulfate
  2. Minimizes environmental stimuli
  3. Keeps emergency equipment readily available in anticipation of complications
  4. Places the client on seizure precautions
  5. Uses a lift sheet to move the client rather than pulling or grasping the client directly
  6. Observes the client for unusual surface projections or depressions over bony areas, as well as for normal joint motion

Hypofunction, Adrenal

OVERVIEW

- A decreased production of adrenocortical steroids (adrenal hypofunction) may occur secondary to inadequate secretion of adrenocorticotropic hormone (ACTH), dysfunction of the hypothalamic-pituitary control mechanism, or complete or partial destruction of the adrenal glands.
- *Primary* hypofunction, also referred to as *Addison's disease,* occurs when a client's physiologic require-

ments for glucocorticoid and mineralocorticoid hormones exceed available supply due to autoimmune factors, tuberculosis, carcinoma, acquired immunodeficiency syndrome (AIDS), hemorrhage, sepsis, radiation, or adrenalectomy.

- *Secondary* hypofunction is the result of failure in the hypothalamic or pituitary portion of the adrenal axis, which causes decreased cortisol and adrenal androgen production:
    1. Most frequent cause is the sudden cessation of long-term, high-dose glucocorticoid therapy
- In clients with *acute* adrenocortical insufficiency (adrenal crisis), manifestations may appear suddenly, without warning, and create a life-threatening situation.

COLLABORATIVE MANAGEMENT

Assessment

- The nurse records the client's
    1. Description of symptoms
    2. Activity level
    3. Salt intake (salt craving)
    4. Past medical history
        a. Radiation to the head or abdomen
        b. Tuberculosis
        c. Intracranial surgery
        d. Medications such as steroids, anticoagulants, or cytotoxic drugs
- The nurse assesses for
    1. Gastrointestinal problems:
        a. Anorexia
        b. Nausea, vomiting, diarrhea
        c. Abdominal pain
        d. Weight loss
    2. Increased or decreased skin pigmentation
    3. Hyperpigmentation of the mucous membranes, surgical scars, areolae, skin folds, and area over knuckles on the hand (not seen in secondary disease)
    4. Decreased body hair
    5. Hypoglycemia (cortisol hypersecretion):
        a. Sweating
        b. Headache
        c. Tachycardia
        d. Tremors

6. Volume depletion (cortisol and aldosterone deficiencies):
    a. Postural hypotension
    b. Dehydration
7. Emotional lability, forgetfulness
8. Low serum cortisol, decreased fasting blood sugar, low sodium, elevated potassium, and increased blood urea nitrogen levels. Eosinophil count and ACTH level are elevated in primary disease.

Planning and Implementation

- The nurse
    1. Carefully measures intake and output
    2. Records the client's weight every day
    3. Takes vital signs frequently to detect postural hypotension and dysrhythmias
    4. Administers cortisone and hydrocortisone to correct glucocorticoid deficiency
    5. Administers supplemental mineralocorticoids, such as fludrocortisone (Florinef), as ordered, to maintain electrolyte balance
- The nurse teaches the client that
    1. Medications should be taken with meals or snacks
    2. The physician is consulted regarding increasing dosage during increased stress
    3. A Medic-Alert bracelet or necklace must be worn at all times

HYPOKALEMIA

OVERVIEW

- Hypokalemia is defined as a serum potassium ion (K^+) level below 3.5 (mmol/L)
- Hypokalemia is potentially life-threatening because every body system can be affected
- Common causes include
    1. Inappropriate or excessive use of diuretics, digitalis, or corticosteroids
    2. Increased secretion of aldosterone
    3. Diarrhea, vomiting
    4. Wound drainage, excessive drainage from ostomies

5. Prolonged nasogastric suction
6. Heat-induced excessive diaphoresis
7. Inadequate potassium intake, such as occurs when the client has nothing by mouth for several days
8. Cushing's syndrome
9. Metabolic acidosis
10. Presence of excess amounts of insulin in the blood, such as during hyperalimentation infusions or during treatment of uncontrolled diabetes
11. Renal disease impairing resorption of potassium
12. Dilution of serum potassium that may occur secondary to water intoxication or intravenous therapy with potassium-poor solutions

COLLABORATIVE MANAGEMENT

Assessment

- The nurse records the client's
    1. Age
    2. Medication use, especially diuretics, corticosteroids, and potassium supplements
    3. Dietary history
- The nurse assesses for
    1. Cardiovascular changes:
        a. Variable pulse rate, more often rapid
        b. Pulse thready and weak
        c. Peripheral pulses difficult to palpate
        d. Postural hypotension
        e. Electrocardiogram abnormalities:
            (1) ST depression
            (2) Inverted or flat T wave
            (3) Prominent U wave
            (4) Dysrhythmias
    2. Respiratory changes:
        a. Shallow, ineffective respirations
        b. Diminished breath sounds and respiratory effort
    3. Neuromuscular changes:
        a. Anxiety, lethargy, confusion, coma
        b. Loss of tactile discrimination
        c. General skeletal muscle weakness
        d. Deep-tendon hyporeflexia
        e. Eventual flaccid paralysis
    4. Gastrointestinal changes:
        a. Decreased motility or peristalsis
        b. Hypoactive to absent bowel sounds

405

c. Nausea, vomiting

d. Abdominal distention

e. Paralytic ileus

f. Constipation

5. Renal changes:

a. Decreased ability to concentrate urine

b. Polyuria

c. Decreased specific gravity

6. Phychosocial:

a. Behavioral changes

b. Lethargy

c. Unable to perform simple problem-solving tasks

Planning and Implementation

✦ NDx: Risk For Injury

- The nurse administers drug therapy, as ordered:

1. Potassium is a severe tissue irritant and is never administered IM or SC.

2. IV potassium may irritate the veins, causing a chemical phlebitis. It must be diluted well and administered slowly; the maximum infusion rate is 5 to 10 mEq/hr and should never exceed 20 mEq/hr under any circumstances.

3. Rapid increases of serum potassium may cause cardiac arrest.

4. Oral potassium has a strong, unpleasant taste. It must not be given on an empty stomach because it may cause nausea and vomiting.

5. Potassium sparing diuretics that may be appropriate for clients needing diuretic therapy include spironolactone (Aldactone), triamterene (Dyrenium), and amiloride (Midamor).

- The nurse

1. Provides foods high in potassium, including avocados, bananas, cantaloupe, raisins, and whole-wheat bread

2. Instructs the client to avoid boiling, poaching, or frying of vegetables and fruits in water

3. Provides frequent rest periods for the client susceptible to skeletal muscle weakness

4. Maintains a hazard-free environment

5. Assists the client with ambulation

- The nurse
  1. Monitors the client's rate and depth of respiration once each hour
  2. Monitors the client's ability to cough deeply
  3. Examines the client's face, oral mucosa, and nail beds for signs of pallor or cyanosis

✦ **NDx:** Constipation

- The nurse
  1. Administers laxatives that add bulk or fiber to stimulate peristalsis
  2. Administers drugs such as metoclopramide (Reglan, Maxeran◆), as ordered
  3. Provides a high-fiber diet and encourages fluids
  4. Encourages physical activity and exercise to promote gastric motility

Continuing Care

- The nurse
  1. Assesses the ability of the client with a chronic condition that increases his or her risk for hypokalemia to live safely in the home care environment based on physical and mental functioning
  2. Provides drug information, as needed
  3. Teaches early recognition of the signs and symptoms of hypokalemia
  4. Provides information on food rich in potassium and how potassium is lost from the body
  5. Teaches the client to measure the rate, rhythm, and quality of his or her peripheral pulses once each day
  6. Refers client to home health care services as needed

HYPOMAGNESEMIA

- Hypomagnesemia is a serum magnesium ion level below 1.6 mg/dL.

- Common causes include
  1. Malnutrition or starvation
  2. Diarrhea or steatorrhea
  3. Celiac disease, Chron's disease
  4. Alcoholism, especially when accompanied by liver disease
  5. Certain drugs:
     a. Diuretics
     b. Aminoglycoside antibiotics
     c. Cisplatin (Platinol)
     d. Amphotericin B
     e. Citrate (blood products)
     f. Ethanol ingestions
  6. Hyperglycemia
  7. Insulin administration
  8. Sepsis
  9. Alkalosis
- Clinical manifestations include
  1. Hyperactive deep-tendon reflexes
  2. Painful paresthesia
  3. Tetanic muscle contractions
  4. Positive Chvostek's and Trousseau's signs
  5. Tetany and seizures
  6. Depression or irritability
  7. Frank psychosis
  8. Confusion
  9. Electrocardiogram changes:
     a. Tall T waves
     b. Depressed ST segments
  10. Dysrhythmias:
     a. Ectopic beats
     b. Ventricular tachycardia
     c. Ventricular fibrillation
  11. Shallow respirations
  12. Hypertension
  13. Decreased gastric motility with anorexia, nausea, and abdominal distention
- Management of hypomagnesemia includes
  1. Stopping drugs that contribute to the development of hypomagnesemia (loop diuretics, aminoglycosides
  2. Intravenous infusion of magnesium sulfate
  3. Increasing the client's intake of foods high in magnesium, such as meats, nuts, legumes, fish, and vegetables

Hyponatremia

OVERVIEW

- Hyponatremia is a serum sodium level below 135 mEq/L (mmol/L).
- Usually associated with fluid volume imbalances.
- Common causes include
    1. Increased sodium excretion
        a. Excessive diaphoresis
        b. Diuretics
        c. Wound drainage (especially gastrointestinal)
        d. Decreased secretion of aldosterone
        e. Hyperlipidemia
        f. Renal disease
    2. Inadequate sodium intake:
        a. Nothing by mouth (NPO)
        b. Low-salt diet
    3. Dilution of serum sodium:
        a. Excessive ingestion of hypotonic fluids
        b. Psychogenic polydipsia
        c. Freshwater drowning
        d. Renal failure (nephrotic syndrome)
        e. Irrigation with hypotonic fluids
        f. Syndrome of inappropriate antidiuretic hormone (SIADH)
        g. Hyperglycemia
        h. Congestive heart failure

🕮 Women's Health Considerations

1. More women develop brain damage and die from coma or seizure activity as a complication of postoperative hyponatremia.

COLLABORATIVE MANAGEMENT

- The nurse assesses for
    1. Neuromuscular changes:
        a. Generalized muscle weakness that is worse in the extremities
        b. Diminished deep-tendon reflexes
        c. Personality changes

      d. Headache

      e. Seizures

  2. Gastrointestinal changes:

      a. Increased motility; abdominal cramping

      b. Nausea

      c. Hyperactive bowel sounds

      d. Diarrhea

  3. Cardiovascular changes:

      a. Normovolemic:

        (1) Rapid pulse rate

        (2) Normal blood pressure

      b. Hypovolemic:

        (1) Rapid pulse rate

        (2) Pulse thready and weak

        (3) Hypotensive

        (4) Central venous pressure normal or low

        (5) Flat neck veins

      c. Hypervolemic:

        (1) Rapid bounding pulse

        (2) Central venous pressure normal or elevated

        (3) Blood pressure normal or elevated

  4. Respiratory changes (secondary to the influence of low serum sodium on cerebral function and circulatory status); late manifestations related to

      a. Skeletal muscle weakness

      b. Shallow, ineffective respiratory movements

      c. Hypervolemia

      d. Pulmonary edema:

        (1) Rapid, shallow respirations

        (2) Moist rales

  5. Renal changes:

      a. Increased urinary output

      b. Decreased specific gravity of urine

- The nurse administers drug therapy, as ordered, for

  1. Hyponatremia with fluid volume deficit: IV saline infusions are given to restore both sodium content and fluid volume

  2. Hyponatremia with fluid volume excess: Diuretics that promote excretion of water rather than sodium:

      a. Osmotic diuretics such as mannitol (Osmitrol)

  3. Hyponatremia as a result of inappropriate or excessive secretion of antidiuretic hormone (ADH) may be treated with agents such as demeclocycline or lithium

- The nurse monitors and maintains diet therapy, as needed:
    1. Increases oral sodium and restricts oral intake of fluids to some extent, in consultation with the dietitian; common food sources of sodium are table salt, soy sauce, cured pork, cottage cheese, and American cheese
    2. Accurately measures intake and output
    3. Reinforces the rationale for fluid restriction

HYPOPARATHYROIDISM

OVERVIEW

- Is directly related to the lack of parathyroid hormone (PTH) or decreased effectiveness of PTH on target tissue
- Always results in hypocalcemia
- Two forms:
    1. *Iatrogenic,* is inadvertently caused by removal of all viable parathyroid tissue during total thyroidectomy or by surgical removal of hyperplastic parathyroid glands
    2. *Idiopathic,* a rare condition that can occur spontaneously in children and adults; an autoimmune basis is suspected

COLLABORATIVE MANAGEMENT

- The nurse questions the client regarding
    1. Neck surgery or radiation therapy to the head or neck area
    2. Signs and symptoms:
        a. Paresthesia
        b. Tetany
        c. Periorbital tingling
        d. Numbness and tingling sensation in the hands and feet
- The nurse assesses the client for
    1. Muscle cramping
    2. Carpopedal spasms
    3. Seizures

4. Mental changes
5. Chvostek's or Trousseau's sign
- The nurse
    1. Ensures compliance with medication regimen, as ordered, to correct hypocalcemia, vitamin D deficiency, and hypomagnesemia
    2. Encourages the client to eat food high in calcium and low in phosphorus
    3. Stresses that therapy for hypocalcemia is lifelong
    4. Advises the client to wear Medic-Alert emblem and to carry a wallet card

HYPOPHOSPHATEMIA

- Hypophosphatemia is a serum phosphate level below 2.7 mg/dL.
- Body functions are not significantly impaired as a result of rapid, wide fluctuations in serum levels.
- Alterations in function are more obvious when hypophosphatemia is chronic.
- Common causes include
    1. Malnutrition or starvation
    2. Ingestion of large amounts of antacids containing aluminum hydroxide (ALternaGEL, Amphojel) and/or magnesium (Bisodol, milk of magnesia)
    3. Hyperparathroidism
    4. Hypocalcemia
    5. Renal failure
    6. Malignancy
    7. Hyperglycemia
    8. Hyperalimentation
    9. Respiratory alkalosis
- Clinical manifestations do not appear until the decrease in serum phosphate levels is severe or prolonged and include
    1. Decreased stroke volume
    2. Decreased cardiac output
    3. Peripheral pulses slow, difficult to find, and easy to obliterate
    4. Weak, ineffective myocardial contractions
    5. Generalized skeletal muscle weakness

6. Ineffective respiratory movements, possibly leading to respiratory failure if skeletal muscle weakness is present
7. Immunosupression
8. Prolonged bleeding time in response to relatively slight trauma or tissue injury
9. Decreased platelet aggregation
10. Increased irritability
11. Seizure activity
12. Coma
13. Decreased bone density, alterations in bone shape, fractures

- Treatment of hypophosphatemia includes
    1. Stopping all drugs, such as antacids, osmotic diuretics, and calcium supplements
    2. Administering oral supplements of phosphates and vitamin D
    3. Administering parenteral phosphate only when the serum phosphate level is less than 1 mg/dL and the client is experiencing serious clinical manifestations
    4. Encouraging the client to eat foods high in phosphorus, such as beef, pork, fish, chicken, whole-grain breads, beans, and other legumes and discouraging calcium rich foods

Hypopituitarism

OVERVIEW

- Hypopituitarism is a deficiency of one or more of the anterior pituitary hormones.
- The clinical features and symptoms vary, depending on the severity of the disease and the number of deficient hormones.
- Growth retardation (in children), metabolic abnormalities, and sexual dysfunction may occur.
- Deficiencies of adrenocorticotropic hormone (ACTH) and thyroid-stimulating hormone (TSH) are life threatening.

COLLABORATIVE MANAGEMENT

Assessment

- The nurse records the client's
    1. Loss of secondary sex characteristics:
        a. Adult males may report
            (1) Loss of facial and body hair
            (2) Episodes of impotence
            (3) Decreased libido
        b. Adult females may report
            (1) Secondary amenorrhea
            (2) Difficulty becoming pregnant
            (3) Painful intercourse
            (4) Decreased libido
- The nurse assesses for
    1. Neurologic manifestations:
        a. Changes in visual acuity and peripheral vision
        b. Bilateral temporal headaches
        c. Diplopia and ocular muscle paralysis secondary to dysfunction of cranial nerves III, IV, and VI
    2. Decrease or loss of facial and/or body hair
    3. Decrease in muscle mass and tone
    4. Testicular atrophy in males
    5. Loss or decreased axillary and pubic hair and atrophy of the breasts in females
    6. Changes in body image and self-esteem
    7. Anxiety and ineffective coping skills
    8. Levels of triiodothyronine (T_3), thyroxine (T_4), testosterone, estradiol, and ACTH that are low or in low-normal ranges
- Management of hypopituitarism focuses on replacement of deficient hormones.
- The nurse
    1. Instructs the client about hormone replacement therapy
    2. Administers androgens (testosterone) intramuscularly for males, as ordered; the nurse
        a. Instructs the client in self-administration
        b. Begins dosage at 50 mg, which is gradually increased to 200 mg, based on age, as ordered
        c. Teaches the client that injections are usually required every 4 to 6 weeks depending on clinical evaluation and recurrence of symptoms

    d. Teaches the side effects of testosterone, which include gynecomastia, baldness, and prostatic hypertrophy

    e. Alerts the client that the maximal effects of treatment include

        (1) Increase in penis size, libido, and muscle mass

        (2) Increased growth of facial, pubic, and axillary hair

        (3) Deepened voice

        (4) Increased bone size and strength

        (5) Increased self-esteem and improved body image

3. Administers human chorionic gonadotropin (hCG) therapy for achieving fertility, as ordered

4. Administers hormone replacement with a combination of estrogen and progesterone administered in a cyclic manner to females, as ordered, and teaches the client about adverse effects of drug therapy, such as hypertension and thrombophlebitis

Hypothyroidism

OVERVIEW

- Hypothyroidism results from inadequate peripheral tissue thyroid hormone levels.
- *Primary* hypothyroidism is a result of pathologic changes in the thyroid gland itself.
- *Secondary* hypothyroidism may result from inadequate pituitary production of thyroid-stimulating hormone.
- *Goiter* is an enlargement of the thyroid gland due to inadequate production of thyroid hormone.
- Myxedema coma is a rare but serious presentation of hypothyroidism, manifested by coma, hypotension, hyponatremia, respiratory failure, and hypoglycemia.
- Hypothyroidism occurs more frequently in women than in men.
- Endemic goiter occurs in areas where the soil and water are deficient in iodine.

COLLABORATIVE MANAGEMENT

Assessment

- The nurse records the client's
    1. Change in sleep habits (usually significantly increased)
    2. Generalized weakness, anorexia, muscle aches, paresthesia, and cold intolerance
    3. Change in bowel pattern (usually constipation)
    4. Past medical history, with special attention to use of drugs such as lithium, aminoglutethimide, sodium or potassium perchlorate, thiocyanates, or cobalt
- The nurse assesses for
    1. Integumentary changes:
        a. Cool, pale or yellowish, dry, coarse, scaly skin
        b. Thick, brittle nails
        c. Decreased hair growth, loss of eyebrow hair
    2. Pulmonary changes:
        a. Hypoventilation
        b. Pleural effusion
        c. Dyspnea
    3. Cardiovascular changes:
        a. Bradycardia
        b. Other dysrhythmias
        c. Enlarged heart
        d. Decreased exercise or activity tolerance
        e. Hypotension
    4. Gastrointestinal changes:
        a. Anorexia
        b. Constipation
        c. Abdominal distention
    5. Musculoskeletal changes:
        a. Muscle aches and pains
        b. Delayed contraction and relaxation of muscles
    6. Neurologic changes:
        a. Slowing of intellectual functions
        b. Slowness or slurring of speech
        c. Impaired memory
        d. Inattentiveness
        e. Lethargy
        f. Confusion
        g. Paresthesia
        h. Decreased deep-tendon reflexes
    7. Physiologic and emotional changes:
        a. Apathy

    b. Agitation
    c. Depression
    d. Paranoia
  8. Metabolic changes:
    a. Decreased basal metabolic rate
    b. Decreased body temperature
    c. Cold intolerance
  9. Reproductive changes:
    a. Females: changes in menses, infertility, decreased libido
    b. Males: decreased libido, impotence
 10. Other changes:
    a. Periorbital edema
    b. Facial puffiness
    c. Nonpitting edema of the hands and feet
    d. Goiter
    e. Anemia
    f. Easy bruising
    g. Decreased serum T_3 and T_4 levels

Planning and Implementation

✦ NDx: Decreased Cardiac Output

- Clients with chronic hypothyroidism may have cardiovascular disease.
- The nurse
  1. Monitors blood pressure, heart rate, and rhythm
  2. Observes closely for signs of hemodynamic compromise:
     a. Hypotension
     b. Decreasing urinary output
     c. Mental status changes
- The nurse teaches the client about lifelong replacement of thyroid hormone:
  1. Administers synthetic hormone preparations: levothyroxine sodium (Synthroid, Eltroxin◆)
  2. Observes closely for chest pain and dyspnea when initiating therapy
  3. Monitors for signs and symptoms of hyperthyroidism that can occur during replacement therapy

✦ NDx: Ineffective Breathing Pattern

- The nurse
  1. Observes and records the rate and depth of respirations

417

2. Auscultates lungs and notes abnormalities, such as decreased breath sounds
3. Recognizes that severe respiratory distress may be associated with myxedema coma
4. Avoids sedating the client as it may contribute to respiratory distress; if sedation must be used, the usual dosage is decreased because hypothyroidism increases sensitivity to these drugs

✦ **NDx:** Altered Thought Processes

* The nurse
    1. Notes the presence and severity of symptoms, such as lethargy, memory deficit, inattentiveness, and difficulty communicating
    2. Orients the client; explains procedures slowly and carefully
    3. Encourage the family to accept the client's mood changes and mental slowness, which should improve with therapy

Continuing Care

* The nurse teaches the client
    1. About the possible need for extra heat or clothing because of cold intolerance if the symptoms have not cleared before discharge
    2. Drug information:
        a. Emphasizes the need for lifelong administration of medication
        b. Reviews the signs and symptoms of hyperthyroidism and hypothyroidism
        c. Contraindications of over-the-counter medications that may interact with the thyroid medication
        d. Importance of wearing a Medic-Alert bracelet or necklace because many thyroid medications potentiate and interact with many other drugs.
        e. Provides the elderly client with additional information about the effects of aging on the thyroid gland
    3. Diet information to prevent constipation
    4. The importance of adequate rest periods before the client assumes a full schedule

IBS

See Irritable Bowel Syndrome.

IDIOPATHIC POLYNEURITIS, ACUTE

See Guillain-Barré Syndrome.

IDIOPATHIC THROMBOCYTOPENIC PURPURA

See Thrombocytopenic Purpura, Autoimmune.

IMMUNODEFICIENCIES

- An immunodeficiency is a deficient response of the immune system that is due to a missing or damaged immune component.
- The client is susceptible to infections, malignancies, and other diseases.
- B-cell, or antibody-mediated, immunity normally protects the host from a variety of bacterial infections and some viral infections through the production of specific antibodies; lack of this protection leads to recurrent infections with encapsulated bacteria and/or a history of treatment failure.

- Types of antibody-mediated immunodeficiency include
  1. Bruton's, or X-linked, agammaglobulinemia:
     a. Congenital antibody-mediated immunodeficiency
     b. Overall good prognosis if hormonal replacement begins early in life, except for clients who have poliomyelitis, chronic echovirus infection, or a lymphoreticular malignancy
     c. Treatment with intravenous (IV) or intramuscular (IM) immune serum globulin
  2. Common variable immunodeficiency, or acquired hypogammaglobulinemia:
     a. Appears in adolescents or young adults
     b. Is characterized by recurrent bacterial infections
     c. Complications include giardiasis, bronchiectasis, gastric carcinoma, lymphoreticular malignancy, and cholelithiasis
     d. Treated by the regular administration of IV or IM immune serum globulin and the use of antibiotics intermittently or chronically
  3. Immunoglobulin A (IgA) deficiency:
     a. May be asymptomatic or have chronic recurrent respiratory tract infections, atopic diseases, and/or collagen-vascular diseases; may have malabsorption syndrome
     b. Treatment limited to appropriate and vigorous treatment of infection
- *Iatrogenic* immunodeficiency is an immunodeficiency or immunosuppressive state induced in the client by medical therapies or procedures:
  1. Drug induced:
     a. Cytotoxic drugs
     b. Corticosteroids
     c. Cyclosporine
  2. Radiation induced

IMPOTENCE

OVERVIEW

- Impotence is the inability to achieve or maintain an erection firm enough for sexual intercourse 25% of the time.

- Causes of psychogenic impotence include anxiety, fatigue, boredom, depression, guilt, and pressure to perform sexually.
- Causes of physiologic impotence include injury, disease, hormonal imbalance, or surgery.
- Impotence occurs in 50% to 60% of diabetic men.

COLLABORATIVE MANAGEMENT

- Assessment of sexual and medical history includes
  1. Psychologic impotence:
     a. Acute onset
     b. Selectivity
     c. Periodicity
     d. Nocturnal erections and emissions
     e. Ability to masturbate
     f. Ability to have an erection and function sexually under certain circumstances
     g. Retention of testicular sensitivity
  2. Physiologic impotence:
     a. Gradual loss of erectile dysfunction in all sexual circumstances
     b. Lack of nocturnal erection and emissions
     c. Some degree of erectile dysfunction in all sexual circumstances
  3. Medical history:
     a. Family history of impotence
     b. Diabetes
- Nonsurgical management includes
  1. Psychosocial intervention
  2. Change or adjustment in medication
  3. Control of underlying disease
  4. Mechanical devices or pharmacologic injection to increase blood flow to the penis
  5. Viagra, a drug that increases blood flow, but should not be given to clients with cardiac disease, especially those clients taking nitrates
- Surgical interventions include
  1. Arterial bypass procedure to improve blood flow to the penis
  2. Penile prosthesis insertion
- Also see Nursing Care to Promote Sexual Health (p. 33).

I

INCONTINENCE, URINARY

OVERVIEW

- Urinary incontinence (UI) is the involuntary loss of urine that is severe enough to cause social or hygienic problems; it may be transient or permanent, and is *not* a normal change of aging.
- It involves abnormalities of bladder contraction, urethral relaxation, and conscious control mechanisms.
- Abnormal bladder contraction:
    1. *Urge* incontinence is the involuntary loss of urine associated with a strong desire to urinate. Clients are unable to suppress the signal from the bladder muscle to the brain that it is time to urinate.
    2. *Overflow* incontinence occurs when the bladder has reached its absolute maximum capacity and some urine must leak out to prevent bladder rupture. The detrusor muscle is underactive and does not send signals to the brain that the bladder is full.
- Abnormalities of urethral relaxation most often result in *stress* incontinence, which is the involuntary loss of urine during activities, such as coughing or sneezing, that increases abdominal and detrusor pressure. Clients are unable to tighten the urethra sufficiently to overcome the increased detrusor pressure; leakage of urine results.
- Abnormalities outside the bladder and urethra most often result in *functional* incontinence, which is leakage of urine caused by factors other than pathology of the lower urinary tract.
- In adult clients younger than 65 years of age, incontinence occurs twice as frequently in women than in men.

✇ Considerations for Elderly Clients

1. The elderly are predisposed to developing incontinence as a result of decreased mobility, sensory deficits, or muscle weakness.
2. Up to 35% of the elderly who live in the community and up to 50% of nursing home residents are incontinent.

COLLABORATIVE MANAGEMENT

Assessment

- The nurse
    1. Questions the client about a history of incontinence:
        a. Onset, recent, or in the past
        b. Intermittent or continuous
        c. Time of occurrence (day or night)
        d. Contributing factors (e.g., sneezing, coughing)
        e. Circumstances surrounding the problem
        f. Voiding patterns and changes
        g. Perception of bladder fullness
        h. Presence of warning signals
    2. History of pregnancies or surgical procedures
    3. Past medical history
    4. Menopause status
    5. Medication history
    6. Stressors and other concerns associated with work, family, or financial status

- The nurse
    1. Palpates the abdominal area for evidence of urinary distention or discomfort
    2. Percusses the abdomen and listens for the dull sound of a distended bladder
    3. Observes for urine leakage while the client strains by coughing or bearing down in the standing position
    4. Catheterizes the client after the client voids to determine the amount of residual urine, if ordered
    5. Inspects the external genitalia of female clients to determine whether there is apparent urethral or uterine prolapse or cystocele
    6. Describes the color, consistency, and odor of any secretions from the genitourinary orifices
    7. Inspects the urinary meatus of male clients for the presence of discharge or other characteristics
    8. Queries the client on the effects of incontinence on socialization, family relationships, and emotional status
    9. Monitors the urine for the presence of red or white blood cells
    10. Reviews the results of the voiding cystourethrogram, which detects the anatomical structure and function of the bladder, as well as the post-voiding residual

423

Planning and Implementation

✦ NDx: Stress Incontinence

Nonsurgical Management

- The nurse
    1. Administers medications as ordered:
        a. Phenylpropanolamine, an alpha-adrenergic agonist
        b. Tricyclic antidepressants: imipramine (Tofranil, Novo-Pramine◆)
        c. Estrogen for postmenopausal women
    2. Collaborates with the dietitian to develop a dietary plan to assist the obese client to lose weight, and to encourage the client to avoid alcohol and caffeine (bladder stimulants)
    3. Teaches the woman how to do Kegel exercises to strengthen the muscles of the pelvic floor; biofeedback devices may be used to help the client detect effectiveness of the exercises
    4. Instructs the client in the correct use of vaginal cones:
        a. The lightest cone is inserted into the vagina with the string to the outside for a 1-minute test period.
        b. If the client is able to hold the first cone in place without it slipping out while she walks around, she proceeds to the second cone and repeats the procedure.
        c. Treatment is begun with the heaviest cone that the client can hold in her vagina for the 1-minute test period.
        d. The treatment period is for 15 minutes twice a day; when the client can hold the cone comfortably in her vagina for 15 minutes, she proceeds to the next heaviest weight.
- Other treatments include behavior modification, psychotherapy, and electrical devices for the inhibition of bladder contraction.
- A new reusable product, the Reliance insert, is a tampon-like device inserted into the urethra. The client inflates the attached balloon, which prevents urine flow.

Surgical Management

- Preoperatively, the nurse
    1. Provides instruction and clarifies events surrounding the surgery

2. Prepares the client for any diagnostic testing

- Operative procedures for women are used to elevate the bladder and urethra into a normal intra-abdominal position, increase the length of the urethra, and decrease hypermobility of the bladder neck:

    1. *Anterior vaginal repair* (Kelly procedure) to elevate the urethral position and repair any cystocele
    2. *Retropubic suspension* to elevate the urethral position and provide longer-lasting results
    3. *Needle bladder neck suspension* (Pereyra or Stamey procedure) to elevate the urethra and provide a longer-lasting result without a long operative time
    4. *Pubovaginal sling procedure* in which a sling made of synthetic material is placed under the urethrovesical junction to elevate the bladder neck
    5. *An artifical sphincter,* a mechanical device that opens and closes the urethra, is placed around the anatomic urethra; the procedure is used for men more often than for women

- Postoperatively, the nurse

    1. Assesses and intervenes to prevent and detect complications
    2. Secures the urethral catheter to prevent unnecessary movement or traction on the bladder neck
    3. Monitors the suprapubic catheter, if present, for leakage of urine and serosanguineous drainage

✦ NDx: Urge Incontinence

- Interventions for urge incontinence include behavioral interventions and medication; surgery is not recommended.
- The nurse

    1. Administers medications as ordered:
        a. Anticholinergic agents: propantheline bromide (Pro-Banthine, Propanthel◆), or oxybutynin (Ditropan) and dicyclomine hydrochloride (Bentyl, Formulex◆, Spasmoban◆)
        b. Tricyclic antidepressants: imipramine (Tofranil, Novo-Pramine◆), desipramine (Norpramin), nortriptyline (Pamelor)
    2. Instructs the client to avoid foods that have a bladder-stimulating effect, such as caffeine and alcohol

425

3. Instructs the client to space fluids throughout the day and to limit fluids after dinner
- Bladder training is an educational program to help clients to gain control of the bladder:
    1. Regular schedule of voiding is established.
    2. The client is instructed to void during the established time frame and to ignore any urge to urinate that occurs between the mandated interval.
    3. Once the client is comfortable with the initial interval, the time interval is increased by 15 to 30 minutes.
- Habit training is a variation of bladder training that is useful for cognitively impaired clients; the caregiver assists the client to void every 2 hours.
- Exercise therapy, such as Kegel exercises and vaginal cone therapy, is also useful.
- Electrical stimulation with a variety of intravaginal and intrarectal devices has been used to treat both stress and urge incontinence.

✦ NDx: Overflow Incontinence

- Surgery may be needed to relieve the obstruction of the bladder outlet.
    1. Removal of the prostate and repair of genital prolapse
- The nurse
    1. Administers bethanechol chloride, as ordered, for the short-term management of urinary retention
    2. Uses the Credé technique, Valsalva maneuver, or double-voiding technique to assist in promoting bladder contraction
    3. Teaches intermittent self-catheterization to clients with long-term problems of incomplete bladder emptying

✦ NDx: Functional Incontinence

- The primary focus of the intervention is to treat reversible causes of incontinence; when that is not possible, the goal is to contain the urine and protect the client's skin.
- The nurse
    1. Teaches the client how to use applied devices, such as the intravaginal pessaries for women and urethral clamps for men

426

2. Uses absorbent pads and briefs to collect urine and keep the client's skin and clothing dry
3. Inserts a Foley catheter or begins an intermittent catheterization program as indicated

Continuing Care

- The nurse
    1. Considers the personal, physical, emotional, and social resources of the client
    2. Considers who the primary caretaker will be and what circumstances or factors exist in the environment that will influence the effectiveness of the plan
    3. Assists the client to control or manage fears and anxieties related to incontinence while in public
- The nurse teaches the client about
    1. Causes of incontinence and treatment options available
    2. Prescribed medications (purpose, dosage, method, and route of administration, and expected and potential side effects)
    3. Importance of weight reduction and dietary modification
    4. Options available for external devices or incontinence pads and assists the client to make a selection that considers lifestyle and resources
    5. Demonstrates the technique of self-catheterization and ensures that a return demonstration is correct

INFECTION

OVERVIEW

- Infection is caused by the invasion of the body by microorganisms.
- Infectious diseases include those that are thought to be communicable (e.g., hepatitis and influenza) and those that are not communicable (e.g., pancreatitis and cellulitis).
- A *pathogen* is any microorganism that is capable of producing disease in a human (host).

427

- *Pathogenicity* is the ability to cause disease.
- *Virulence* refers to the frequency with which the disease occurs in persons exposed to the organism (degree of communicability) and the ability to invade and damage a host; it also refers to the severity of the disease.
- In *colonization* the microorganisms are present in the tissues of the host yet cause neither symptomatic nor subclinical disease.
- Microorganisms that behave as parasites live at the expense of their human host.
- Factors that must be present for transmission of infection are the reservoir host, pathogen, portal of entry, mode of transmission, and portal of exit.
- Prevention of the spread of infection is dependent on breaking the chain of infection at any point.
- Host factors that increase the risk of infection include
  1. Congenital or acquired immunodeficiencies (e.g., acquired immunodeficiency syndrome [AIDS])
  2. Alteration of normal flora by antibiotic therapy
  3. Age (especially infants and elderly clients)
  4. Pregnancy, diabetes, corticosteroid therapy, and adrenal insufficiency
  5. Defective phagocytic function, circulatory disturbances, and neutropenia
  6. Break in skin or mucous membrane integrity
  7. Interference with the flow of urine, tears, or saliva
  8. Impaired cough reflex or ciliary action
  9. Malnutrition
  10. Smoking, alcohol consumption, and inhalation of toxic chemicals
  11. Invasive therapy, chemotherapy, radiation therapy, steroid therapy, and surgery
- Modes of transmission of infection are commonly
  1. Direct contact
  2. Indirect contact
  3. Droplet spread
  4. Common vehicle (contaminated food, water)
  5. Vectors (tics, mosquitoes)
  6. Oral-fecal
  7. Airborne
- The portal of exit is usually through the portal of entry.
- Human defenses against infection include
  1. Intact skin
  2. Mucous membranes

428

3. Respiratory tract
4. Gastrointestinal tract
5. Genitourinary tract
6. Phagocytosis
7. Inflammation
8. Antibody-mediated and cell-mediated immune system

- A nosocomial infection is an infection acquired while the client is in the hospital.
- Infection or the spread of infection can be controlled by
    1. Hand washing
    2. Hygiene
    3. Sanitation
    4. Disinfection/sterilization
    5. Barriers
- Certain diseases must be reported to the Centers for Disease Control and Prevention (CDC).
- New isolation guidelines from CDC in 1996 include Standard, Airborne, Droplet, and Contact Precautions:
    1. *Standard* precautions should be used in the care of *all* clients. These precautions combine body substance and universal precautions, and acknowledge that all body secretions, excretions, and moist membranes and tissues (excluding perspiration) are potentially infectious.
    2. *Airborne* precautions are used for clients known or suspected to have serious infections transmitted by small droplet nuclei that are expelled during coughing or sneezing. Tuberculosis (TB), measles (rubeola), and chickenpox are examples of airborne diseases. Health care workers must wear HEPA or N-95 respirators to filter inspired air when in the room of a client with known or suspected TB.
    3. *Droplet* precautions are used for clients with known or suspected serious infections transmitted by large droplets. Examples include influenza, mycoplasma pneumonia, and pertussis.
    4. *Contact* precautions are used to prevent the transmission of organisms that are spread primarily by close or direct contact. Examples include scabies, pediculosis, and *Clostridium difficile.*
- Typical complications of infection are relapse, cellulitis, pneumonia, abscess formation, systemic complications, and systemic sepsis.

Considerations for Elderly Clients

- The nurse
  1. Assesses for atypical manifestations of infection, such as confusion and unusual behavior; fever and pain may not be present.
  2. Monitors for renal function when the client receives antibiotic therapy
  3. Observes for and reports adverse side effects of antibiotic therapy because the elderly client is at risk for these complications
  4. Monitors for diarrhea and obtains a specimen for culture, as ordered
  5. Keeps the client well hydrated unless this is contraindicated

COLLABORATIVE MANAGEMENT
Assessment

- The nurse records the client's
  1. Exposure to a person with similar clinical symptoms or to contaminated food or water and date of exposure
  2. Contact with animals
  3. Travel history
  4. Sexual history
  5. Intravenous (IV) drug use
  6. Transfusion history
  7. Order of onset of symptoms
- Common clinical manifestations are associated with specific sites of infection; the nurse assesses for
  1. Gastrointestinal tract manifestations:
     a. Fever
     b. Nausea and vomiting
     c. Diarrhea
     d. Abdominal distention
  2. Genitourinary tract manifestations:
     a. Dysuria
     b. Frequency
     c. Urgency
     d. Hematuria
     e. Fever
     f. Purulent discharge
     g. Pelvic or flank pain
  3. Respiratory tract manifestations:
     a. Cough

    b. Congestion
    c. Rhinitis
    d. Sore throat
    e. Fever
    f. Chest pain
4. Skin manifestations:
    a. Redness
    b. Warmth
    c. Swelling
    d. Drainage
    e. Pain
5. Generalized infection manifestations:
    a. Fever
    b. Malaise
    c. Fatigue
    d. Muscle aches
    e. Joint pain
6. Psychosocial dysfunction:
    a. Anxiety and frustration
    b. Social isolation
7. Abnormal laboratory results:
    a. Positive culture findings
    b. Serologic testing
    c. White blood cell count
    d. Erythrocyte sedimentation rate

Planning and Implementation

✦ NDx: Hyperthermia

- Effective antibiotic therapy requires
  1. Appropriate antibiotic
  2. Sufficient dosage
  3. Proper rate of administration
  4. Sufficient duration
- The nurse
  1. Obtains an allergy history before giving antibiotics
  2. Monitors the client for side effects of antibiotics, including nausea, vomiting, and rash
  3. Applies a hypothermia blanket and monitors for shivering
  4. Sponges the client with tepid water or uses ice packs
  5. Monitors for signs of dehydration, such as increased thirst, decreased skin turgor, and dry mucous membranes

431

6. Encourages fluid intake
7. Records strict measurement of intake and output

- Aspirin and acetaminophen are generally not given unless the client is extremely uncomfortable or if fever presents a significant risk (if the client has a history of heart failure, febrile seizures, or head injury).

✦ NDx: Fatigue

- The nurse
    1. Collaborates with the dietitian and client to identify a diet that the client can tolerate and that meets calorie and protein requirements
    2. Ensures bed rest during the acute phase of the illness
    3. Collaborates with the client to develop a progressive program for return to a normal level of activity
    4. Encourages frequent rest periods

✦ NDx: Social Isolation

- The nurse
    1. Educates the client and family about the mode of transmission of the infection and mechanisms that prevent the spread of organisms from the client to others
    2. Encourages family and friends to visit the client; provides information and instructions on isolation techniques and other precautions needed to prevent transmission of the disease
    3. Ensures that the client has access to a telephone and radio
    4. Visits with the client frequently (every hour or more if time permits) to say hello and check if the client needs anything

Continuing Care

- The nurse
    1. Emphasizes the importance of a clean home environment
    2. Ensures that the client has proper storage facilities at home for medications and knows how to recognize signs of improper storage
    3. Explains the importance of hand-washing facilities in the home and provides supplies and instruction as needed

4. Instructs the client about the disease, method of transmission, and how to prevent its transmission
5. Explains the importance of compliance regarding taking medications at home:
   a. Timing of doses
   b. Completion of planned number of days of therapy
   c. Side effects of medications
   d. Allergic manifestations
   e. Importance of notifying the physician if an adverse or allergic reaction occurs
6. Teaches the client with infusion devices for administration of medications:
   a. Care of the device
   b. Indications of device malfunction
   c. Indications of infection of the device or the site of insertion

INFECTIONS, CHLAMYDIAL

OVERVIEW

- *Chlamydia trachomatis* is the most commonly transmitted bacteria in the United States, with more than 5 million acute infections estimated annually.
- *C. trachomatis* invades columnar epithelial tissues in the reproductive tract and causes clinical manifestations similar to those of gonorrhea.
- The incubation period ranges from 1 to 3 weeks, although the pathogen may be present in the genital tract for months or years without producing symptoms.

COLLABORATIVE MANAGEMENT
Assessment

- The nurse assesses for
  1. Men: urethritis, dysuria, frequency of urination, mucoid discharge that is more watery and less copious than gonorrheal discharge
  2. Women: 75% are asymptomatic, mucopurulent cervicitis, change in vaginal discharge, dysuria, urinary frequency, soreness in the affected area

- The nurse also assesses for
  1. Sexual history:
     a. History of sexually transmitted diseases (STDs)
     b. Sexual partner with history of STDs
     c. Sexual partner with suspicious symptoms
  2. Risk factors associated with *C. trachomatis:*
     a. Pregnancy
     b. Sexual activity during adolescence
     c. Use of nonbarrier method of birth control
     d. History of multiple sexual partners
  3. Exclusion of gonorrhea on Gram's stain and culture
  4. Diagnostic tests such as enzyme-linked immunoassay and a direct fluorescent antibody test
- Complications include
  1. Men: epididymitis, prostatitis, infertility, and Reiter's syndrome
  2. Women: salpingitis, pelvic inflammatory disease, ectopic pregnancy, and infertility

Interventions

- The treatment of choice is doxycycline (Vibramycin, Novodoxylin◆) or tetracycline (Tetracyn, Nu-tetra◆).
- Client education includes
  1. Transmission and treatment
  2. Signs and symptoms
  3. Complications of untreated chlamydial infections
  4. Avoid sexual activity
  5. Partner treatment
  6. Use of condoms

INFECTIONS, EAR

See Otitis Media.

INFECTIONS, SKIN

OVERVIEW

- The majority of *cutaneous bacterial* infections are caused by *Staphylococcus* or *Streptococcus.*
- *Folliculitis* is a superficial staphylococcal infection involving the upper portion of the hair follicle and is associated with mild discomfort.
- *Furuncles* (boils) are caused by *Staphylococcus,* but the infection occurs deeper in the hair follicle.
- *Cellulitis* is a generalized nonfollicular infection with either *Staphylococcus* or *Streptococcus,* involving deeper connective tissue.
- *Viral* skin infections include *herpes simplex* virus (HSV) infections (type I virus, or classic cold sores; and type II virus, or genital herpes), *herpes zoster* (shingles), and herpetic whitlow.
- Many *fungal* infections may affect the skin.
- Superficial fungal (dermatophyte) infections, or tinea, include
    1. Tinea pedis (athlete's foot)
    2. Tinea manus (hands)
    3. Tinea cruris (groin)
    4. Tinea corporis (ringworm)
    5. Tinea capitis (scalp)
    6. Tinea barbae (beard)
- *Candidiasis* is an opportunistic yeast infection of the skin and mucous membranes.

COLLABORATIVE MANAGEMENT

Assessment

- The nurse records the client's
    1. Recent history of skin trauma
    2. Past or current history of staphylococcal or streptococcccal infections
    3. Lesions appearing on the lips, oral cavity, and/or genitals
    4. Past history of similar lesions
    5. Prodromal symptoms of burning, tingling, and/or pain
    6. Previous exposure to chickenpox

I

7. History of shingles
8. Anatomic location of dermatophyte infection
9. Social and environmental factors
10. History of recent antibiotics or immunosuppressive drugs
11. Medical history, including diabetes or cancer
12. Nutritional deficiencies

- The nurse assesses for clinical manifestations of common skin infections such as
    1. Redness
    2. Warmth
    3. Edema
    4. Tenderness
    5. Pain
    6. Itching
    7. Stinging
    8. Localized areas of inflammation
    9. Blisters
    10. Pustules
    11. Papules
    12. Vesicles
    13. Scaling
    14. Single or multiple lesions

Interventions

- The nurse
    1. Teaches the client to bathe daily with antibacterial soap for bacterial infection
    2. Applies warm compresses to furuncles or cellulitis
    3. Applies astringent compresses such as Burow's solution to viral lesions
    4. Allows the skin to dry between treatments
    5. Provides optimal client positioning to promote air circulation
    6. Teaches the client to avoid tight garments
    7. Uses proper hand washing to prevent cross-contamination
    8. Maintains strict isolation for resistant *Staphylococcus*
    9. Teaches the client to avoid sexual contact when recurrent herpes lesions are present
    10. Teaches the client and family to avoid sharing contaminated personal items of clients with dermatophyte infections

11. Applies antibacterial ointment (e.g., neomycin, gentamicin, chloramphenicol, and povidone-iodine) and cream (e.g., silver sulfadiazine), as ordered

12. Applies antifungal ointment and cream, such as clotrimazole, nystatin, ciclopirox, miconazole, econazole, tolnaftate, haloprogin, and undecylenic acid, as ordered, which are the treatments of choice for dermotophyte and yeast infections

13. Applies antifungal powder, such as nystatin and tolnaftate, as ordered

14. Administers antifungal oral preparation, such as nystatin and clotrimazole, as ordered

15. Administers anti-inflammatory steroid preparations, as ordered, ranging from low to potent fluorinated agents

16. Applies an antiviral ointment, such as acyclovir, as ordered, which is the treatment of choice for viral infections

- Incision and drainage of *furuncles* is the primary surgical procedure that is done for skin infections.

INFECTIOUS POLYNEURITIS

See Guillain-Barré Syndrome.

INFECTIVE ENDOCARDITIS

See Endocarditis, Infective.

INFLAMMATORY DISEASE, PELVIC

See Pelvic Inflammatory Disease.

INFLUENZA

- Influenza (flu) is a highly contagious, acute viral respiratory infection caused by one of several viruses.
- Typical symptoms include severe headache, muscle aches, fever, chills, fatigue, weakness, anorexia, and respiratory symptoms, such as sore throat, cough, and rhinorrhea.
- Treatment is symptomatic and includes
    1. Bed rest
    2. Increased oral fluid intake, unless contraindicated
    3. Acetaminophen (Tylenol) or aspirin
    4. Saline gargles
    5. Antihistamines
- As a preventive measure, it is recommended that people older than 65 years of age and those with chronic illness or immune compromise receive the influenza vaccination annually.

INSUFFICIENCY, AORTIC (AORTIC REGURGITATION)

- In aortic insufficiency, the aortic valve leaflets do not close properly during diastole, and the annulus may become dilated, loose, or deformed.

- Regurgitation of blood from the aorta into the left ventricle occurs during diastole; the left ventricle dilates to accommodate the greater blood flow and hypertrophies.
- Nonrheumatic causes include infective endocarditis, congenital anatomic aortic valvular abnormalities, hypertension, and Marfan's syndrome, a generalized, systemic connective tissue disease.
- Clients with aortic insufficiency remain asymptomatic for many years owing to the compensatory mechanisms of the left ventricle.
- Signs and symptoms include
    1. Palpitations (severe disease)
    2. Dyspnea
    3. Orthopnea
    4. Paroxysmal nocturnal dyspnea
    5. Nocturnal angina with diaphoresis
    6. Bounding pulse
    7. Widened pulse pressure
    8. High-pitched, blowing, decrescendo diastolic murmur
- Aortic valve replacement surgery is the treatment of choice; the valve is excised during cardiopulmonary bypass surgery then replaced with a prosthetic (synthetic) or biologic (tissue) valve.
- The postoperative client requires lifetime anticoagulation therapy to prevent thrombus formation on the valve.
- For preoperative and postoperative care, see "Surgical Management" under Coronary Artery Disease.

INSUFFICIENCY, MITRAL, AND MITRAL REGURGITATION

- Mitral insufficiency is a pathologic process that occurs from thickening of the mitral valve in the left heart.
- The fibrotic and calcific changes cause the mitral valve to fail to close completely, allowing backflow of blood from the left ventricle into the left atrium during ventricular systole.

- During diastole, regurgitant output is returned from the left atrium to the left ventricle, in addition to the normal blood amount, increasing the volume of blood to be ejected during systole.
- Rheumatic heart disease is the predominant factor, usually coexisting with mitral stenosis.
- Signs and symptoms include
  1. Fatigue and weakness
  2. Dyspnea on exertion
  3. Orthopnea
  4. Atrial fibrillation
  5. Neck vein distention
  6. Pitting edema
  7. High-pitched, systolic murmur
- Drug therapy is instituted to maintain normal cardiac output.
- The reparative surgical procedure is mitral annuloplasty, which is performed during cardiopulmonary bypass surgery; mitral valve leaflets and annuli are reconstructed to narrow the valve orifice.
- The postoperative client requires lifetime anticoagulation therapy to prevent thrombus formation on the valve.
- For preoperative and postoperative care, see care of the client undergoing a coronary artery bypass grafting procedure under Coronary Artery Disease.
- The nurse
  1. Provides health teaching information regarding
     a. Medications
     b. Oral hygiene
     c. Plan of work, activity, and rest to conserve energy
     d. Importance of antibiotics before any procedures (e.g., dental work, surgery)
  2. Refers the client to community resources, such as the American Heart Association

INTESTINAL OBSTRUCTION

See Obstruction, Intestinal.

IRON DEFICIENCY ANEMIA

See Anemia, Iron Deficiency.

IRRITABLE BOWEL SYNDROME

OVERVIEW

- Irritable bowel syndrome (IBS), also known as spastic bowel and mucous colitis, is the most common digestive disorder facing Americans today, entailing a change in bowel habits without an inflammatory process or changes in bowel mucosa.
- Factors such as depression, fear, food, drugs, toxins, colonic distention, or anxiety may precipitate exacerbations.
- Changes in gastrointestinal motility result in diarrhea, constipation, or diarrhea alternating with constipation
- More than two thirds of those affected are women.

Transcultural Considerations

The incidence of IBS is higher among Caucasians and Jews than in other groups.

COLLABORATIVE MANAGEMENT

Assessment

- The nurse assesses for
    1. Pain in the lower left quadrant of the abdomen that increases after eating and is relieved by a bowel movement
    2. Nausea associated with mealtime and defecation
    3. Diarrhea or constipation
    4. Belching, gas, anorexia, and bloating
    5. Fatigue, anxiety, and headache
    6. Difficulty in concentrating
    7. Tympanic bowel sounds
    8. Anxiety

Interventions

- The nurse
    1. Administers bulk-forming laxatives such as psyllium hydrophilic mucilloid (Metamucil) or calcium polycarbophil (Mitrolan), as ordered
    2. Administers antidiarrheal agents, such as diphenoxylate hydrochloride with atropine sulfate (Lomotil), loperamide (Imodium), or camphorated tincture of opium (Paregoric), as ordered, to decrease cramping and frequent stools
    3. Administers anticholinergic receptor blocking agents, such as dicyclomine hydrochloride (Bentyl, Bentylol◆) and propantheline bromide (Pro-Banthine, Propanthel◆), as ordered, to help relieve cramping and intestinal spasm
    4. Consults with the dietitian to teach the client to add 30 to 40 g of fiber to the diet daily
    5. Encourages the client to eat regular meals and chew food slowly
    6. Teaches the client to drink 8 to 10 cups of liquid per day
    7. Helps the client identify and eliminate offending or upsetting foods
    8. Assists the client in learning relaxation techniques
    9. Encourages the client to implement a regular exercise program to promote bowel elimination and reduce stress

Continuing Care

- The nurse instructs the client
    1. To establish regular bowel patterns and to defecate regularly
    2. To implement a regular exercise program
    3. To follow a high-fiber diet with adequate liquid intake and regular mealtimes
    4. To avoid alcohol, caffeine, and other gastric irritants
    5. To follow instructions regarding medications

ITP

See Thrombocytopenic Purpura, Autoimmune.

JOINT DISEASE, DEGENERATIVE

OVERVIEW

- Degenerative joint disease (DJD), also known as osteoarthritis, is characterized by the progressive deterioration and loss of articular cartilage in peripheral and axial joints.
- Weight-bearing joints, the vertebral column, and the hands are the sites primarily affected.

 Transcultural Considerations

Native Americans are affected more often than non–Native American groups.

COLLABORATIVE MANAGEMENT

Assessment

- The nurse records the client's risk factors:
    1. Occupation and nature of work
    2. Family history of arthritis
    3. Involvement in sports
    4. History of trauma
    5. Age
    6. Weight
- The nurse assesses for
    1. Joint pain, which, early in the disease process, diminishes after rest and intensifies after activity; later, pain occurs with slight motion or even at rest
    2. Crepitus, a continuous grating sensation
    3. Joint enlargement
    4. Heberden's nodes (at the distal interphalangeal joints) or Bouchard's nodes (at the proximal interphalangeal joints), if the hands are involved
    5. Intra-articular and periarticular effusions, if the knees are involved
    6. Skeletal muscle atrophy adjacent to the involved area
    7. Compression of the spine manifested by radiating pain, stiffness, and muscle spasms in one or both extremities

8. Level of mobility
9. Ability to perform activities of daily living (ADL)
10. Anger, depression, and body image changes

Planning and Implementation

♦ NDx: Chronic Pain

Nonsurgical Management

- The nurse administers drug therapy, as ordered:
    1. Acetaminophen (Tylenol, Atasol♦)
    2. Nonsteroidal anti-inflammatory drugs such as ibuprofen (Motrin, Advil, Nuprin, Amersol♦), naproxen (Naprosyn, Apo-Naproxen♦), or Ansaid
    3. Salicylates in small doses (aspirin, Ancasal♦)
    4. Corticosteroid injections into single joints
    5. Muscle relaxants for severe muscle spasms
- The nurse
    1. Immobilizes the affected joint with a splint or brace, as prescribed
    2. Recommends 10 hours of sleep at night and a 1- or 2-hour nap in the afternoon
    3. Places the affected joints in functional positions:
        a. Avoids large pillows under the head or knees
        b. Uses a bed or foot cradle, if needed
        c. Has the client lie prone twice per day, if feasible
    4. Applies and or teaches the importance of a moist heating pad, a hot shower, hot packs or compresses, paraffin dips, diathermy, and ultrasound
    5. Implements cold applications for acutely inflamed joints
    6. Encourages the obese client to reduce weight
    7. Applies a transcutaneous electrical nerve stimulator (TENS), as ordered
    8. Teaches imagery, music therapy, and relaxation techniques to reduce pain

Surgical Management

- An *osteotomy* is a procedure in which the bone is cut to promote realignment.
- A *total joint replacement* (TJR) is used when all other measures of pain relief have failed; hips and knees are most commonly replaced. TJR is contraindicated in the presence of infection, advanced osteoporosis, or severe inflammation.

- *Total hip replacement* (THR):
  1. The nurse provides preoperative care:
     a. Reinforces the information concerning the surgery, including the implications of cemented or noncemented prostheses
     b. Obtains urine and sputum cultures and recommends dental examinations
     c. Teaches the client to use a povidone-iodine (Betadine) scrub the night before or the morning before surgery
     d. Administers intravenous antibiotics, as ordered, which are started before surgery
  2. Intraoperative care often includes
     a. A specially cleaned operating room
     b. Laminar airflow units that may be used as an added precaution against infection
     c. A minimum of movement into and out of the operating room
  3. The nurse provides postoperative care:
     a. Provides routine postoperative care
     b. Places the client in a supine position with the head slightly elevated
     c. Places the affected leg in a neutral position by using a cradle boot or other device
     d. Turns the client toward either side as long as the legs remain abducted
     e. Observes for signs of hip dislocation, including increased pain, shortening of the affected leg, and leg rotation
     f. Observes for signs of infection and bleeding
     g. Performs frequent neurovascular assessments
     h. Follows the physician's orders related to activities, mobilization, pain management, and weight-bearing
     i. Applies thigh-high antiembolism stockings and sequential compression devices
     j. Administers anticoagulants, such as aspirin (Ecotrin, Ancasal◆), warfarin (Coumadin, Warfilone◆), enoxaparin (Lovenox), or heparin (Hepalean◆), to prevent thrombi
     k. Teaches leg exercises, including plantar flexion and dorsiflexion, circumduction of the feet, gluteal and quadriceps setting, and straight leg raises

J

l. Assesses respiratory status for signs of pulmonary emboli, atelectasis, and pneumonia

m. Teaches the use of incentive spirometry every 1 to 2 hours for the first 2 or 3 days

n. Provides follow-through on the exercise program developed by the physical therapist

o. Assists the client to use assistive-adaptive devices

- *Total knee replacement* (TKR):
    1. The nurse provides preoperative care
    2. The nurse provides postoperative care:
        a. Provides routine postoperative care
        b. Provides care similar to that for hip replacement
        c. Monitors and maintains the continuous passive motion (CPM) machine, which is often applied immediately after surgery and used intermittently for 8 hours per day (to provide passive flexion and extension)
        d. Observes for bleeding, especially if the CPM machine is used

- *Total shoulder replacement:*
    1. Total shoulder replacement is not as successful as other replacement surgeries; the Neer prosthesis is the most commonly used.
    2. The nurse provides postoperative care:
        a. Maintains the affected arm in a sling and swathe for 2 or 3 days until an exercise program is begun
        b. Monitors the CPM machine, which may be used instead of the sling
        c. Performs frequent neurovascular assessments

- *Total elbow replacement:*
    1. Total elbow replacement is successful in increasing range of motion.
    2. Infection is a frequent complication.
    3. The CPM device is often used.

- *Finger and wrist replacements:*
    1. A bulky dressing is used for 3 to 5 days after surgery, followed by a dynamic splint, brace, or cast.
    2. The arm is elevated as much as possible.
    3. A splint or short arm cast may be applied.

- *Total ankle and toe replacement:*
    1. When an ankle is replaced, an arthrodesis, or bone fusion, is usually performed for added stability.
    2. Treatment involves one or more osteotomies and fusions, which are immobilized by wires and a cast.

    ◆ **NDx:** Impaired Physical Mobility

- The nurse reinforces the exercise program developed by physical therapy:
    1. Encourages consistency
    2. Teaches the client to stop if pain is increased with exercise
    3. Instructs the client to decrease the number of repetitions when inflammation is severe
    4. Teaches that exercises should be active rather than passive
    5. Teaches that ADL or household tasks do not substitute for an exercise program

Continuing Care

- The nurse
    1. Helps the client and family to identify and correct hazards in the home before discharge
    2. Ensures that the client can correctly use all assistive-adaptive devices before discharge
    3. Provides a detailed plan of care at the time of discharge for clients to be transferred to a rehabilitation or long-term-care facility
    4. Reviews the prescribed exercise regimen and ensures client mastery by observing correct performance on return demonstration
    5. Teaches joint protection techniques:
        a. Turning doorknobs counterclockwise
        b. Using two hands instead of one to hold objects
        c. Sitting in a chair with a high, straight back
        d. Not bending at the waist; bending the knees instead while keeping the back straight
        e. Using a small pillow for sleep only
    6. Provides drug information, as necessary
    7. Instructs the client to check with the Arthritis Foundation about "new" treatments that propose to cure the disease
    8. Stresses the importance of follow-up visits with the health care provider(s) and therapist(s)

J

KERATITIS

See Corneal Disorders.

KERATOCONUS

See Corneal Disorders.

KERATOSES, ACTINIC

See Cancer, Skin.

KIDNEY DISEASE, POLYCYSTIC

OVERVIEW

- Polycystic kidney disease (PKD) is an inherited kidney disorder of the renal parenchyma that occurs bilaterally.
- The nephron is the primary site of cyst development; cysts develop in the glomeruli and tubules, resulting in less effective glomerular filtration, tubular reabsorption, and tubular secretion.
- The kidneys become grossly enlarged; cysts become progressively larger, and other abdominal organs may be displaced.

COLLABORATIVE MANAGEMENT

Assessment

- The nurse records the client's
    1. Family history of PKD
    2. Current health status
    3. Age of parents at development of clinical manifestations and related complications
    4. Family history of sudden death from a strokelike phenomenon
    5. History of constipation
    6. Changes in urine or frequency of urination
    7. History of hypertension
    8. History of headaches

- The nurse assesses for
    1. Protruding and distended abdomen
    2. Enlarged kidney on palpation
    3. Abdominal pain
    4. Tender tissue and flank pain
    5. Hematuria or cloudy urine
    6. Dysuria
    7. Severe headache
    8. Hypertension
    9. Edema
    10. Uremic symptoms
    11. Anger, resentment
    12. Futility, sadness

Interventions

- The nurse
    1. Administers analgesics for comfort, as ordered, avoiding aspirin-containing products
    2. Administers antibiotics, as ordered, for the infectious process
    3. Applies dry heat to the abdomen or flank
    4. Teaches relaxation techniques

- *Nephrectomy* (kidney removal) is performed when pain, infection, and bleeding are not controlled by medical management. (See Carcinoma, Renal, for care of the client undergoing a nephrectomy.)
- Preoperative care includes the administration of blood and fluids to achieve hemodynamic stabilization.
- The nurse
    1. Administers antihypertensive agents, as ordered, including vasodilators, beta-blockers, and calcium channel blockers

449

2. Administers diuretics, as ordered, to clients with renal insufficiency
3. Monitors intake and output
4. Records daily weights
5. Provides a low-sodium diet initially
6. Maintains protein restriction as renal insufficiency progresses
7. Provides counseling, support, and teaching about health maintenance
8. Discusses coping strategies used successfully in past
9. Refers the client to support groups
10. Refers the client to professional counseling services
11. Encourages the client to verbalize feelings or frustrations

- The nurse teaches the client and family
    1. How to measure and monitor blood pressure and body weight
    2. Dietary restrictions, such as a low-sodium or protein-restricted diet
    3. Desired effects and adverse effects of prescribed medications, including antihypertensive drugs and diuretics
    4. Measures for preventing constipation and their rationale
    5. Resources that are available for research and education, such as the Polycystic Kidney Research Foundation

KNEE INJURIES

See Trauma, Knee.

KNEE TRAUMA

See Trauma, Knee.

LABYRINTHITIS

- Labyrinthitis is an infection of the labyrinth, part of the inner ear.
- Clinical manifestations include hearing loss, tinnitus, spontaneous nystagmus to the affected side, nausea, vertigo, and vomiting.
- The most common complication is meningitis.
- Treatment includes
    1. Systemic antibiotics, such as ampicillin (Omnipen, Apo-Ampi◆)
    2. Bed rest in a darkened room
    3. Antiemetics, such as chlorpromazine (Thorazine, Novo-Chlorpromazine◆)
    4. Antivertiginous medications
    5. Psychologic support to cope with hearing loss

L

LACERATIONS, EYE

- The most common areas involved in lacerations of the eye are the eyelids and cornea.
- *Eye lacerations:*
    1. Bleed heavily and look more severe than they actually are
    2. Are treated by closing the eye and applying a small ice pack, checking visual acuity, and cleaning and suturing the eyelid
- *Corneal lacerations:*
    1. The ocular contents may prolapse through the laceration.
    2. The laceration is manifested by severe eye pain, photophobia, tearing, and decreased visual acuity.
    3. The penetrating object is *never* removed from the eye; it may be holding ocular structures in place.
    4. Treatment includes surgical repair under general anesthesia and antibiotic ointment. An *enucleation* may be needed if the ocular contents have protruded through the laceration.
    5. Complications include scarring, which may alter vision.

LANDRY'S PARALYSIS

See Guillain-Barré Syndrome.

LARYNGEAL TRAUMA

See Trauma, Laryngeal.

LARYNGITIS

* Laryngitis is an inflammation of mucous membranes lining the larynx with or without edema of the vocal cords.
* Laryngitis is commonly associated with upper respiratory tract infections.
* Etiologic factors include exposure to irritating inhalants and pollutants, overuse of the voice, and inhalation of volatile gases.
* Clinical manifestations include acute hoarseness, dry cough, and dysphagia; aphonia may occur.
* Management includes
    1. Steam inhalation
    2. Voice rest
    3. Increased fluid intake
    4. Throat lozenges
    5. Antibiotics
    6. Bronchodilators
* Clients with recurrent bouts of laryngitis require further evaluation.

Leiomyoma, Uterine

OVERVIEW

- Uterine leiomyomas, also called myomas and fibroids (fibroid tumors), are the most frequently occurring benign pelvic tumors.
- Leiomyomas develop from the uterine myometrium and are attached to it by a pedicle or stalk.
- Leiomyomas are classified according to their position in the layers of the uterus and anatomic position.
- The most common types are
    1. *Intramural:* contained in the uterine wall within the myometrium
    2. *Submucosal:* protrude into the cavity of the uterus
    3. *Subserosal:* may grow laterally and extend into the broad ligament

🖉 Considerations for Elderly Clients

Fibroids are more common in women in their older reproductive years and postmenopausally if the woman takes hormone replacement therapy.

➤ Transcultural Considerations

Leiomyomas are seen two to five times more frequently in African-American women than Caucasians.

COLLABORATIVE MANAGEMENT

Assessment

- The nurse records the client's history of abnormal bleeding.
- The nurse assesses for
    1. Complaints of a feeling of pelvic pressure
    2. Constipation
    3. Urinary frequency or retention
    4. Increased abdominal size
    5. Dyspareunia (painful intercourse)
    6. Infertility
    7. Abdominal pain occurring with torsion of the fibroid or pedicle

8. Uterine enlargement on abdominal, vaginal, or rectal examination

Planning and Implementation

✦ NDx: Potential for Hemorrhage

Nonsurgical Management

- The client who has no symptoms or who desires child-bearing is observed and examined for changes in the size of the leiomyoma every 4 to 6 months.
- If the woman is postmenopausal, the fibroids usually shrink.

Surgical Management

- Surgical treatment depends on whether future child-bearing is desired, the age of the woman, the size of the fibroid, and associated symptoms.
- A *myomectomy* (removal of the leiomyomas with preservation of the uterus) is done to preserve childbearing capabilities.
- *Hysterectomy* is the usual surgical management in the older woman who has multiple symptomatic leiomyomas.
- A *total hysterectomy* involves the removal of the uterus by either a vaginal or abdominal approach.
- A *subtotal hysterectomy,* removal of the uterus except the cervix, is rarely performed.
- *Panhysterectomy,* or *total abdominal hysterectomy,* includes the removal of the uterus, ovaries, and fallopian tubes.
- A *radical hysterectomy* involves removal of the uterus, lymph nodes, the upper third of the vagina, and the surrounding tissues.
- Preoperative care includes routine measures and a complete psychologic evaluation.
- The nurse
    1. Explores the client's feelings about the loss of the uterus, including childbearing, self-image and femininity, or sexual functioning
    2. Identifies the support system
    3. Discusses the client's fear of rejection from her sexual partner
- Postoperative care for the client undergoing abdominal hysterectomy is similar to that of any other client having abdominal surgery:

    1. Assessment for vaginal bleeding
    2. Assessment for bleeding at incision site
    3. Maintenance of a Foley catheter
- The nurse provides postoperative care for a client with a vaginal hysterectomy:
  1. Assesses for vaginal bleeding
  2. Provides perineal care:
     a. Sitz baths
     b. Heat lamps
     c. Ice packs
  3. Maintains a Foley or suprapubic catheter
- Complications
  1. Abdominal hysterectomy:
     a. Intestinal obstruction
     b. Thromboembolism
     c. Atelectasis
     d. Pneumonia
     e. Wound dehiscence
  2. Vaginal hysterectomy:
     a. Hemorrhage
     b. Urinary tract problems, especially infection and retention
  3. Both types of hysterectomy:
     a. Pulmonary embolism
     b. Depression
     c. Decreased libido

L

🕃 Considerations for Elderly Clients

Older women are more at risk for all postoperative complications, particularly pulmonary embolism. Obese women are more at risk for thromboembolism.

Continuing Care

- The appropriate health teaching depends on the specific treatment.
- The nurse instructs the client who has had an abdominal or vaginal hysterectomy
  1. To avoid or limit stair climbing for 1 month
  2. To avoid tub baths and sitting for long periods
  3. To avoid strenuous activity or lifting anything weighing more than 5 pounds (2.3 kg)
  4. To expect certain physical changes, including cessation of menses, inability to become pregnant,

weakness and fatigue in the convalescence period, and absence of menopausal symptoms unless the ovaries are removed

5. To participate in moderate exercise, such as walking
6. To consume foods that aid in healing, such as foods high in protein, iron, and vitamin C
7. To avoid sexual intercourse for 3 to 6 weeks
8. To observe for signs of complications, including infection
9. To expect emotional reactions and changes

LEPROSY

- Leprosy, or Hansen's disease, is a chronic, highly contagious, systemic mycobacterial infection of the peripheral nervous system complicated by secondary skin involvement.
- Clinical manifestations are directly related to the degree of individual resistance to mycobacteria.
- *Localized* leprosy (high immunity) is characterized by one or two isolated, erythematous, anesthetic plaques that are hairless and scaly in texture.
- *Generalized* leprosy (low immunity) involves widespread, faintly erythematous macules, papules, nodules, and plaques with concomitant peripheral nerve damage.
- Treatment is aimed at controlling bacterial proliferation and minimizing associated deformities; clients are treated as outpatients to prevent spread.
- The drug of choice is dapsone, a sulfone.

LEUKEMIA

OVERVIEW

- The leukemias are a group of malignant disorders involving abnormal overproduction of specific cell types, usually at the immature stage, in bone marrow.

456

- Leukemia may be either acute or chronic.
- The two major types of leukemia include
  1. Lymphocytic or lymphoblastic, involving cells within the committed lymphoid maturational pathways (acute and chronic)
  2. Myelocytic or myelogenous, involving cells within the myeloid maturational pathways (acute and chronic)
- Acute myelogenous leukemia (AML) is the most common type seen in adults.
- The basic pathologic defect in leukemia is malignant transformation of stem cells or early committed precursor leukocytes, producing an abnormal proliferation of a specific type of leukocyte in the bone marrow that shuts down normal bone marrow production of erythrocytes, platelets, and functionally mature leukocytes.

COLLABORATIVE MANAGEMENT

L

Assessment

- The nurse records the client's
  1. Age
  2. Environmental exposure
  3. Previous illness and exposure to ionizing radiation or medications
  4. History of infections, including influenza, cold, pneumonia, bronchitis, and unexplained fever
  5. Overt bleeding episodes
  6. History of weakness or fatigue
  7. Associated symptoms
- The nurse assesses for
  1. Integumentary manifestations:
     a. Ecchymosis
     b. Petechiae
     c. Pallor of the conjunctiva, the nail beds, and the palmar creases around the mouth
  2. Gastrointestinal manifestations:
     a. Bleeding gums
     b. Anorexia
     c. Weight loss
     d. Enlarged liver and spleen
  3. Renal manifestations: hematuria
  4. Cardiovascular manifestations:
     a. Tachycardia at basal activity levels
     b. Orthostatic hypotension

  c. Palpitations
  d. Increased capillary filling times
 5. Respiratory manifestations:
  a. Abnormal breath sounds
  b. Dyspnea on exertion
 6. Neurologic manifestations:
  a. Fatigue
  b. Headache
  c. Papilledema
 7. Hematologic manifestations:
  a. Decreased hemoglobin, hematocrit, and platelet count
  b. Altered (usually elevated) white blood cell count
  c. Abnormal coagulation studies
  d. Abnormal bone marrow findings
 8. Musculoskeletal manifestations:
  a. Bone pain
  b. Joint swelling and pain

Planning and Implementation

✦ NDx: Risk for Infection

- The nurse employs infection control measures:
  1. Washes hands frequently and thoroughly between client contacts
  2. Wears a mask (with clients with upper respiratory infections)
  3. Places the client in a private room, if able
  4. Uses aseptic technique for dressing changes
- The nurse
  1. Monitors for signs of infection
  2. Provides meticulous skin care to maintain skin integrity
  3. Provides pulmonary toilet to prevent respiratory infections
  4. Administers chemotherapeutic drugs, as ordered, to interrupt or halt infectious processes and to control infection:
     a. Induction chemotherapy includes administration with agents such as cytosine arabinoside with daunorubicin
     b. Consolidation therapy consists of another course of the same drugs or a different combination of chemotherapeutic agents

c. Maintenance therapy includes transfusion of red blood cells, platelets, and granulocytes

---

🗑 Women's Health Considerations

- Pregnancy may increase a woman's risk of developing leukemia, although current data are inconclusive.
- The nurse administers
    1. Antibacterial agents (antibiotics including aminoglycosides and a systemic penicillin), as ordered
    2. Antifungal agents when fungal infections are present (amphotericin B and ketoconazole), as ordered
    3. Antiviral agents used prophylactically (e.g., acyclovir), as ordered
- A bone marrow transplant is the treatment of choice for clients with closely matched donors and who are experiencing temporary remission. A suitable donor is identified after human leukocyte antigen (HLA) typing. The marrow is harvested from the donor and administered by intravenous infusion through a central catheter to the client.
- The client must undergo a conditioning regimen before transplantation that may include intensive chemotherapy and sometimes radiotherapy, usually total body irradiation.
- The nurse monitors for complications of bone marrow transplantation:
    1. Infection due to loss of natural immunity
    2. Severe thrombocytopenia
    3. Failure to engraft
    4. Graft-versus-host disease (GVHD)
    5. Veno-occlusive disease
- The immunosuppressive agents required to prevent GVHD increase the client's susceptibility to infection.
- Isolation procedures are required for bone marrow recipients.

✦ NDx: Risk for Injury

- The nurse
    1. Protects the client from situations that could lead to bleeding
    2. Examines stool, urine, nasogastric drainage, and vomiting for blood loss

3. Measures any blood loss as accurately as possible
4. Measures the client's abdominal girth each shift
5. Monitors laboratory values daily

✦ **NDx:** Fatigue

- The nurse
    1. Increases dietary intake with small, frequent meals high in protein and carbohydrates
    2. Provides blood transfusions, as ordered, to increase the oxygen-carrying capacity of the blood
    3. Conserves the client's energy by providing rest periods and eliminating or postponing activities

Continuing Care

- The nurse teaches the client and family
    1. Measures to protect the client from infection
    2. The importance of meticulous mouth care
    3. The need to report signs of infection immediately to the physician
    4. The necessity of maintaining a healthy diet
    5. The importance of maintaining medical follow-up despite unpleasant side effects
    6. Resources for psychosocial and financial support for role and self-esteem adjustment
    7. Safety and bleeding precautions
    8. Care of the central catheter if still in place at discharge

LIVER ABSCESSES

See Abscesses, Hepatic.

LIVER CANCER

See Cancer, Liver.

LIVER, FATTY

- Fatty liver is caused by the accumulation of triglycerides and other fats in the hepatic cells.
- The most common cause is chronic alcoholism.
- Other causes include malnutrition, diabetes mellitus, obesity, pregnancy, prolonged parenteral nutrition, and exposure to toxic drugs.
- The client usually has no symptoms; the typical finding is hepatomegaly (an enlarged liver).
- The nurse assesses for
    1. Right upper abdominal pain
    2. Ascites
    3. Edema
    4. Jaundice
    5. Fever
    6. Signs of cirrhosis (see Cirrhosis)
- Liver biopsy confirms the diagnosis.
- Interventions are aimed at removing the underlying cause of the infiltration and dietary restrictions.

LIVER TRANSPLANTATION

See Transplantation, Liver.

LIVER TRAUMA

See Trauma, Liver.

LOCKJAW

See Tetanus.

LOU GEHRIG'S DISEASE

See Amyotrophic Lateral Sclerosis.

LUNG CANCER

See Cancer, Lung.

LUPUS ERYTHEMATOSUS

OVERVIEW

- *Systemic lupus erythematosus* (SLE) is a chronic progressive, systemic, inflammatory disease that can cause major body organs and systems to fail; it has no cure.
- *Discoid lupus erythematosus* (DLE) affects only the skin; it is uncommon.
- Lupus is thought to be an autoimmune process, characterized by spontaneous remissions and exacerbations.

➤ Transcultural Considerations

- One in 700 women between the ages of 15 and 64 have the disease.
- One in 250 African Americans in this age group are affected.

COLLABORATIVE MANAGEMENT

Assessment

- The nurse assesses for
    1. Dry, scaly, raised rash on the face or upper body (may be the only indicator of DLE)
    2. Articular involvement; *initial* joint changes are similar to those of rheumatoid arthritis, but deformities are not uncommon

462

3. Avascular necrosis
4. Muscle atrophy
5. Myalgia
6. Fever
7. Various degrees of weakness, fatigue, anorexia, and weight loss
8. Renal involvement, such as changes in urinary output, proteinuria, hematuria, and fluid retention
9. Pulmonary effusions
10. Pericarditis
11. Neurologic changes, such as psychoses, seizures, paresis, migraine headaches, and cranial nerve palsies
12. Raynaud's phenomenon
13. Abdominal pain
14. Liver enlargement
15. Sjögren's syndrome
16. Body image changes
17. Social isolation

Interventions

- The nurse administers drug therapy, as ordered:
  1. Topical steroid preparations
  2. Hydroxychloroquine (Plaquenil) to decrease the inflammatory response
  3. Chronic steroid therapy to treat the systemic disease process
  4. Intravenous steroids for acute exacerbations
  5. Antineoplastic agents, including cyclophosphamide (Cytoxan, Procytox◆) and azathioprine (Imuran)
- The nurse teaches measures for skin protection:
  1. Avoiding exposure to sunlight and other forms of ultraviolet light:
     a. Wearing long sleeves and wide-brimmed hats
     b. Using sun-blocking agents with a sun protection factor of 30 or higher
  2. Cleaning skin with a mild soap and avoiding harsh, perfumed substances
  3. Using cosmetics with moisturizers
  4. Using a mild shampoo and avoiding permanents and frosting
- The nurse reinforces measures for joint protection and energy conservation (see Arthritis, Rheumatoid)
- The nurse provides health teaching:
  1. Protection of the skin

2. Importance of monitoring for fever (the first sign of an exacerbation)
3. Importance of joint protection and energy conservation
4. Importance of follow-up visits with the physician(s)
5. Use of the Lupus Foundation and Arthritis Foundation as resources
6. Drug information, as needed

LYME DISEASE

- Lyme disease is transmitted by infected deer ticks.
- The disease can be prevented by avoiding heavily wooded areas or areas with thick underbrush, by wearing long-sleeved tops and long pants, and by using an insect repellent on skin and clothes when in an area where infected ticks are likely to be found.
- The disease is manifested by a spreading circular rash, malaise, fever, chills, swollen glands, headache, and muscle or joint aches.
- Cardiac symptoms may include low-grade heart block, bradycardia, tachycardia, chest pain, and syncope.
- Neurologic manifestations include meningitis, cranial neuropathy, and encephalitis.
- Lyme disease is treated with oral antibiotics such as tetracycline (Achromycin), which may alleviate arthritic, cardiac, and neurologic manifestations.
- Testing for Lyme disease should not be done until 4 to 6 weeks after being bitten by a tick because it is not reliable before that time.

LYMPHOMA, HODGKIN'S

See Hodgkin's Lymphoma.

MACULAR DEGENERATION

See Degeneration, Macular.

MALABSORPTION SYNDROME

- Malabsorption syndrome is associated with a variety of disorders and intestinal surgical procedures in which one or multiple nutrients are not digested or absorbed.
- Physiologic mechanisms limit absorption because of one or more abnormalities.
  1. Bile salt deficiencies
  2. Enzyme deficiencies
  3. Bacteria
  4. Disruption of the mucosal lining of the small intestine
  5. Alteration in lymphatic or vascular circulation
  6. Decreased gastric or intestinal surface area

- Clinical manifestations of malabsorption include steatorrhea, weight loss, fatigue, decreased libido, easy bruising, anemia, bone pain, and edema.
- Interventions focus on avoiding dietary substances that aggravate malabsorption and supplementing nutrients and surgical or nonsurgical management of the primary causative disease.

MALNUTRITION

OVERVIEW

- Protein-calorie malnutrition (PCM) is a multinutrient problem in which protein catabolism exceeds protein intake and synthesis and results in negative nitrogen balance, weight loss, decreased muscle mass, and weakness.

- Causes of PCM include inadequate nutrition intake, increased nutrient losses, or increased nutrient requirements.

COLLABORATIVE MANAGEMENT

- The nurse records the client's
  1. Normal daily food intake
  2. Eating behaviors
  3. Change in appetite
  4. Weight changes
  5. Current and past medical history
  6. Economic status
- Clinical manifestations include
  1. Reddened, dry skin
  2. Difficulty or pain on swallowing
  3. Nausea, vomiting, or heartburn
  4. Low hemoglobin and hematocrit
  5. Serum albumin level less than 3.5 g/dL
  6. Serum transferrin level less than 200 mg/dL
- Treatment includes
  1. High-calorie, high-protein diet
  2. Small, frequent feeding (six meals per day)
  3. Nutritional supplements or partial enteral nutrition
  4. Total enteral nutrition (complications include fluid imbalance, increased osmolarity, dehydration, diarrhea, and electrolyte imbalance)
  5. Parenteral nutrition:
     a. Total parenteral nutrition (TPN)
     b. Partial parenteral nutrition (PPN)
     c. Major complications include fluid and electrolyte imbalance

Continuing Care

- In collaboration with the nurse, the dietitian teaches the client about the need for a high-calorie, high-protein diet and nutritional supplements.
- The client may need continued enteral or parenteral nutrition in the home setting.

MASTOIDITIS

- Mastoiditis is a secondary disorder resulting from an untreated or inadequately treated chronic or acute otitis media.
- Clinical manifestations include swelling behind the ear and pain with minimal movement of the tragus, pinna, and/or head.
- Otoscopic examination reveals a reddened, dull, thick, immobile tympanic membrane with or without perforation, low-grade fever, malaise, and anorexia.
- Treatment includes antibiotics and/or surgical removal of the infected tissue, such as a *tympanoplasty,* or a simple or modified radical *mastoidectomy.*
- Complications of surgery include damage to the abducens and facial nerves (cranial nerves VI and VII, respectively), meningitis, brain abscess, chronic purulent otitis media, and wound infection.

M

MD

See Dystrophy, Muscular.

MELANOMA

See Cancer, Skin.

MELANOMA, OCULAR

OVERVIEW

- Melanoma of the eye is a unilateral tumor that occurs most frequently in the uveal tract.
- Symptoms are not readily obvious, and the lesion may be found during a routine eye examination.
- The problem is manifested by blurred vision, changes in visual acuity, increased intraocular pressure, change in color of the iris, and sudden change in peripheral vision.

COLLABORATIVE MANAGEMENT

- Treatment includes
    1. *Enucleation* (removal of the entire eyeball) and insertion of a ball implant to maintain conformity of the eye socket until a prosthesis is fitted (approximately 1 month)
    2. Radiation therapy:
        a. Complications include radiation tumor vasculopathy, radiation retinopathy, and cataract formation.
        b. Cycloplegic eyedrops (Cyclogyl) and an antibiotic-steroid combination (tobramycin, dexamethasone) are ordered.
- Nursing management includes
    1. Closely monitoring the client for hemorrhage, reporting any change in vital signs and/or the presence of bright red drainage on the dressing to the physician
    2. Teaching the client strategies to
        a. Insert antibiotic-steroid ointment into the culde-sac once each day
        b. Insert and remove the eye prosthesis

MÉNIÈRE'S SYNDROME

OVERVIEW

• Ménière's syndrome refers to overproduction or decreased resorption of endolymphatic fluid.

COLLABORATIVE MANAGEMENT

• The nurse assesses for
  1. Duration, intensity, and time between episodes of the classic triad of symptoms:
     a. Tinnitus, a continuous, low-pitched roar or a humming sound, is present much of the time but worsens just before and during a severe attack.
     b. Hearing loss, initially for low-frequency tones, worsens to include all levels after repeated episodes. Permanent hearing loss develops as the number of attacks increases.

     c. Vertigo, described as periods of whirling that might cause the client to fall to the ground, may be so intense that even while lying down, the client holds the bed or ground in an attempt to prevent the whirling. The severe vertigo usually lasts only 3 to 4 hours and is followed by a sense of dizziness.
  2. Presence of a feeling of fullness in the ear before an attack
  3. Nausea and vomiting
  4. Nystagmus (rapid eye movements)
  5. Severe headache
• The nurse
  1. Instructs the client to make slow head movements.
  2. Teaches dietary changes, such as salt and fluid restriction
  3. Teaches the importance of smoking cessation
  4. Administers nicotinic acid, as ordered, which is useful for its vasodilator effect
  5. Administers antihistamines, as ordered, such as diphenhydramine (Benadryl, Allerdryl◆) and dimenhydrinate (Dramamine, Gravol◆)
  6. Administers antiemetics, as ordered, such as chlorpromazine (Thorazine, Novo-Chlorpromazine◆),

droperidol (Inapsine), and trimethobenzamide (Tigan, Arrestin)

7. Administers diazepam (Valium, Apo-Diazepam◆) as ordered, to calm the anxious client and help control vertigo, nausea, and vomiting

- Surgical treatment is controversial because the remaining hearing in the affected ear is sacrificed.
- *Labyrinthectomy* involves the resection of the vestibular nerve or total removal of the labyrinth.
- An endolymphatic drainage and shunt may be performed early in the course of the disease to relieve vertigo.

MENINGITIS

OVERVIEW

- Meningitis is an inflammation of the arachnoid and pia mater of the brain and spinal cord.
- Bacterial meningitis occurs most frequently and is most often caused by *Streptococcus pneumoniae* and *Neisseria meningitidis;* viral meningitis is usually self-limiting; cryptococcal meningitis is the most common fungal meningitis.

COLLABORATIVE MANAGEMENT

Assessment

- The nurse records the client's
  1. Past medical history, including information about viral or respiratory diseases; head trauma; ear, nose, and/or sinus infection; heart disease; diabetes mellitus; cancer; immunosuppressive therapy; neurologic surgery and/or procedures
  2. Exposure to communicable disease
- The nurse assesses for
  1. Level of consciousness, orientation, cognition, and memory
  2. Pupil size and reaction to light, photophobia, nystagmus, abnormal eye movement
  3. Motor strength
  4. Severity of headache

5. Nuchal ridigity: positive Kernig's sign and Brudzinski reflex
6. Dysfunction of cranial nerves III, IV, VI, VII, and VIII
7. Nausea, vomiting
8. Fever, chills
9. Generalized aches and pains
10. Seizure activity
11. Syndrome of inappropriate antidiuretic hormone (SIADH) production
12. Fluid and electrolyte imbalance, particularly hyponatremia
13. Changes in color and temperature of extremities
14. Presence of all peripheral pulses
15. Presence of a red macular rash (meningococcal meningitis)
16. Results of cerebrospinal fluid (CSF) analysis

Interventions

- The nurse

  1. Assesses and records the client's vital signs and neurologic checks at least every 4 hours
  2. Performs neurologic and vascular assessments every 4 hours
  3. Administers medications as ordered
     a. Antibiotics
     b. Analgesics
  4. Maintains isolation precautions per hospital policy
  5. Implements routine seizure precautions
  6. Monitors for complications, such as shock and septic complications

METABOLIC ACIDOSIS

See Acidosis, Metabolic.

METABOLIC ALKALOSIS

See Alkalosis, Metabolic.

MG

See Myasthenia Gravis.

MIGRAINE HEADACHE

See Headache, Migraine.

MITRAL INSUFFICIENCY

See Insufficiency, Mitral, and Mitral Regurgitation.

MITRAL REGURGITATION

See Insufficiency, Mitral, and Mitral Regurgitation.

MITRAL STENOSIS

See Stenosis, Mitral.

Mitral Valve Prolapse

See Prolapse, Mitral Valve.

MS

See Sclerosis, Multiple.

Mucous Colitis

See Irritable Bowel Syndrome.

Multiple Sclerosis

See Sclerosis, Multiple.

Muscle Pulls

See Strains.

Muscular Dystrophy

See Dystrophy, Muscular.

Myasthenia Gravis

OVERVIEW

- Myasthenia gravis (MG) is a chronic, neuromuscular, autoimmune disease that involves a decrease in the number and effectiveness of acetylcholine (ACh) receptors at the neuromuscular junction.

🕸 Considerations for Elderly Clients

1. Although before the age of 40 women are affected two to three times more often than men, in later life the incidence in the sexes is about equal.
2. Men have more associated thymomas (encapsulated thymus gland tumors).

COLLABORATIVE MANAGEMENT

Assessment

- The nurse records the client's
    1. Rapid onset of fatigue
    2. Muscular weakness that increases on exertion or as the day wears on and improves with rest (with a temporary increase in weakness sometimes noted after vaccination, menstruation, and exposure to extremes in environmental temperature)
    3. Inability to perform activities of daily living (ADL)
    4. Ptosis, diplopia
    5. Respiratory distress
    6. Choking, dysphagia
    7. Weakness of voice
    8. Difficulty holding head up
    9. Paresthesia or aching in weakened muscles
- The nurse assesses for
    1. Progressive paresis of affected muscle groups that is resolved by rest, at least in part
    2. Symptoms related to involvement of the levator palpebrae or extraocular muscles
        a. Ocular palsies
        b. Ptosis
        c. Diplopia
        d. Weak or incomplete eye closure

3. Involvement of muscles for facial expression, chewing, and speech
   a. The client's smile may turn into a snarl
   b. The jaw hangs
   c. Difficulty chewing and swallowing may lead to severe nutritional deficits
4. Proximal limb weakness; the client has difficulty climbing stairs, lifting heavy objects, and/or raising arms overhead
5. Mild or severe neck weakness
6. Difficulty sustaining a sitting or walking posture
7. Respiratory distress
8. Bowel and bladder incontinence
9. Weakness of the pelvic and shoulder girdles (seen in Eaton-Lambert syndrome, a special form of MG often observed in combination with small cell carcinoma of the lung)
10. Body image disturbance
11. Feelings of loss, fear, helplessness, and grief
12. Usual coping methods
13. Positive ACh receptor antibodies
14. Significant improvement after Tensilon testing

Interventions

- The nurse
  1. Performs a respiratory assessment at least every 8 hours
  2. Monitors for respiratory distress: dyspnea, shortness of breath, air hunger, confusion
  3. Assesses tidal volume and vital capacity every 2 to 4 hours
  4. Encourages the client to turn, cough, and deep breathe every 2 hours
  5. Monitors arterial blood gases as the client's condition indicates
  6. Performs chest physiotherapy, including postural drainage, percussion, and vibration
  7. Has intubation equipment readily available

Nonsurgical Management

- The nurse
  1. Assesses motor strength before and after periods of activity
  2. Provides assistance with mobilization as necessary

3. Teaches the client to plan activities early in the day or during the energy peaks that follow the administration of medications
4. Plans rest periods for the client to avoid excessive fatigue
5. Performs active and passive range-of-motion (ROM) exercises
6. Uses heel and elbow protectors as needed
7. Assesses the need for an eggcrate or alternating pressure mattress
8. Recognizes that medications *must* be given on time to maintain blood levels
9. Administers anticholinesterase drugs such as neostigmine, pyridostigmine (Mestinon), or ambenonium (Mytelase), as ordered, to increase the response of muscles to nerve impulses, thus improving strength:
   a. The drug is given with a small amount of food to minimize gastrointestinal (GI) side effects; meals are provided 45 minutes to 1 hour after taking medication.
   b. Drugs containing magnesium, morphine or its derivatives, curare, quinine, quinidine, procainamide, hypnotics, and sedatives are avoided because they may increase weakness.
10. Avoids antibiotics such as neomycin, kanamycin, streptomycin, polymyxin B, and certain tetracyclines that have been shown to increase myasthenic symptoms
11. Recognizes that edrophonium produces a temporary improvement in myasthenic crisis but no improvement or a worsening of symptoms in cholinergic crisis
12. Administers corticosteroids, such as prednisone (Deltasone), used in conjunction with anticholinesterase drugs; worsening of symptoms may be seen for the first 7 to 10 days
13. Observes for side effects of corticosteroids, such as electrolyte imbalance, weight gain, acne, GI upset, and hyperglycemia
14. Administers immunosuppressive agents with drugs such as azathioprine (Imuran), methotrexate (Mexate), and cyclophosphamide (Cytoxan), as ordered, which have resulted in some clinical improvement

- Plasmapheresis is a method by which autoantibodies are removed from the plasma. Immunosuppressive drugs are administered concurrently to decrease the formation of additional antibodies. Nursing management includes maintaining the intravenous line or shunt, monitoring vital signs, and assessing neurologic signs.
- The nurse observes for myasthenic crisis, an exacerbation of the myasthenic symptoms caused by undermedication with anticholinergic drugs or infection.
- The nurse monitors for respiratory compromise; anticholinesterase drugs may be withheld.
- The nurse observes for cholinergic crisis, an acute exacerbation of muscle weakness caused by over-medication with cholinergic (anticholinesterase) drugs.

Surgical Management

- Thymectomy is an alternative method of treatment.
- The nurse provides preoperative care:
  1. Provides routine preoperative care
  2. Administers pyridostigmine (Mestinon), as ordered, to keep the client stable throughout surgery
  3. Gives steroids before surgery but tapers them postoperatively
  4. Administers antibiotics, as ordered

- The nurse provides postoperative care:
  1. Monitors the client in the intensive care unit
  2. Provides routine postoperative care
  3. Observes for signs of pneumothorax or hemothorax, such as chest pain, sudden shortness of breath, diminished or absent breath sounds, and restlessness or a change in vital signs
  4. Provides routine chest tube care
  5. Observes for signs and symptoms of wound infection
- The nurse
  1. Assesses the client's ability to perform ADL to establish his or her abilities and limitations
  2. Encourages the client to perform activities as independently as possible; provides assistance as needed
  3. Plans activities to follow the administration of medication to maximize independence and successful attempts at self-care
  4. Documents and monitors the client's response to or tolerance of activity

5. Collaborates with physical and occupational therapists to identify the need for adaptive-assistive devices

- The nurse
    1. Assesses cranial nerves III, IV, VI, and VII to determine deficits and abilities
    2. Provides orientation to the surroundings and explains the need for assistance with ADL and mobility if the client has visual impairments
    3. Applies artificial tears to the client's eyes to keep the corneas moist and free from abrasion
    4. Alternates patches on each eye to treat diplopia

✦ NDx: Impaired Verbal Communication

- The nurse
    1. Assesses cranial nerves V, VII, IX, X, and XII to determine the client's ability to communicate
    2. Instructs the client to speak slowly; attempts to lip read; repeats information to verify that it is correct
    3. Collaborates with the speech therapist to develop a communication system that the client can use, such as eye blinking, use of flash cards, and/or a word board

- The nurse
    1. Weighs the client daily
    2. Maintains a calorie count
    3. Assesses the client's gag reflex and ability to chew and swallow without undue fatigue or aspiration
    4. Provides frequent oral hygiene
    5. Obtains a dietary consultation to identify food preferences and dislikes
    6. Provides small, frequent meals and high-calorie snacks
    7. Administers anticholinesterase medications 45 minutes to 1 hour before meals, as ordered
    8. Observes the client for choking, nasal regurgitation, and aspiration
    9. Gives tube feedings, if necessary
    10. Establishes a bowel program to treat diarrhea or constipation

- The nurse
    1. Establishes a trusting and therapeutic relationship with the client and family by listening, providing emotional support, and just "being there" for them

2. Reinforces the client's abilities
3. Keeps the client and family informed of progress
4. Encourages the client and family to talk about the future
5. Refers the client and family to local and national support groups

Continuing Care

- The nurse
    1. Identifies and suggests correction of hazards in the home prior to discharge
    2. Ensures that the client can correctly use all assistive-adaptive devices ordered for home use
    3. Provides drug information, including informing the client to avoid such medications as morphine, quinine, quinidine, procainamide, mycin-type antibiotics, and drugs containing magnesium
    4. Encourages the client to become certified in cardiopulmonary resuscitation

- The nurse emphasizes specific points concerning the disease process:
    1. Its episodic nature
    2. Factors that predispose the client to exacerbation, such as infection, stress, surgery, and hard physical exercise
    3. Symptoms of myasthenic crisis and cholinergic crisis
    4. Lifestyle adaptations that may be indicated, such as avoiding heat (sauna, sunbathing), crowds, overeating, and erratic changes in sleep habits

Myopia

See Refractive Errors.

NASAL CANCER

See Cancer, Nasal and Sinus.

NASAL FRACTURE

See Fracture, Nasal.

NEARSIGHTEDNESS

See Refractive Errors.

NEPHROSCLEROSIS

- Changes in the afferent and efferent arterioles and glomerular capillary loops of the kidney nephron cause nephrosclerosis.
- Changes include thickening of the vessel walls and narrowing of the vessel lumen, resulting in decreased renal blood flow and interstitial tissue changes.
- Ischemia and fibrosis develop over time.
- Nephrosclerosis is associated with benign essential hypertension or malignant hypertension, atherosclerosis, and diabetes mellitus.
- Control of blood pressure and preservation of renal function are goals of treatment, which includes antihypertensive agents.

Neuroma, Acoustic

- An acoustic neuroma is a benign, but destructive, tumor of the vestibular, or acoustic, cranial nerve. Damage to hearing, facial movements, and sensation may result.
- Clinical manifestations begin with tinnitus and progress to gradual sensorineural hearing loss; constant mild vertigo occurs later.
- Diagnosis is made by computed tomographic scanning, audiograms, and cerebrospinal fluid analysis (which shows increased pressure and protein).
- Surgical removal of the neuroma by means of a craniotomy is necessary, and hearing is permanently affected. Extreme care to preserve the function of the facial nerve (cranial nerve VII) is taken. (See "Surgical Management" under Tumors, Brain for care of the client having a craniotomy.)

Obesity

OVERVIEW

- Obesity is defined as body fat greater than 22% to 25% for men and greater than 35% for women.
- It involves complex interrelationships of major factors, including genetic, environmental, psychologic, social, cultural, pathologic, and physiologic.
- Complications include diabetes mellitus, hypertension, altered lipid metabolism, cardiac disease, sleep apnea, cholelithiasis, chronic back pain, early degenerative arthritis, susceptibility to infections, and certain cancers.

➤ Transcultural Considerations

1. The prevalence of obesity among African Americans, Hispanic Americans, Pacific Islanders, Na-

tive Americans, and Native Alaskans and Hawaiians is substantially higher than in Caucasians, especially among women.

2. The percentage of obese African American women is almost double that of Caucasian women.

COLLABORATIVE MANAGEMENT

- Assessment of the client includes
  1. Economic status
  2. Usual food intake
  3. Eating behaviors
  4. Cultural background
  5. Attitude toward food and current weight
  6. Appetite
  7. Medications
  8. Physical activity
  9. Height and weight

🕦 Women's Health Considerations

1. Women are more vulnerable to complications of being overweight or obese.
2. Women whose fat stores are primarily in their abdominal or truncal area are at the highest risk for complications.

- Management includes
  1. Dietary management
  2. Drug therapy
     a. Sympathomimetic amines may be given to increase energy expended and heat loss.
     b. Side effects include potential for abuse, sleep disturbances, heart palpitations, increased blood pressure, dry mouth, and depression.
     c. Other drugs include fluoxetine and mazindol.
  3. Exercise program
  4. Behavioral treatment including reinforcement techniques and cognitive restructuring
- Surgery is indicated for the client who repeatedly fails at dietary management or is morbidly obese.
  1. Maxillomandibular fixation or jaw wiring
  2. Permanently encircling the esophagus with a band
  3. Intestinal bypass to connect the stomach and jejunum

    4. Gastroplasty or stapling or banding the stomach
- Postoperative care after gastroplasty or intestinal bypass includes
    1. Routine postoperative care
    2. Monitoring the patency of the nasogastric tube and recording the amount of drainage
    3. Providing clear liquids slowly, as ordered, on the third postoperative day if bowel sounds are present and the client is passing flatus; increasing the diet as tolerated

Continuing Care

- The client is given a list of community resources, such as Weight Watchers, Overeaters Anonymous, and Take Off Pounds Sensibly (TOPS).
- In collaboration with the nurse, the dietitian provides health teaching regarding the diet and the importance of maintaining a healthy eating pattern.

OBSTRUCTION, BOWEL

See Obstruction, Intestinal.

OBSTRUCTION, INTESTINAL

OVERVIEW

- Partial or total intestinal obstruction can be either mechanical or nonmechanical (paralytic).
- *Mechanical obstruction* can be due to
    1. Disorders outside the intestine (adhesions and hernias)
    2. Blockage of the intestinal lumen (tumors, inflammation, strictures, or fecal impaction)

- The most common causes of mechanical obstruction include adhesions and hernias.
- *Nonmechanical obstruction* (paralytic or adynamic ileus) involves decreased muscular activity of the intestine, resulting in a slowing of the movement of intestinal contents.
- Distention results from the intestine's inability to absorb and mobilize intestinal contents; increased peristalsis occurs, leading to additional distention, edema of the bowel, and increased capillary permeability.
- Paralytic, or adynamic, ileus is the most common cause of intestinal obstruction because it can be caused by physiologic, neurogenic, or chemical imbalances.
- *Strangulated obstruction* results when there is obstruction with compromised blood flow.
- Complications of intestinal obstruction include
    1. Fluid and electrolyte imbalance
    2. Hypovolemia
    3. Metabolic acidosis or alkalosis
    4. Renal insufficiency
    5. Peritonitis
    6. Septic shock
- Mechanical obstruction of the small intestine is most often caused by adhesions; obstruction in the colon is related to tumors, diverticulitis, or volvulus.
- Paralytic ileus is associated with trauma, abdominal surgery, hypokalemia, myocardial infarction, or vascular insufficiency.

COLLABORATIVE MANAGEMENT

Assessment

- The nurse records the client's
    1. Past medical history, including abdominal surgical procedures, radiation therapy, or bowel diseases, such as Crohn's disease, ulcerative colitis, diverticular disease, gallstones, hernias, and tumors
    2. Diet history
    3. Bowel elimination patterns, including the presence of blood in the stool
    4. Familial history of colorectal cancer

- The nurse assesses (for mechanical intestinal obstruction)
    1. Intermittent upper abdominal cramping (characteristic of mechanical obstruction)
    2. Peristaltic waves
    3. High-pitched bowel sounds (borborygmi) in *early* obstructive process
    4. Absent bowel sounds in *later* stages
    5. Abdominal distention (hallmark sign)
    6. Nausea and vomiting
        a. Obstruction above the ileum causes early and profuse vomiting of partially digested food and chyme, changing to watery contents containing bile and mucus.
        b. Obstruction in the large intestine produces vomitus with an orange-brown color and a foul odor caused by bacterial overgrowth, which may be fecal contamination.
    7. Obstipation (characteristic of total small and large mechanical obstruction)
- The nurse assesses (for nonmechanical intestinal obstruction)
    1. Constant, diffuse abdominal discomfort; severe pain in intestinal vascular insufficiency or infarction
    2. Decreased bowel sounds in *early* obstruction
    3. Absent bowel sounds in *later* obstruction
    4. Vomiting of gastric contents and bile
    5. Singultus (hiccups) (common with all types of intestinal obstruction)

Planning and Implementation

✦ **NDx:** Altered (Gastrointestinal) Tissue Perfusion

Nonsurgical Management

- The nurse
    1. Maintains the client on nothing-by-mouth (NPO) status.
    2. Monitors drainage from the nasogastric tube, such as the Salem sump or Anderson suction tube, which sit distally in the stomach and are connected to low continuous suction (commonly used).

3. Monitors drainage from the intestinal tube, such as the Miller-Abbott, Cantor, or Harris tube, which is used for small intestine obstructions. (These tubes, weighted with mercury-filled balloons, act as a food bolus, stimulating peristalsis advancing through the intestinal tract, and are less commonly used.)
4. Assists with intestinal tube progression by helping the client change position every 2 hours and by advancing the tube 3 to 4 inches at specified times, as ordered.
5. Avoids taping the intestinal tube to the nose until the desired position is reached in the intestine.
6. Monitors intestinal tube drainage, which occurs by gravity, and instills 10 mL of air, as ordered, if the drainage stops; *does not* irrigate the tube with fluid.
7. Maintains low intermittent or continuous suction, as ordered, when the tube has reached the desired location.
8. Provides frequent mouth care for the client with an intestinal tube.

- Obstruction caused by fecal impaction resolves after disimpaction and enema.
- Intussusception (telescoping of bowel) may resolve during hydrostatic pressure changes during a barium enema.

Surgical Management

- Surgical management is required for complete mechanical obstruction and for many cases of incomplete mechanical obstruction.
- An exploratory laparotomy is performed to locate the obstruction and determine the nature of the problem.
- The specific surgical procedure performed is dependent on the cause and location of the obstruction. Examples of procedures include lysis of adhesions; colon resection with anastomosis for obstruction due to tumor or diverticulitis; and embolectomy or thrombectomy for intestinal infarction.
- Nursing care for abdominal surgery is similar to that described under Cancer, Colorectal.

✦ NDx: Fluid Volume Deficit

- The nurse
  1. Administers intravenous (IV) fluid because of vascular fluid losses from lack of normal reabsorption in the intestine, increased intestinal secretions, nasogastric suction, and NPO status (normal saline solutions with potassium replacement are used according to electrolyte results)
  2. Provides blood products in case of strangulated obstruction because of blood loss into the bowel or peritoneal cavity
  3. Provides ice chips only with a physician's order
  4. Monitors vital signs and other measures of fluid status (urinary output, skin turgor, mucous membrane)
  5. Assesses the client for edema
  6. Administers total parenteral nutrition, as ordered
  7. Provides frequent mouth care

✦ NDx: Pain

- The nurse
  1. Reports changes in pain to the physician, including pain that significantly increases or changes from a colicky, intermittent type to constant discomfort (changes could indicate perforation or peritonitis)
  2. Usually withholds opioid analgesics (if given, the drug is usually meperidine hydrochloride [Demerol], as ordered)
  3. Provides a position of comfort, including semi-Fowler's, which helps to relieve the pressure of abdominal distention and facilitates thoracic excursion and normal breathing patterns

Continuing Care

- Client and family education depends on the specific cause and treatment of the obstruction.
- The nurse instructs the client to report signs that may indicate recurrent obstruction, including abdominal pain or distention, nausea, vomiting, or constipation (for nonmechanical obstruction after surgery or trauma).

- The nurse instructs the client to develop a structured bowel regimen, including a high-fiber diet, daily exercise, and psyllium hydrophilic mucilloid (e.g., Metamucil) with copious amounts of water (for prevention of recurrences of fecal impaction).
- The nurse teaches the client postoperatively about incision care, drug therapy, and activity restriction.

OBSTRUCTION, UPPER AIRWAY

- Upper airway obstruction is a life-threatening emergency, defined as any interruption in airflow through the nose, pharynx, larynx, or mouth into the lungs.
- The obstruction may be caused by laryngeal edema, peritonsillar abscess, laryngeal carcinoma, cerebral vascular accident, thickened secretions, tongue occlusion, smoke inhalation injury, tracheal and laryngeal trauma, foreign body aspiration, and anaphylaxis.
- Assessment includes increasing anxiety, sternal retractions, seesawing chest, abdominal movements, air hunger, and the universal distress sign for airway obstruction (hands to the neck).
- Management depends on the cause, including
    1. Hyperextension of the neck
    2. Suctioning of oral secretions
    3. Heimlich maneuver for a foreign body
    4. Cricothyroidotomy as an emergency procedure
    5. Endotracheal intubation
    6. Tracheostomy

OCCUPATIONAL PULMONARY DISEASE

See Pulmonary Disease, Occupational.

OCULAR MELANOMA

See Melanoma, Ocular.

ORAL CANCER

See Cancer, Oral.

OSTEOARTHRITIS

See Joint Disease, Degenerative.

O

OSTEOMALACIA

OVERVIEW

- Osteomalacia is a reversible metabolic disease in which there is a defect in the mineralization of bone as a result of vitamin D deficiency.

🌀 Considerations for Elderly Clients

1. The homebound or institutionalized elderly are at increased risk of developing osteomalacia.

COLLABORATIVE MANAGEMENT

Assessment

- The nurse records the client's
    1. Age
    2. Exposure to sunlight
    3. Skin pigmentation (dark skin is at greater risk than light skin)
    4. Dietary habits
    5. Current medical problems and prescribed and over-the-counter medications
    6. History of fracture(s) and when the fracture occurred
- The nurse assesses for
    1. Muscle weakness in the lower extremities, which may progress to a waddling and unsteady gait
    2. Bone pain and muscle cramps
    3. Bone tenderness
    4. Skeletal malalignment, such as long-bone bowing or spinal deformity
    5. Indications of hypocalcemia or hypophosphatemia
    6. Anxiety regarding the suspected diagnosis or the possible occurrence of a fracture or deformity
    7. Changes in x-ray findings, such as the presence of radiolucent bands called Looser's lines or zones (pseudo-fractures)

Interventions

- The nurse encourages increased dietary intake of vitamin D through dietary intake, sun exposure, and drug supplementation.
- Refer to the text on Osteoporosis for additional nursing care and diagnoses.

OSTEOMYELITIS

OVERVIEW

- *Osteomyelitis* is the term used to describe any infection of the bone.

- Acute or chronic osteomyelitis may occur.
- Common causes of osteomyelitis include trauma, infection elsewhere in the body, drug abuse, or long-term catheters.

🕮 Considerations for Elderly Clients

1. Clients with diabetes mellitus or peripheral vascular disease who have foot ulcers commonly acquire osteomyelitis.
2. Multiple organisms are responsible for osteomyelitis in these clients.

COLLABORATIVE MANAGEMENT

Assessment

- The nurse assesses for
  1. Fever
  2. Swelling, tenderness, and erythema around the site of infection
  3. Draining ulcers on the feet or hands
  4. Bone pain that is described as a constant, localized, pulsating sensation that intensifies with movement
  5. An elevated white blood cell count and erythrocyte sedimentation rate
  6. A positive result on a blood culture

Interventions

- The nurse
  1. Administers intravenous (IV) antibiotic(s) specific for the involved organism(s) for 4 to 6 weeks (may require up to 3 months of oral antibiotics)
  2. Administers ciprofloxacin (Cipro), a potent oral antibiotic used as an alternative to IV drug therapy; the client is cautioned not to take antacids because they decrease absorption of the antibiotic
  3. Irrigates the wound with antibiotic solution
  4. Implements drainage precautions for all open wounds
  5. Covers the wound and uses strict aseptic technique when changing dressings

- Wounds may be managed through the window of a cast, which must remain dry during dressing or irrigation procedures.
- Hyperbaric oxygen therapy may be used to increase tissue perfusion.
- *Sequestrectomy* is performed to debride the infected bone and allow revascularization of tissue.
- *Bone grafts* are used to obliterate bone defects.
- *Bone segment transfers* are used when the infected bone is extensively resected and consist of reconstruction with microvascular bone transfers.
- *Muscle flaps* arc used to treat relatively small bony defects.
- *Amputation* of the affected limb may be required if the surgical procedure is ineffective or inappropriate.

OSTEOPOROSIS

OVERVIEW

- Osteoporosis is an age-related metabolic disease in which bone demineralization results in decreased density and subsequent fractures, most commonly in the wrist, hip, and vertebral column.
- There are two types of osteoporosis
    1. *Type I* occurs in women between the ages of 55 and 65 years and is related to a decrease in serum estrogen.
    2. *Type II* occurs mainly in women older than 65 years of age, but also in men.
- Vertebral fractures occur in both types.
- Wrist fractures are associated with postmenopausal osteoporosis; hip fractures are seen more frequently with senile osteoporosis.

 Transcultural Considerations

1. Caucasian women are affected more often than African American women.

2. Postmenopausal women of any culture or race are at high risk for the development of osteoporosis.

COLLABORATIVE MANAGEMENT

Assessment

- The nurse records the client's
    1. Age, sex, race, body build, height, and weight
    2. Usual exposure to sunlight
    3. Cigarette, alcohol, and caffeine use
    4. Daily calcium and vitamin D intake
    5. Usual exercise pattern
    6. Current medical problems and prescribed and over-the-counter medications
    7. History of falls, fractures, and/or other injuries
    8. Family history of osteoporosis
    9. Daily routine
- The nurse assesses for
    1. Classic dowager's hump (kyphosis of the dorsal spine) by inspection and palpation of the vertebral column
    2. Back pain after lifting, bending, or stooping
    3. Back pain that increases with palpation, particularly of the lower thoracic and lumbar vertebrae
    4. Back pain with tenderness and voluntary restriction of spinal movement, which indicates compression fracture(s), usually of T8–L3
    5. Fractures in the distal end of the radius or at the upper third of the femur
    6. Constipation, abdominal distention, and respiratory compromise from movement restriction and spinal deformity
    7. Body image disturbance, especially if the client is severely kyphotic
    8. Impaired social interactions, which may have been self-curtailed because of changes in appearance or an inability to sit in restaurants, theaters, and so forth

Interventions

- The nurse administers drug therapy, as ordered
    1. Estrogens, calcium supplements, and vitamin D, if necessary, for prevention and treatment

2. Alendronate (Fosamax), a bone resorption inhibitor, used in the prevention of osteoporosis
3. Sodium fluoride, used clinically or investigationally with extreme caution, with estrogen and calcium, to stimulate new bone formation and to inhibit bone loss
4. Androgens to decrease bone resorption (may cause masculinization and/or liver disease in postmenopausal women)
5. Calcitonin to inhibit bone loss (expensive and must be administered by injection)

- The nurse
  1. Teaches the client to increase his or her dietary intake of calcium and vitamin D
  2. Teaches the client to avoid alcohol and caffeine
  3. Teaches the client to increase dietary protein, vitamin C, and iron to promote bone healing in clients with fractures
  4. Creates a hazard-free environment

- The nurse
  1. Teaches exercises to strengthen the abdominal and back muscles to improve posture and provide support for the spine (in collaboration with physical therapy)
  2. Encourages abdominal isometrics, deep breathing, and pectoral stretching to increase pulmonary capacity
  3. Encourages extremity exercises
     a. Isometric
     b. Resistive
     c. Active range of motion (ROM) to improve joint mobility and increase muscle tone
  4. Encourages daily walking, both slow and fast, and bicycling
  5. Teaches the client to avoid recreational activities that could cause vertebral compression, such as bowling and horseback riding

- The nurse administers drug therapy for pain relief, as ordered
  1. Analgesics, opoids, and non-narcotics for the acute phase
  2. Muscle relaxants to ease the discomfort of muscle spasms
  3. Anti-inflammatory agents for pain and spinal nerve root inflammation

494

    a. Monitors the client (particularly the elderly) for problems associated with nonsteroidal anti-inflammatory drugs, such as GI bleeding and congestive heart failure
- Back braces may be used to immobilize the spine during the acute phase and to provide spinal column support. (Because elderly clients tolerate these devices poorly, the nurse carefully ensures proper fit and assesses client tolerance.)
- Surgery may be needed to reduce or alleviate pain when medications and orthotics are ineffective.

Continuing Care

- The nurse
  1. Helps the client and family to identify and correct hazards in the home prior to discharge
  2. Ensures that the client can correctly use all assistive-adaptive devices ordered for home use
  3. Teaches measures to prevent falls, such as use of orthotic and ambulatory aids
  4. Reviews the prescribed exercise regimen
     a. Strengthening, ROM, and weight-bearing exercises
     b. Schedules follow-up physical therapy appointments
  5. Obtains a dietary consultation to help the client select personal food preferences high in essential nutrients
  6. Provides drug information
     a. Using sunlight exposure as a source of vitamin D
     b. Taking all medication in the correct dosage
     c. What to do if a dose is missed or if complications or side effects occur
  7. Emphasizes the importance of follow-up visits with the physician(s)
  8. Refers to home health agency and support groups

OTITIS MEDIA

OVERVIEW

- Otitis media is an infection in the middle ear that causes an inflammatory process within the mucosa.
- This inflammatory process leads to swelling and irritation of the bones, or ossicles, within the middle ear, resulting in the formation of purulent inflammatory exudate.
- Otitis media may be *acute, chronic,* or *serous.*

COLLABORATIVE MANAGEMENT

- The nurse assesses for (for acute or chronic otitis media)
    1. Ear pain (is relieved if the tympanic membrane ruptures)
    2. Feeling of fullness in the ear
    3. Slightly retracted tympanic membrane initially; later is red, thickened, and bulging, with a loss of landmarks; exudate may be seen behind the membrane; if the disease progresses, the membrane spontaneously perforates, and pus or blood drains from the ear
    4. Conductive hearing loss
    5. Headache
    6. Malaise
    7. Fever
    8. Nausea and vomiting
    9. Slight dizziness or vertigo
- The nurse
    1. Ensures bed rest to limit head movement and thus decrease pain
    2. Applies localized heat and occasionally the application of cold
    3. Administers systemic antibiotic therapy
    4. Administers analgesics, as ordered, such as acetylsalicylic acid (aspirin, Entrophen◆) or acetaminophen (Tylenol, Abenol◆) or treats severe pain with opioid analgesics such as meperidine (Demerol)
    5. Administers oral and nasal decongestants, as ordered

- *Myringotomy* is the surgical precedure performed after initial antibiotic therapy and the tympanic membrane continues to bulge. It is usually performed with anesthesia, often in the physician's office.
- Postoperative care consists of antibiotic eardrops, such as neomycin sulfate or bacitracin.
- Care must be taken to keep the external ear and canal free from other substances while the incision is healing; the client should avoid showering and washing his or her hair.

OTOSCLEROSIS

OVERVIEW

- Otosclerosis is a disease of the labyrinthine capsule of the middle ear, resulting in the development of irregular areas of new bone formation.
- It has a familial tendency; the incidence of disease in women is twice that in men.

COLLABORATIVE MANAGEMENT

- The nurse assesses for
    1. Slowly progressive conductive hearing loss
        a. The loss is bilateral, although the progression of the disease is different in each ear, which gives the effect of one "good" ear and one "bad" ear.
        b. Initial hearing loss is of the lower frequencies but progresses to all frequencies.
    2. Roaring or ringing type of constant tinnitus
    3. Normal tympanic membrane; occasionally, the eardrum has a pinkish discoloration
- Treatment is directed toward improving hearing through amplification with a hearing aid.
- Surgical procedures used to correct hearing loss include a partial or complete *stapedectomy* (removal of stapes) with a prosthesis.

OVARIAN CANCER

See Cancer, Ovarian.

OVARIAN CYSTS

See Cysts, Ovarian.

OVARIAN FIBROMA

See Fibroma, Ovarian.

OVARIAN TUMORS, EPITHELIAL

See Tumors, Epithelial Ovarian.

OVERHYDRATION

OVERVIEW

- Overhydration is not an acutal disease but a clinical manifestation of a physiologic problem in which fluid intake or retention exceeds fluid need.
- There are two types of overhydration

498

1. *Isotonic,* or hypervolemia, which occurs as a result of excess fluid in the extracellular fluid compartment (ECF) and rarely has serious consequences if mild to moderate; may result in circulatory overload and interstitial edema if severe
2. *Hypotonic,* or water intoxication, in which all body fluid compartments experience expansion, with effects related to specific electrolyte dilution

COLLABORATIVE MANAGEMENT
Assessment

- The nurse assesses for
  1. Cardiovascular changes
     a. Increased pulse rate, bounding pulse
     b. Full peripheral pulses
     c. Elevated blood pressure, decreased pulse pressure
     d. Elevated central venous pressure
     e. Distended neck and hand veins
     f. Engorged venous varicosities
  2. Respiratory changes
     a. Increased respiratory rate with shallow respirations
     b. Dyspnea that increases with exertion or in the supine position
     c. Moist rales or crackles on auscultation
  3. Integumentary changes
     a. Pitting edema
     b. Skin pale and cool to touch
  4. Neuromuscular changes
     a. Altered level of consciousness
     b. Headache
     c. Visual disturbances
     d. Skeletal muscle weakness
     e. Paresthesia
  5. Gastrointestinal changes (increased motility)
  6. Manifestations of isotonic overhydration
     a. Liver enlargement
     b. Ascites formation
     c. Decreased hemoglobin, hematocrit, and serum protein values
  7. Manifestations of hypotonic overhydration
     a. Polyuria

O

b. Diarrhea

c. Nonpitting edema

d. Cardiac dysrhythmias associated with electrolyte dilution

e. Projectile vomiting

f. Decreased complete blood count (CBC) and protein and electrolyte levels

Interventions

- The nurse administers drug therapy, as ordered
    1. Diuretics (provided that renal failure is not the cause of the overhydration)
        a. Osmotic diuretics are used first to avoid initiating or exacerbating electrolyte disturbances.
        b. High-ceiling (loop) diuretics are given if osmotic diuretics are not effective.
- The nurse monitors the client for response to medications, especially weight loss and increased urinary output.
- The nurse
    1. Recognizes that diet therapy may be of value in controlling fluid volume through restrictions of both fluids and sodium
    2. Measures intake and output
    3. Weighs the client at the same time and on the same scale each day
- The nurse observes the client for pulmonary edema and depression of vital organ function.

Continuing Care

- The nurse
    1. Teaches the client about specific food or fluid restrictions
    2. Reviews the signs and symptoms of the specific imbalance for which the client is at risk, as well as what specific information should be reported immediately to the primary health care provider

PAGET'S DISEASE

OVERVIEW

- Paget's disease is a metabolic disorder of bone remodeling, or turnover, in which increased resorption or loss results in bone deposits that are weak, enlarged, and disorganized.
- Three phases of the disease are
    1. *Active,* in which a prolific increase in osteoclasts causes massive bone destruction and deformity
    2. *Mixed,* in which the osteoblasts react in a compensatory manner to form new bone, and bone is disorganized and chaotic in structure
    3. *Inactive,* in which the newly formed bone becomes sclerotic and ivory hard
- Common sites include the vertebrae, the femur, the skull, the sternum, and the pelvis.

➤ Transcultural Considerations

1. There may be a link between the disease and ethnic origin.
2. Paget's disease occurs more frequently in Europe and less often in Asia and Scandinavia.

COLLABORATIVE MANAGEMENT

Assessment

- The nurse assesses for
    1. Bone pain, described as aching, deep, and aggravated by weight-bearing and pressure; severe bone pain may indicate complications such as osteogenic sarcoma
    2. Back pain and headache
    3. Arthritis at the joints of affected bones
    4. Nerve impingement, particularly in the lumbosacral area of the vertebral column
    5. Posture, stance, and gait to identify gross bony deformities
    6. Flexion contracture of the hips
    7. Size and shape of the skull, which is soft, thick, and enlarged

P

8. Deafness and vertigo
9. Cranial nerve compression
10. Warm and flushed skin
11. Apathy, lethargy, and fatigue
12. Pathologic fractures
13. Hyperparathyroidism and gout
14. Congestive heart failure
15. Hydrocephalus from bony enlargement of the skull, which blocks the cerebrospinal fluid
16. Increase in serum alkaline phosphatase
17. Ability to cope with pain and the effects of having a chronic disorder
18. Fear associated with the potential development of bone cancer

Interventions

- The nurse administers drug therapy, as ordered:
    1. Nonsteroidal anti-inflammatory drugs (NSAIDs), such as ibuprofen (Motrin, Apo-Ibuprofen◆) and indomethacin (Indocin, Apo-Indomethacin◆) given for pain
    2. Calcitonin (calcitonin-salmon [Calcimar]), effective in initiating a remission of the disease, with the usual duration of therapy 6 months followed by a 6-month course of etidronate disodium (Didronel)
    3. Mithramycin (Mithracin), a potent anticarcinogen and antibiotic reserved for clients with marked hypercalcemia or severe disease and neurologic compromise
    4. Alendronate (Fosamax), a bone resorption inhibitor and calcium regulator, which corrects hypercalcemia and decreases the risk of fractures
- The nurse
    1. Applies heat and massage
    2. Reviews the exercise program developed in collaboration with physical therapy
    3. Applies and teaches the application of orthotic devices for support and immobilization
    4. Provides the client with the address of the Paget's Disease Foundation and the local chapter of the Arthritis Foundation
- A partial or total joint replacement may be needed to treat secondary arthritis and uncontrolled pain.

P_{AIN}

OVERVIEW

- Pain has both sensory and behavioral components and is strongly influenced by various physiologic, psychologic, and sociologic factors.
- One's pain threshold or sensation of pain is the amount or degree of noxious stimulus that leads a person to interpret a sensation as painful.
- *Pain tolerance* refers to the ability of the client to endure the intensity of pain; it is more a function of psychologic and social variables than of biologic characteristics.
- The factors that tend to *decrease* the threshold for and tolerance of pain include discomfort, insomnia, fatigue, anxiety, fear, anger, sadness, depression, and past experience with pain.
- Factors that tend to *increase* the threshold for and tolerance for pain are typically relief of symptoms, sleep or rest, understanding, diversion, and elevation of mood.
- *Psychogenic* or *psychosomatic* pain is pain that is believed to arise from mental or emotional factors.
- Demographic factors, such as gender and sociocultural, background, and personality characteristics, strongly influence the client's ability to process pain sensations and react to them.

P

Considerations for Elderly Clients

1. The perception of cutaneous (skin) pain may diminish, but the perception of visceral pain may increase.
2. Older adults usually receive less analgesia than young adults.
3. Older adults hold various beliefs about pain, including that it is "normal," that they might get addicted to pain medication if they take it, and pain signifies a serious illness or impending death.

1. Many studies have shown a relationship between pain and culture, but the findings have not been consistent.
2. Health care providers tend to stereotype some ethnic groups, such as Mexican-American women who usually moan or cry when they are in pain.

- Pain is generally classified into three types:

1. *Acute* pain is usually temporary, of sudden onset, easily localized, and confined to the affected area.
2. *Postoperative* pain is poorly understood and not always well managed:
   a. It has a sensory component related to tissue destruction and location and also a major psychosocial component.
   b. Intrathoracic and upper intra-abdominal surgical approaches are generally associated with severe pain.
   c. Superficial surgery of the head and neck, chest wall, or limb is often associated with minimal pain.
3. *Chronic* pain:
   a. It affects an estimated 25% of the people in the United States and is defined as pain that persists or recurs for indefinite periods, usually for more than 6 months.
   b. It can be subdivided into 3 types: chronic non-malignant pain, chronic pain syndrome, and chronic malignant pain.
   c. It frequently involves deep somatic and visceral structures and is usually diffuse, poorly localized, and difficult to describe.
   d. It is associated with cancer, connective tissue diseases, peripheral vascular diseases, musculoskeletal disorders, and post-traumatic insults.
   e. It has physiologic and psychosocial ramifications, which are influenced by the client's ability to cope, the availability of family support and social resources, and the severity of the physiologic and emotional consequences.
   f. It may interfere with activities of daily living (ADL) and personal relationships and may cause emotional and financial burdens.

🅔 Considerations for Elderly Clients

1. Clients who are anxious or disoriented may not be able to verbalize the degree of pain they are experiencing; the nurse assesses for nonverbal indications of pain, such as grimacing, crying, or changes in behavior (confusion, combativeness).
2. Demerol may cause cerebral irritability in older people, leading to seizures, memory loss, hallucinations, paranoia, and depression.
3. NSAIDs should be used with caution because of the side effects of sodium and water retention, which can lead to congestive heart failure.

COLLABORATIVE MANAGEMENT

Assessment

- The nurse records
   1. Chronology of events:
      a. Length of time the client has experienced pain
      b. Precipitating factors
      c. Aggravating factors
      d. Localization of pain
      e. Character and quality of pain
      f. Duration of pain
   2. Adjustments in the life of the client or family
   3. The client's beliefs about the cause of the pain and what should be done about it

- The nurse assesses for
   1. Changes in vital signs:
      a. Tachycardia
      b. Blood pressure changes
   2. Diaphoresis
   3. Restlessness, apprehension
   4. Splinting or holding painful body parts while moving
   5. Location of pain:
      a. Localized (confined to site of origin)
      b. Projected (along a specific nerve or nerves)
      c. Radiating (diffuse around the site of origin, not well localized)
      d. Referred (perceived in an area distant from the site of painful stimuli)
      e. Superficial or deep
   6. Character and quality of pain

P

505

7. Intensity of pain
8. Pattern of pain
9. Psychosocial factors

Planning and Implementation

✦ NDx: Pain

- The nurse
    1. Administers appropriate drug therapy, as ordered:
        a. Codeine (Roxicodone)
        b. Hydromorphone (Dilaudid)
        c. Oxycodone (Percodan, Tylox, Percocet)
        d. Acetylsalicylic acid (aspirin, Ancasal◆)
        e. Morphine (Roxanol, Statex◆)
        f. Meperidine (Demerol): Use with caution in clients with renal disease or the elderly
        g. Acetaminophen (Tylenol, Ace-Tabs◆)
        h. NSAIDs
    2. Assesses and evaluates the effectiveness of drug therapy
- Pain management for the client with a substance abuse problem consists of
    1. Following the principles of opioid use
    2. Use of nonopioid therapies, including medications, cutaneous stimulation techniques, and cognitive behavioral techniques
    3. Consultation with other health team members (substance abuse counselor, pharmacist, social worker)
- Intraspinal analgesics are generally used during surgery and in the immediate postoperative period:
    1. *Epidural analgesia,* the instillation of a pain-blocking agent, usually morphine or fentanyl, into the epidural space
    2. *Intrathecal analgesia,* the instillation of a pain-blocking agent into the space between the arachnoid mater and pia mater of the spinal cord
- Complications associated with intraspinal analgesia include catheter displacement, pruritus, nausea, vomiting, infection, respiratory depression, and urinary retention.
- Patient-controlled analgesia (PCA) allows the client to control the dosage of analgesia received.
    1. PCA is achieved through the use of a PCA infusion pump, which delivers the desired amount of medication through a conventional intravenous

route or through an implantable intravenous catheter inserted in subcutaneous tissue.

2. Drug security with PCA is ensured through a locked syringe pump system or drug reservoir system programmed to deliver a certain amount of drug within a specified interval.

- The nurse implements methods of cutaneous stimulation, such as transcutaneous electrical nerve stimulation (TENS) or hot and cold compresses when appropriate, as ordered. These methods may be used for acute or chronic pain.
- The nurse teaches the client that
    1. Benefits of cutaneous stimulation techniques are highly unpredictable
    2. Pain relief is generally sustained only as long as the stimulation continues
    3. Trials may be necessary to establish the desired effects
    4. Stimulation itself may aggravate pre-existing pain or may produce new pain
    5. TENS involves the use of a battery-operated device capable of delivering small electrical current to the skin and underlying tissues:
        a. Electrodes connected to a small box are placed over the painful sites.
        b. Voltage or current is regulated by adjusting a dial to the point at which the client perceives a prickly, "pins-and-needles" sensation.
        c. The client can continue to participate in ADL.
        d. The client's skin at the electrode sites may become irritated, and sites should be rotated.
- Alternative methods to relieve pain, such as cognitive and behavioral strategies, may be helpful (visual, auditory, or environmental distractions).

P

✦ **NDx:** Chronic Pain

Nonsurgical Management

- The nurse
    1. Administers drug therapy, as ordered:
        a. Nonopioid analgesics:
            (1) Acetylsalicylic acid (aspirin, Ancasal◆)
            (2) Acetaminophen (Tylenol, Ace-Tabs◆)
            (3) NSAIDs, such as ibuprofen (Motrin, Amersol◆)

　　　　(4)　Carbamazepine (Tegretol, Mezepine◆)
　　　　　　and phenytoin (Dilantin) to treat certain
　　　　　　neuralgias
　　b. Opioid analgesics:
　　　　(1)　Meperidine (Demerol)
　　　　(2)　Codeine
　　　　(3)　Morphine sulfate
　　　　(4)　Oxycodone (Percodan, Tylox)
　　　　(5)　Hydromorphone (Dilaudid)
　　c. Antidepressants:
　　　　(1)　Amitriptyline (Elavil)
　　　　(2)　Imipramine (Tofranil)
　　　　(3)　Doxepin (Sinequan)
　　　　(4)　Trazodone (Desyrel)

- *Physical dependency* is associated with the long-term administration of opioids; it is a physiologic adaptation of the body tissue so that continued administration of the drug is necessary for normal tissue function.
- *Drug tolerance* is characterized by a gradual resistance of the body to the effects of an opioid, including its pain-relieving properties.
- *Addiction* is used to describe persistent drug craving and abuse of a drug for recreational purposes.
- *Adjuvant therapy* involves the use of medication and additional therapies, such as TENS and cognitive-behavioral strategies.
- Continuous intravenous opioid analgesia is recommended for the management of cancer-related pain and other progressive pain syndromes.
- The nurse
  1. Monitors the client's vital signs hourly until an adequate and safe level of the drug is achieved
  2. Monitors the client for adequate pain relief
- Continuous subcutaneous opioid analgesia is used for clients with compromised venous access or whose central venous lines are being used for other fluids:
  1. Morphine is the most common drug used.
  2. The catheter is usually placed in the subclavicular tissue underneath the clavicle or the abdomen.
- The nurse
  1. Observes for leakage of fluid and edema around the insertion site
  2. Monitors the client for adequate pain relief

- Long-term intraspinal analgesia may be used for the management of chronic intractable pain and involves the use of a permanent epidural catheter.
- Transdermal opioid administration involves administration of fentanyl (Duragesic) by means of a skin patch placed on the chest, preferably on an area without hair.
- The nurse
    1. Teaches the client to report side effects, such as dizziness, sedation, nausea, and decreased respiratory rate
    2. Tells the client it may take up to 24 hours before pain relief is apparent
- Absorption of transdermal analgesia is affected by higher body temperature; in the presence of a temperature of 102° F or higher, drug absorption from the skin may accelerate and lead to side effects.
- The nurse teaches the client about cognitive and behavioral strategies to help reduce the pain:
    1. Imagery
    2. Relaxation
    3. Hypnosis
    4. Biofeedback
    5. Acupuncture

Surgical Management

- The purpose of surgery is to interrupt the pain pathways in situations in which pain is intractable or severely debilitating.
- *Nerve blocks* are usually indicated for patients whose pain is confined to a specific area or nerve distribution. The procedure involves the destruction of a nerve root or roots by the use of a chemical agent such as phenol or alcohol.
- *Rhizotomy* involves the destruction of sensory nerve roots where they enter the spinal cord:
    1. A *closed rhizotomy* is performed by inserting a percutaneous catheter to destroy the sensory nerve roots with a neurolytic chemical, coagulation, or cryodestruction (freezing).
    2. *Open rhizotomy* requires a laminectomy; the nerve roots are isolated and destroyed.
- *Cordotomy* involves transection of the pain pathways at the midline portion of the spinal cord before nerve impulses ascend to the spinothalamic tract.

P

- The nurse provides postoperative care, including assessing the neurologic deficit and teaching the client how to protect the surgical area from harm.

Continuing Care

- The nurse
  1. Involves the client and family in continuing health care behaviors that will relieve pain and improve psychologic well-being and overall functional status
  2. Teaches administration of drug therapy and use of other pain-reduction modalities
  3. Collaborates with the physician to assess the need for a referral to a specialized pain clinic

PAIN, BACK

OVERVIEW

- Back pain is second only to headache as the most common complaint of people in most countries.
- The areas of the back most commonly affected by back pain are the cervical and lumbar vertebrae.
- *Cervical back pain* is usually related to a herniation of the nucleus pulposus in an intervertebral disk (ruptured disk) between the fifth and sixth vertebrae or to nerve compression caused by osteophyte formation; it may also occur from muscle strain or ligament sprain.
- *Lumbosacral (low back) pain* (LBP) is typically caused by a herniated nucleus pulposus (usually between the fourth and fifth lumbar or fifth lumbar and first sacral vertebrae), ligament sprain, disk injury from hyperflexion, or muscle sprain or spasm.
- If back pain continues for 3 months, or if repeated episodes occur, the client is diagnosed as having *chronic* back pain.
- Risk factors for *acute* back pain include
  1. Trauma (twisting or hyperflexion during lifting)
  2. Obesity
  3. Congenital spinal problems, such as scoliosis
  4. Smoking (causes premature disk degeneration)
- Risk factors for *chronic* back pain include

1. Poor posture
2. Wearing high-heeled shoes

🎓 Considerations for Elderly Clients

1. In elderly clients, back pain is usually caused by degenerative joint disease.
2. Cervical pain is also common in clients with advanced rheumatoid arthritis who experience cervical disk subluxation, most often at the C1–2 level (first and second cervical vertebrae).
3. Physiologic changes associated with aging, such as spinal stenosis, vertebral malalignment, and vascular changes, also contribute to back pain in the elderly.

COLLABORATIVE MANAGEMENT

Assessment

- The nurse assesses the client for
    1. Posture and gait
    2. Vertebral alignment and swelling
    3. Muscle spasm
    4. Pain radiating down the arm or leg
    5. Tenderness of the back and involved extremity
    6. Sensory changes: paresthesia, numbness
    7. Muscle tone and strength
    8. Limitations in movement
    9. Reaction to illness
    10. Vertebral changes on x-ray, computed tomography scan, or magnetic resonance imaging

Interventions

Nonsurgical Management

- Treatment of *acute* LBP is a 1- or 2-day period of rest and the Williams position (semi-Fowler's bed position with the knees flexed). A bed board may be useful for clients with a muscle injury; for clients with a herniated disk, a flat position may aggravate the pain.
- Muscle relaxants such as cyclobenzaprine hydrochloride (Flexeril) and nonsteroidal anti-inflammatory drugs, such as aspirin or ibuprofen (Motrin, Amersol◆) are often given.
- Epidural steroid injections may be administered in some cases.

- Traction is becoming less popular as treatment for acute pain. The purpose of traction is to separate the vertebrae and relieve pressure on the impinged nerve.
- For care of the client in cervical traction, see Trauma, Spinal Cord. For other types of traction, see Fractures.
- Other approaches for *chronic* back pain include a custom-fitted lumbosacral brace or corset for LBP, moist heat, ice, massage, transcutaneous electrical nerve stimulation (TENS), distraction, imagery, music therapy, and deep-heat therapy, such as ultrasound or diathermy.
- The nurse
  1. Collaborates with the physical therapist to develop an individualized exercise program.
  2. Collaborates with the dietitian to plan and implement a calorie-restricted diet plan, if appropriate.

Surgical Management

- *Conventional* operative procedures include
  1. A *diskectomy,* in which the spinal nerve is usually lifted to remove the offending portion of the disk.
  2. A *laminectomy,* which is the removal of one or more vertebral laminae, plus osteophytes, and the herniated nucleus pulposus through a 3-inch (7.5-cm) incision.
  3. A *spinal fusion,* which stabilizes the spine if repeated laminectomies are performed.
- Clients undergoing the conventional operative procedures require a hospital stay of 2 to 4 days, depending on the procedure.
- *Alternative* operative procedures have varying degrees of popularity but have shortened hospital stays. Spinal cord complications are also less likely with these procedures—percutaneous lumbar diskec-tomy, and microdiskectomy, and laser-assisted laparoscopic lumbar diskectomy.
- *Percutaneous lumbar diskectomy* includes
  1. The insertion of a metal cannula adjacent to the affected disk under fluoroscopy and the threading of a special cutting tool through the cannula for removal of pieces of the disk that are compressing the nerve root (laser surgery may be used)
  2. A risk of infection and nerve root injury
  3. A hospital stay of 2 or 3 days
- *Microdiskectomy* includes

1. Microscopic surgery through a 1-inch (2.5-cm) incision
2. The possible complications of infection, dural tears, and missed disk fragments

- *Laser-assisted laparoscopic lumbar diskectomy* includes
    1. A laser with modified standard disk instruments inserted periumbilically through the laparoscope
    2. Risks include infection and nerve root injury
    3. Clients are discharged from the hospital in 24 to 48 hours

- The nurse provides preoperative care:
    1. Provides routine preoperative care
    2. Warns the client that various sensations may be experienced in the affected leg or both legs (for lumbar surgery) because of manipulation of nerves and muscles during surgery
    3. Teaches the client what to expect postoperatively and how to move in bed
    4. Addresses the need for a postoperative brace, autologous blood donation, and bone grafting if the client is having a spinal fusion

- The nurse provides postoperative care:
    1. Takes vital signs and neurologic checks every 4 hours during the first 24 hours
    2. Assesses for fever and hypotension
    3. Checks the dressing for any drainage (clear drainage may indicate a cerebrospinal fluid leak)
    4. Measures intake and output (an inability to void may indicate damage to sacral spinal nerves)
    5. Administers intramuscular opioid analgesics or monitors patient-controlled anesthesia during the first 12 to 24 hours
    6. Recognizes that most clients may be out of bed with assistance the evening of surgery; bed rest for 24 to 48 hours may be necessary for clients with a spinal fusion
    7. Logrolls the client every 2 hours
    8. Provides routine postoperative care
    9. Ensures that a brace or other type of thoracolumbar support is worn when the client is out of bed (for spinal fusion)

P

Continuing Care

- The nurse teaches the client and family about

513

1. The prescribed exercise program (client mastery is ensured by observing correct performance on return demonstration, in collaboration with physical therapy)
2. Restrictions on lifting and bending and on activities
3. Principles of body mechanics
4. The use of a firm mattress or bed board, if appropriate
5. Drug information
6. Weight-reduction diet, if needed
7. Use of moist heat
8. Possibility of recurrence of back pain

PALSY, BELLS

See Paralysis, Facial.

PANCREATIC ABSCESSES

See Abscesses, Pancreatic.

PANCREATIC CARCINOMA

See Cancer, Pancreatic.

PANCREATIC PSEUDOCYSTS

See Pseudocysts, Pancreatic.

PANCREATITIS, ACUTE

OVERVIEW

- Acute pancreatitis is an inflammatory process of the pancreas resulting in autodigestion of the organ by its own enzymes, including trypsin, elastase, phospholipase A, lipase, and kallikrein.
- The extent of the inflammation and tissue destruction ranges from mild involvement, characterized by edema and inflammation, to severe, necrotizing hemorrhagic pancreatitis, characterized by diffusely bleeding pancreatic tissue with fibrosis and tissue death.
- Activation of the inflammatory process occurs after insult or injury, causing obstruction of the pancreatic duct and resulting in the production and release of pancreatic enzymes.
- Following pancreatic duct obstruction, increased pressure within the pancreas and the pancreatic ducts may cause the duct to rupture, allowing spillage of trypsin and other enzymes into the pancreas parenchymal tissue.
- Many factors, including alcohol, can cause injury to the pancreas; biliary tract disease with gallstones; postoperative trauma from surgical manipulation after biliary tract, pancreatic, gastric, and duodenal procedures; drug toxicities, including opiates, sulfonamides, thiazides, steroids, and oral contraceptives; and other medical diseases.
- Complications include adult respiratory distress syndrome (ARDS), pleural effusions, shock, and coagulation defects.

COLLABORATIVE MANAGEMENT

Assessment

- The nurse records the client's
  1. History of abdominal pain related to alcohol ingestion or high fat intake
  2. Individual and family history of alcoholism, pancreatitis, or biliary tract disease
  3. Previous abdominal surgeries or diagnostic procedures

4. Medical history, including peptic ulcer disease, renal failure, vascular disorders, hyperparathyroidism, and hyperlipidemia
5. Recent viral infection
6. Use of prescription and over-the-counter drugs

- The nurse assesses for
  1. Abdominal pain (the most frequent symptom), including a sudden onset, mid-epigastric, or left upper quadrant location with radiation to the back; aggravated by a fatty meal, ingestion of a large amount of alcohol, or lying in the recumbent position
  2. Weight loss, with nausea and vomiting
  3. Jaundice
  4. Discoloration of the abdomen and periumbilical area (Cullen's sign)
  5. Bluish discoloration of the flanks (Turner's sign)
  6. Absent or decreased bowel sounds
  7. Abdominal tenderness, rigidity, and guarding
  8. Dull sound on abdominal percussion indicating ascites
  9. Elevated temperature with tachycardia and decreased blood pressure
  10. Adventitious breath sounds, dyspnea, or orthopnea
  11. Elevated serum amylase and lipase levels

Planning and Implementation

✦ **NDx:** Pain

Nonsurgical Management

- The nurse
  1. Withholds food and fluids in the acute period; hydration is maintained with intravenous fluids
  2. Maintains nasogastric intubation to decrease gastric distention and suppress pancreatic secretion
  3. Administers meperidine hydrochloride (Demerol), as ordered, the drug of choice for pain because it less frequently causes spasm of the smooth musculature of the pancreatic ducts and the sphincter of Oddi
  4. Administers antacids, as ordered, to neutralize gastric secretions
  5. Administers histamine receptor-blocking drugs, as ordered, such as ranitidine (Zantac), to decrease hydrochloric acid production

6. Administers anticholinergics, as ordered, such as dicyclomine HCl (Bentyl, Lomine◆), to decrease vagal stimulation and decrease gastrointestinal motility
7. Helps the client assume a fetal position to decrease abdominal pain
8. Provides frequent oral hygiene
9. Encourages the client to express the emotions and responses he or she is feeling
10. Provides reassurances and diversional activities

Surgical Management

- Surgical management is usually not indicated for acute pancreatitis.
- The client with complications such as pancreatic pseudocyst and abscess may require surgical drainage.

✦ **NDx:** Altered Nutrition: Less than Body Requirements

- The nurse
  1. Withholds food and fluids in the early stages of the disease
  2. Administers total parenteral nutrition (TPN), as ordered, for severe nutritional depletion
  3. Provides small, frequent high-carbohydrate and high-protein feedings with limited fats, when tolerated
  4. Provides supplemental liquid diet preparations and vitamins and minerals to boost caloric intake, if needed

Continuing Care

- Client and family health teaching is aimed at preventing further episodes and preventing disease progression to chronic pancreatitis.
- The nurse
  1. Encourages alcohol abstinence to prevent further pain and extension of the inflammation and insufficiency
  2. Teaches the client to notify the physician for acute abdominal pain or symptoms of biliary tract disease, such as jaundice, clay-colored stools, and dark urine
  3. Emphasizes the importance of follow-up visits with the physician(s)

4. Refers the client with an alcohol abuse problem to support groups such as Alcoholics Anonymous
5. Encourages the client to avoid caffeine-containing beverages and foods

Pancreatitis, Chronic

OVERVIEW

- Chronic pancreatitis is a progressive, destructive disease of the pancreas.
- Inflammation and fibrosis of the tissue contribute to pancreatic insufficiency and diminished organ function.
- The disease usually develops after repeated episodes of alcohol-induced acute pancreatitis, also known as *chronic calcifying pancreatitis.*
- Chronic pancreatitis is characterized by protein precipitates that plug the ducts and lead to ductal obstruction, atrophy, and dilation, causing metaplasia and ulceration, resulting in fibrosis of the pancreatic tissue.
- The pancreas becomes hard and firm because of cell atrophy and pancreatic insufficiency.
- *Chronic obstructive pancreatitis* develops from inflammation, spasm, and obstruction of the sphincter of Oddi.
- Inflammatory and sclerotic lesions develop in the head of the pancreas and around the ducts, causing an obstruction and backflow of pancreatic secretions and enzymes.
- *Pancreatic insufficiency* is characterized by the loss of exocrine function, which causes a decreased output of enzymes and bicarbonate; loss of endocrine function results in diabetes mellitus.

COLLABORATIVE MANAGEMENT

Assessment

- The nurse records the client's
  1. History of abdominal pain related to alcohol ingestion or high fat intake, with specific information about alcohol intake, including time, amount, and relationship of alcohol to pain development

2. Individual and family history of alcoholism, pancreatitis, or biliary tract disease
3. Previous abdominal surgeries or diagnostic procedures
4. Medical history, including peptic ulcer disease, renal failure, vascular disorders, hyperparathyroidism, and hyperlipidemia
5. Recent viral infections
6. Use of prescription or over-the-counter drugs

- The nurse assesses for
  1. Abdominal pain (major clinical manifestation)—continuous, burning, or gnawing dullness with intense and relentless exacerbations
  2. Abdominal tenderness
  3. Left upper quadrant mass, indicating a pseudocyst or abscess
  4. Dullness on abdominal percussion, indicating pancreatic ascites
  5. Steatorrhea, foul-smelling stools that may increase in volume as pancreatic insufficiency progresses
  6. Weight loss and muscle wasting
  7. Jaundice and dark urine
  8. Signs and symptoms of diabetes mellitus
  9. Elevated serum alkaline phosphatase and amylase levels

Interventions

Nonsurgical Management

- The nurse
  1. Administers opioid analgesia with meperidine hydrochloride (Demerol, the drug most often used), as ordered; the client may become dependent on opioids with long-term use
  2. Teaches the client to avoid irritating substances
- The nurse
  1. Withholds food and fluids to avoid recurrent pain exacerbated by eating
  2. Administers TPN, as ordered, for severe nutritional depletion
  3. Provides small, frequent high-carbohydrate and high-protein feedings with limited fats, when tolerated
  4. Administers pancreatic enzyme replacement, as ordered, such as pancreatin (Viokase) and pancrelipase (Cotazym or Pancrease) given to

P

aid in digestion and absorption of fat and protein

5. Administers insulin or oral hypoglycemic agents to control diabetes

6. Administers histamine receptor antagonists to decrease gastric acid

- The nurse
    1. Provides a low-fat diet to limit fat intake, decreasing the incidence of fatty stools
    2. Provides nutritional support with TPN, as ordered
    3. Administers intravenous fluids to maintain hydration with fat-soluble vitamin replacement, as ordered
    4. Cleans the skin after each stool

Surgical Management

- Surgical management is not the primary intervention for chronic pancreatitis; surgery may be indicated for intractable pain, incapacitating pain relapses, or complications such as pseudocyst and abscess.
- Surgical procedures include
    1. *Incision* and *drainage* for abscesses or pseudocysts
    2. *Cholecystectomy* or *choledochotomy* for underlying biliary tract disease
    3. *Sphincterotomy* (incision of the sphincter) for fibrosis
    4. *Pancreatojejunostomy* (the pancreatic duct is opened and anastomosed to the jejunum, relieving obstruction) to relieve pain and preserve pancreatic tissue and function
    5. *Partial pancreatectomy* may be performed for advanced pancreatitis or disabling pain
    6. *Vagotomy* with gastric antrectomy to alter nerve stimulation and decrease pancreatic secretion
- For preoperative and postoperative care, see Cancer, Pancreatic, for care of the client undergoing a Whipple procedure.

Continuing Care

- Health teaching is aimed at preventing further exacerbations.
- The nurse teaches the client to
    1. Avoid known precipitating factors, such as alcohol, caffeinated beverages, and irritating foods
    2. Comply with diet instructions: bland, low-fat, frequent meals with avoidance of rich, fatty foods

3. Follow written instructions and prescriptions for pancreatic enzyme therapy:
   a. How and when to take enzymes
   b. Importance of maintaining therapy
   c. Importance of notifying the physician of increased steatorrhea, abdominal distention, cramping, and skin breakdown
4. Comply with elevated glucose management, including either oral hypoglycemic drugs or insulin injections and monitoring of blood glucose levels
5. Keep follow-up visits with the physician(s)
- The nurse refers the client to financial counseling, social services, vocational rehabilitation, home health services, and Alcoholics Anonymous.

Paralysis Agitans

See Parkinson's Disease.

P

Paralysis, Facial

OVERVIEW

- Facial paralysis, or *Bell's palsy,* is an acute paralysis of cranial nerve VII, with maximal paralysis reached within 2 to 5 days.
- Pain behind the face or ear may precede paralysis by a few hours or days.
- The disorder is characterized by an inability to close the eye, wrinkle the forehead, smile, whistle, or grimace; the face appears mask-like and sags.

COLLABORATIVE MANAGEMENT

- The nurse
  1. Administers prednisone (Deltasone, Winpred◆), as ordered
  2. Administers analgesics for pain

521

3. Protects the eye from corneal abrasion or ulceration by patching and administering artificial tears
4. Provides emotional support
5. Provides small, frequent soft meals, in collaboration with the dietitian
6. Teaches the client to use warm, moist heat, massage, and facial exercises, such as whistling, grimacing, and blowing air out of the cheeks three or four times a day

- About 80% of clients recover fully within a few weeks or months.

PARALYSIS, LANDRY'S

See Guillain-Barré Syndrome.

PARKINSON'S DISEASE

OVERVIEW

- Parkinson's disease, also referred to as paralysis agitans, is a debilitating, neurologic disorder involving the basal ganglia and substantia nigra.
- Although the cause is not known, it may be related to a genetic defect of chromosome 4.
- The disease is characterized by resting tremors, decreased postural reflexes, rigidity, bradykinesia, masklike facial expression, and slow, shuffling gait.

COLLABORATIVE MANAGEMENT
Assessment

- The nurse records the client's
  1. Time and progression of symptoms
  2. Bradykinesia, problems performing two activities at once
  3. History of slight tremor, fatigue, and manual dexterity

4. Changes in handwriting, which typically becomes small and can be accomplished only slowly
- The nurse assesses for
   1. Rigidity, which is present early in the disease process and progresses over time:
      a. Cogwheel rigidity, manifested by a rhythmic interruption of the muscles of movement
      b. Plastic rigidity, mildly restrictive movements
      c. Lead-pipe rigidity, total resistance to movement
   2. Mask-like facies (wide-open, fixed, staring eyes caused by rigidity of the facial muscles)
   3. Difficulty chewing and swallowing
   4. Changes in the client's speech pattern:
      a. Soft, low-pitched voice
      b. Dysarthria
      c. Echolalia (automatic repetition of what another person says)
      d. Repetition of sentences
   5. Changes in posture and gait:
      a. Stooped posture with a flexed trunk
      b. Truncal rigidity
      c. Movement of the body as a unit
      d. When standing, fingers abducted and flexed at the metacarpophalangeal joint and the wrist slightly dorsiflexed
      e. Slow and shuffling gait, with short, hesitant steps; propulsive gait (slow to initiate but accelerating almost to a trot)
      f. Bradykinesia to the point at which the client is unable to move
      g. Difficulty stopping quickly
      h. Tremors at rest, absent during sleep
   6. Orthostatic hypotension
   7. Excessive perspiration
   8. Oily skin
   9. Flushing, changes in skin texture
   10. Gastrointestinal dysfunction, such as severe constipation
   11. Emotional lability, depression, and paranoia

Interventions

- The nurse
   1. Collaborates with physical and occupational therapy to plan and implement an active and passive range-of-motion and muscle-stretching program

2. Encourages the client to ambulate as tolerated, to avoid sitting for long periods, and to reposition the body frequently
3. Teaches the client to perform breathing exercises
4. Instructs the client with orthostatic hypotension to change position slowly, especially when moving from a sitting to a standing position

- The nurse administers drug therapy, as ordered:
  1. Levodopa (L-dopa), carbidopa-levodopa combination (Sinemet), or amantadine hydrochloride (Symmetrel)
  2. Bromocriptine mesylate (Parlodel) is especially useful for clients who experience side effects while receiving levodopa
- The nurse monitors the client for drug toxicity and side effects, as evidenced by confusion, decreased effectiveness of the medication, and hallucinations.
- *Stereotactic pallidotomy* can be a very effective treatment for Parkinson's disease; using a probe, the target area in the brain receives a mild electrical stimulation to decrease tremor and rigidity.
- Experimental surgical treatment (brain graft surgery) consists of transplanting small pieces of the client's own adrenal gland into the caudate nucleus of the brain; fetal tissue transplant is also being tried. Both surgeries are considered palliative.
- The nurse
  1. Assesses the client's ability to perform activities of daily living (ADL) to establish his or her abilities and limitations
  2. Encourages the client to perform activities as independently as possible; provides assistance as needed
  3. Allows sufficient time for the client to complete activities
- Collaborates with physical and occupational therapy to identify the need for assistive-adaptive devices
- The nurse
  1. Encourages the client to speak slowly and clearly and to pause and take deep breaths at appropriate intervals during each sentence
  2. Eliminates unnecessary environmental noise to maximize the listener's ability to hear and understand the client

3. Asks the client to repeat words not understood; watches the client's lips and nonverbal expressions for cues to meaning of conversations
4. Instructs the client to organize his or her thoughts before speaking
5. Encourages the client to use facial expressions and gestures (if possible) to augment communication
6. Collaborates with speech-language pathologist to identify alternative methods of communication, such as a communication board, mechanical voice synthesizer, or computer, for a client unable to communicate verbally

- The nurse
  1. Assesses the client's ability to chew and swallow food as well as to feed self independently
  2. Records food and fluid intake
  3. Collaborates with the dietitian for caloric calculation and diet planning
- The nurse
  1. Emphasizes the client's abilities or strengths and provides positive reinforcement
  2. Assists the client to set realistic goals that can be achieved
  3. Assists the client with grooming and hygiene

P

PE

See Embolism, Pulmonary.

PEDICULOSIS

- Pediculosis is infestation by human lice and includes *pediculosis capitis* (head lice), *pediculosis corporis* (body lice), and *pediculosis pubis* (pubic or crab lice).
- The oval-shaped lice measure approximately 2 to 4 mm in length.

- The female louse lays hundreds of eggs, called *nits,* which are deposited at the base of the hair shaft.
- The most common symptom is pruritus, which may or may not be accompanied by excoriation.
- The treatment is chemical killing with agents such as lindane (Kwell, Kwellada◆) or topical malathion.
- Clothing and bed linens must be thoroughly washed in hot water.

PELVIC INFLAMMATORY DISEASE

OVERVIEW

- Pelvic inflammatory disease (PID) is the major gynecologic health problem in the United States affecting over 1 million women each year.
- PID is an infectious process that involves one or more pelvic structures, although the most common site is the fallopian tubes.
- PID is the leading cause of infertility.
- PID is a complex disease in which organisms from the lower genital tract migrate from the endocervix through the endometrial cavity to the fallopian tubes.
- Resultant infections include endometritis, salpingitis, oophoritis, parametritis, and peritonitis, which can cause adhesions and strictures.
- Three sexually transmitted disease (STD) organisms most often cause PID—*Neisseria gonorrhoeae, Chlamydia trachomatis,* and *Mycoplasma hominis.*
- Sexually active women with multiple partners are at increased risk.
- Other risk factors include age less than 20, contraceptive choice, use of vaginal douches, smoking, history of sexually transmitted diseases (STDs), and history of PID.

➔ Transcultural Considerations

1. In the early 1990s, the largest increases in STDs were among inner city, poor, non-Caucasian populations.

526

2. Controversy over differences due to race or environment accounting for incidence of PID.

COLLABORATIVE MANAGEMENT

Assessment

- The nurse records the client's
  1. Medical history
  2. Menstrual history
  3. Obstetric history
  4. Sexual history
  5. Previous episodes of PID or other STDs
  6. Contraceptive use, such as intrauterine devices
  7. History of reproductive surgeries
- The nurse assesses for
  1. Lower abdominal tenderness with rigidity or rebound pain
  2. Chills
  3. Fever
  4. Malaise
  5. Purulent vaginal discharge
  6. Tachycardia
  7. Dysuria
  8. Irregular vaginal bleeding
  9. Uterine or cervical tenderness on pelvic examination
  10. Anxiety and fear
  11. Positive cultures, increased white blood cell count
  12. Findings of laparoscopy, which provides an immediate, accurate diagnosis based on direct inspection

P

Planning and Implementation

✦ **NDx:** Pain

Nonsurgical Management

- The nurse
  1. Provides analgesia, as ordered
  2. Provides sitz baths
  3. Applies heat to the lower back or abdomen
  4. Maintains bed rest in a semi-Fowler's position
  5. Administers antibiotic therapy, as ordered

Surgical Management

- Surgical intervention is an abdominal laparotomy to remove an abscess or pelvic mass for a small number of clients.

- The nurse
    1. Assesses the client's knowledge of PID and its relationship to infertility
    2. Encourages the client to express her feelings and questions
    3. Encourages the family and significant others to provide the client with emotional support

Continuing Care

- The client with PID is typically managed at home.
- Health teaching is focused on providing information about PID, including
    1. Identification of recurrences
    2. Meticulous perineal hygiene
- Treatment of the sexual partner for STDs is necessary
- The nurse
    1. Provides counseling about complications of PID, including infertility, increased risk of ectopic pregnancy, and development of chronic pelvic pain
    2. Teaches contraceptive measures, including oral contraceptives and barrier methods
    3. Teaches lifestyle changes, including decreased frequency of sexual intercourse with multiple partners
    4. Emphasizes the importance of follow-up visits with the health care provider(s)

PEPTIC ULCER DISEASE

See Ulcers, Peptic.

PERICARDITIS

OVERVIEW

- Pericarditis is an inflammation or alteration of the pericardium, the membranous sac enclosing the heart.

- There are two types of pericarditis:
    1. *Acute pericarditis,* which is caused by viruses, bacteria, post–myocardial infarction syndrome, postpericardiotomy syndrome, metastatic tumors, systemic connective tissue diseases, idiopathic causes
    2. *Chronic constrictive pericarditis,* which is caused by tuberculosis, radiation therapy, trauma, renal failure, and metastatic cancer, with the pericardium becoming rigid, preventing adequate ventricular filling, and resulting in cardiac failure

COLLABORATIVE MANAGEMENT

- Assessment findings include
    1. Substernal precordial pain that can radiate to the left neck, shoulder, and back; pleuritic pain aggravated by breathing, coughing, and swallowing
    2. Pericardial friction rub
    3. Acute pericarditis:
        a. Elevated white blood cell count
        b. ST-T wave elevation on electrocardiography (ECG)
        c. Fever (infectious cause)
    4. Chronic constrictive pericarditis:
        a. Right-sided heart failure, including dyspnea, exertional fatigue, and orthopnea
        b. Pericardial thickening on echocardiogram and computed tomography scan
        c. Inverted or flat T waves on ECG
        d. Atrial fibrillation
- Treatment depends on the type of pericarditis.
- For acute pericarditis, the nurse
    1. Administers analgesics or anti-inflammatory agents, as ordered
    2. Administers corticosteroid therapy, as ordered
    3. Administers antibiotics, as ordered
    4. Encourages rest
- For chronic constrictive pericarditis, the definitive treatment is surgical excision of the pericardium (pericardiectomy)
- Complications of pericarditis include
    1. Pericardial effusions
    2. Cardiac tamponade, manifested by jugular venous distention, paradoxical pulse (systolic BP 10

P

mmHg higher or more on expiration than on inspiration), decreased cardiac output, and muffled heart sounds

PERIPHERAL ARTERIAL DISEASE

See Arterial Disease, Peripheral.

PERIPHERAL NERVE TRAUMA

See Trauma, Peripheral Nerve.

PERIPHERAL VASCULAR DISEASE

See Arterial Disease, Peripheral.

PERIPHERAL VENOUS DISEASE

See Venous Disease, Peripheral.

PERITONITIS

OVERVIEW

- Peritonitis is an inflammation of the peritoneal cavity; it may be localized or generalized.
- *Primary peritonitis* results from an acute bacterial infection from another body source that is carried to the peritoneum by the vascular system.
- *Secondary peritonitis* is caused by bacterial invasion as a result of perforation or rupture of an abdominal viscus; it also results from a severe chemical reaction to pancreatic enzymes, digestive juices, or bile released into the peritoneal cavity.
- Complications of peritonitis include shock, respiratory problems, and paralytic ileus.

COLLABORATIVE MANAGEMENT

Assessment

- The nurse records the client's
  1. History of abdominal pain, which is aggravated by movement and respiratory effort and relieved by knee flexion
  2. Abdominal distention
  3. Anorexia
  4. Nausea or vomiting
  5. Elevated temperature with chills
  6. Inability to pass flatus or feces
  7. Medical history, including the date of the last menstrual period
- The nurse assesses for
  1. Pain, which may be sharp and localized or poorly localized and referred to either the shoulder or thoracic areas
  2. Abdominal rigidity ("board-like") or distention with rebound tenderness
  3. Absent bowel sounds
  4. Fever with tachycardia
  5. Dehydration as evidenced by dry mucous membranes, poor skin turgor, and decreased urinary output
  6. Compromised respiratory status

7. Elevated white blood cell count

Interventions

- The nurse
    1. Administers intravenous (IV) fluids and broad-spectrum antibiotics, as ordered
    2. Gives the client nothing by mouth (NPO)
    3. Monitors and records drainage from the nasogastric (NG) tube used for gastric and intestinal decompression
- Surgical management may be necessary to identify and repair the underlying cause of the peritonitis.
- Surgery is focused on controlling the contamination, removing foreign material from the peritoneal cavity, and draining fluid collections.
- During surgery, the peritoneum is irrigated with antibiotic solutions, and drainage catheters are inserted.
- Postoperatively, the nurse
    1. Monitors the client's
        a. Level of consciousness
        b. Vital signs
        c. Fluid and electrolyte status
        d. Intake and output
    2. Maintains the client in a semi-Fowler's position
    3. Provides meticulous wound care
    4. Assists the client to gradually increase activity level

Continuing Care

- The nurse provides written and oral postoperative instructions:
    1. The necessity to report any redness, tenderness, swelling, drainage, or odor from the wound
    2. Care of the incision and dressing
    3. The need to report temperature higher than 101° F (38.2° C) to the physician
    4. Pain medication administration and monitoring
    5. Dietary limitations, if necessary
    6. Activity limitations, including avoidance of heavy lifting until healing has occurred

PERITONSILLAR ABSCESSES

See Abscesses, Peritonsillar.

PHARYNGITIS

- Pharyngitis is an infection of the mucous membranes of the pharynx, usually preceding or occurring with acute rhinitis or sinusitis.
- Causes of acute pharyngitis include bacteria, viruses, and physical and chemical influences.
- Pharyngitis is most commonly caused by a virus; the most common bacterial cause is group A *beta-hemolytic streptococcus.*
- Pharyngitis is characterized by soreness and dryness in the throat, pain, difficulty swallowing, dysphagia, and fever.
- Viral sore throats usually have a gradual onset and are accompanied by rhinorrhea, headache, mild hoarseness, and low-grade fever.
- Bacterial infection is associated with an abrupt onset, dysphagia, arthralgias, myalgias, malaise, and fever.
- Viral and bacterial pharyngitis may be associated with mild to severe hyperemia, with or without enlarged erythematous tonsils and with or without exudate.
- Nasal discharge varies from thin and watery to purulent.
- Management of *viral pharyngitis* includes
  1. Rest
  2. Increased fluid intake
  3. Analgesics for pain
  4. Warm saline throat gargles
  5. Mild antiseptic throat lozenges
- Management of *bacterial pharyngitis* includes antibiotics and supportive care measures.

P

PHEOCHROMOCYTOMA

OVERVIEW

- A pheochromocytoma is a catecholamine-producing tumor that arises in the chromaffin cells of the adrenal medulla.
- Most of these tumors are benign, but they can occur in a malignant form.

COLLABORATIVE MANAGEMENT

- The nurse assesses for
    1. Paroxysmal hypertensive episodes, which vary in length from a few minutes to several hours
    2. Palpitations
    3. Severe headache
    4. Profuse diaphoresis
    5. Flushing
    6. Apprehension or a feeling of impending doom
    7. Pain in the chest or abdomen
    8. Nausea and vomiting
    9. Heat intolerance
    10. Weight loss
    11. Tremors
    12. Elevated vanillylmandelic acid and free catecholamines during a 24-hour urine collection
- Surgery is performed to remove the tumor and the affected adrenal glands.
- The nurse provides preoperative care:
    1. Identifies factors that contribute to hypertensive crisis
    2. Provides a diet rich in calories, vitamins, and minerals
    3. Ensures adequate hydration
    4. Administers alpha-adrenergic blocking agents, as ordered, to decrease the risk of hypertension during surgery
- The nurse provides postoperative care:
    1. Provides the same care as that for an adrenalectomy (see Hyperfunction, Adrenal)
    2. Monitors for hypotension and hypovolemia
    3. Monitors for shock and hemorrhage

- The tumor is managed with alpha- and beta-adrenergic blocking agents if inoperable.
- Clients who are managed medically must be instructed in the correct technique to monitor their own blood pressure.

PHLEBITIS

- Phlebitis is an inflammation of the superficial veins caused by an irritation, commonly intravenous therapy.
- Phlebitis is manifested as a reddened, warm area radiating up an extremity.
- The client may also experience pain, soreness, and swelling of the extremity.
- Treatment involves application of warm, moist soaks, which dilate the vein and promote circulation.

PID

See Pelvic Inflammatory Disease.

P

PKD

See Kidney Disease, Polycystic.

PMS

See Premenstrual Syndrome.

PNEUMOCONIOSIS

See Pulmonary Disease, Occupational.

PNEUMOCONIOSIS AND CHRONIC BRONCHITIS

See Pulmonary Disease, Occupational.

PNEUMONIA

OVERVIEW

- Pneumonia is an infection of pulmonary tissue, including the interstitial spaces, the alveoli, and the bronchioles.
- Pathogens penetrate the airway mucosa and multiply in the alveolar spaces, causing white blood cell migration into the alveoli and a thickening of the alveolar wall.
- The edema associated with inflammation stiffens the lung, decreasing compliance and vital capacity.
- The pneumonic process causes a shunt-type ventilation-perfusion defect, resulting in arterial hypoxemia.
- Pneumonia presents as diffuse patches throughout both lungs or consolidates in one lobe.
- Prevention is aimed at immunizing against the causative agents whenever possible, and reducing the risks of exposure.

 Transcultural Considerations

Of the over 64-year-old group, the highest levels of vaccination were in women and Caucasians.

536

- Community-acquired pneumonias are caused by *Mycoplasma pneumoniae*, *Legionella pneumophila*, *Streptococcus pneumoniae*, and *Haemophilus influenzae*.
- Nosocomial pneumonias are caused by *Staphylococcus aureus*, *Klebsiella pneumoniae*, *Pseudomonas aeruginosa*, and fungi.
- *Pneumocystis carinii* is the most frequent cause of pneumonia in the immunocompromised patient

---

🔊 Considerations for Elderly Clients

1. Pneumonia and influenza are the third leading cause of death among people over 65 years old.
2. Predisposing factors for pneumonia in the elderly include
   a. Chronic airflow limitations
   b. Congestive heart failure
   c. Influenza
   d. Alcoholism
   e. Immobility
   f. Poor nutritional status

COLLABORATIVE MANAGEMENT

Assessment

- The nurse records the client's
  1. Age
  2. Environmental changes
  3. Cigarette and alcohol use
  4. Medications
  5. Drug abuse history
  6. Chronic pulmonary illness
  7. Recent medical history (influenza, pneumonia, viral infections)
  8. Home respiratory equipment use and cleaning regimen
  9. Current symptoms
- The nurse assesses for
  1. General appearance
  2. Breathing pattern
  3. Use of accessory muscles
  4. Cyanosis
  5. Crackles, rhonchi, and wheezes on auscultation
  6. Bronchial breath sounds over areas of density or consolidation
  7. Tactile fremitus

P

8. Dull percussion
9. Character of cough
10. Sputum production, including amount, color, and odor
11. Fever and chills
12. Mental status changes (especially in the elderly)
13. Gastrointestinal symptoms
14. Anxiety
15. Leukocystosis and hypoxia (especially in the elderly)
16. Positive sputum culture
17. Positive chest x-ray

Planning and Implementation

✦ NDx: Ineffective Airway Clearance

- The nurse
    1. Encourages coughing and deep-breathing
    2. Encourages the use of incentive spirometry
    3. Increases fluid intake to thin secretions
    4. Encourages clients to ambulate and gets them out of bed in a chair, as tolerated
    5. Performs nasotracheal suctioning if the client is unable to clear secretions
    6. Administers aerosolized bronchodilators, such as metaproterenol sulfate (Alupent), isoetharine (Bronkosol), and terbutaline sulfate (Brethine), as ordered

✦ NDx: Potential for Sepsis

- The nurse administers antibiotic therapy as determined by sputum analysis, as ordered.

✦ NDx: Impaired Gas Exchange

- The nurse
    1. Instructs the client on the correct use of incentive spirometry (sustained maximal inspiration) and evaluates the client's techniques
    2. Encourages the client to perform 5 to 10 deep breaths each hour while awake

Continuing Care

- The nurse provides health teaching:
    1. Importance of rest
    2. Proper nutrition

3. Adequate fluid intake
4. Avoiding exposure to others with respiratory infections or viruses
5. Risk of increased susceptibility
6. Antibiotic therapy, including prescriptions, as ordered
7. Notification of the physician for chills, fever, dyspnea, hemoptysis, or increasing fatigue if symptoms fail to resolve
8. Encourages the client to quit smoking

- The influenza vaccine is highly recommended for clients older than 65 years of age and for younger people with chronic cardiac disease, severe diabetes, or impaired immune defenses.
- High-risk clients should be given the pneumococcal vaccine, which provides immunity against several strains of pneumococci

PNEUMONITIS, TOXIC

See Pulmonary Disease, Occupational.

PNEUMOTHORAX

- Pneumothorax is an accumulation of atmospheric air in the pleural space, resulting in a rise in intrathoracic pressure and reduced vital capacity.
- Pneumothorax is caused by thoracic injury, including blunt chest trauma.
- Assessment findings include
  1. Diminished breath sounds
  2. Hyperresonance on percussion
  3. Prominence of the involved hemothorax
  4. Pleuritic chest pain
  5. Tachypnea
  6. Subcutaneous emphysema
- Interventions are aimed at rapid removal of trapped atmospheric air, including insertion of a large-bore needle and chest tubes to ensure lung inflation.

Pneumothorax, Tension

- Tension pneumothorax is a complication of blunt chest trauma or mechanical ventilation with positive end-expiratory pressure and occurs as a result of an air leak into the lung or chest wall.
- Air forced into the thoracic cavity causes complete collapse of the affected lung.
- Air entering the pleural space during expiration does not exit during inspiration; therefore, the air accumulates under pressure, compressing the mediastinal vessels and interfering with venous return.
- Assessment findings include
    1. Tracheal deviation to the unaffected side
    2. Respiratory distress
    3. Unilateral absence of breath sounds
    4. Distended neck veins
    5. Cyanosis
    6. Hypertympanic sound over the affected hemothorax
- Initial treatment includes emergency insertion of a large-bore needle into the second intercostal space in the mid-clavicular line on the affected side to relieve pressure.
- Chest tube placement into the fourth intercostal space of the mid-axillary line follows; underwater seal drainage is maintained until the lung is fully expanded.

Polio

See Poliomyelitis.

Poliomyelitis

- Poliomyelitis (polio) is an acute viral disease characterized by destruction of the motor cells of the anterior horn of the spinal cord, the brain stem, and the motor strip of the frontal lobe.
- Polio is transmitted through droplet infection or by the fecal or oral route and the gastrointestinal tract.
- The disease is rare in North America because of immunization during childhood.
- Polio is characterized by fever, chills, excessive perspiration, severe muscle aches and weakness, increased deep tendon reflexes, abdominal tenderness, dysphagia, and irritability.
- Treatment is symptomatic.
- Analgesics are used to relieve pain, and respiratory status is monitored carefully.

Polycystic Kidney Disease

See Kidney Disease, Polycystic.

Polycystic Ovary Syndrome

See Cysts, Ovarian.

POLYNEURITIS AND POLYNEUROPATHY

OVERVIEW

- Both inflammatory and non-inflammatory processes can damage cranial and peripheral nerves.
- *Polyneuritis* implies an inflammatory process, but the terms *polyneuritis* and *polyneuropathy* may be used interchangeably.
- These syndromes are characterized by muscle weakness with atrophy, pain, paresthesia or loss of sensation, impaired reflexes, autonomic manifestations, or a combination of these symptoms.
- The most common type of this disorder is a symmetric polyneuropathy in which the client experiences decreased sensation, along with a feeling that the extremity is asleep. Tingling, burning, tightness, or aching sensations usually start in the feet and progress to the level of the knee before being noted in the hands ("glove and stocking" neuropathy).
- Factors associated with polyneuropathy include diabetes; renal or hepatic failure; alcoholism; vascular disease, vitamin B_1, B_6, and B_{12} deficiency; and exposure to heavy metals or industrial solvents.

COLLABORATIVE MANAGEMENT

- Assessment includes
  1. Light touch and pain in the distal extremities
  2. Position sense and kinesthetic sensation
  3. Sensitivity to vibration by placing a tuning fork on a bony prominence
  4. Any signs of injury
  5. Indications of autonomic dysfunctions, such as orthostatic hypotension, abnormal sweating, and miosis
- Treatment consists of removal or treatment of the underlying cause and symptomatic therapy:
  1. Supplementing the diet with vitamins
  2. Health teaching, including the importance of foot care and inspecting the extremities for injuries
  3. Importance of wearing shoes at all times and of purchasing well-fitting shoes

542

4. Teaching the client how to recognize potential hazards, such as exposure to extremes of environmental temperature
5. Discouraging smoking
6. Establishing a trusting nurse-client relationship

POLYNEURITIS, IDIOPATHIC ACUTE

See Guillain-Barré Syndrome.

POLYNEURITIS, INFECTIOUS

See Guillain-Barré Syndrome.

POLYNEUROPATHY

See Polyneuritis and Polyneuropathy.

POLYPS, CERVICAL

- Cervical polyps are pedunculated (on stalks) tumors arising from the mucosa and extending to the cervical os.
- The polyps result from a hyperplastic condition of the endocervical epithelium or inflammation and are the most common neoplastic growth of the cervix.
- Clinical findings include
  1. Premenstrual or postmenstrual bleeding

2. Postcoital bleeding
   3. Small, single, or multiple bright-red polyps that are soft with fragile consistency and may bleed when touched
- Polyps are easily removed in the physician's office.
- Immediate post-procedure instructions include avoidance of
   1. Tampons
   2. Douching
   3. Sexual intercourse

POLYPS, GASTROINTESTINAL

- Gastrointestinal tract polyps are small growths covered with mucosa and attached to the intestinal surface; most are benign but have the potential to become malignant.
- Adenomas require medical consultation because of their malignant potential.
- Pedunculated polyps are stalk-like, with a thin stem attaching them to the intestinal wall.
- Polyps are usually asymptomatic but can cause rectal bleeding, intestinal obstruction, and intussusception.
- Polyps can usually be removed by *polypectomy* with an electrocautery snare that fits through a colonoscope, eliminating the need for abdominal surgery.
- Postoperatively, the nurse monitors for
   1. Abdominal distention and pain
   2. Rectal bleeding
   3. Mucopurulent rectal drainage
   4. Fever
- The nurse instructs the client to follow up with a repeated colonoscopy or sigmoidoscopy, as ordered.

POSTPOLIO SYNDROME

- Postpolio syndrome is a new onset of weakness, pain, and fatigue in persons who had poliomyelitis 30 or more years previously.

- Physical and emotional stressors are contributing factors.
- Treatment is symptomatic and includes lifestyle modifications to preserve energy and physiologic function.
- Adaptive and orthotic devices may be needed.

PPS

See Postpolio Syndrome.

PREMENSTRUAL SYNDROME

- Premenstrual syndrome (PMS) is a collection of symptoms that are cyclic in nature, occurring each month during the luteal phase of the menstrual cycle, followed by relief with menses and a symptom-free phase.
- The cause is not well understood, but many theories have been reported in the literature.
- Clinical manifestations are highly variable and include
    1. Dermatologic: acne, urticaria, herpes
    2. Respiratory: sinusitis, asthma, rhinitis, colds
    3. Urologic: oliguria, cystitis, enuresis, urethritis
    4. Ophthalmologic: conjunctivitis, styes, glaucoma
    5. Neurologic: headaches, migraine, syncope, vertigo, numbness of hands and feet, epilepsy (if susceptible)
    6. Metabolic: edema, breast tenderness
    7. Emotional and psychologic: depression, irritability, tension, panic attacks, changes in libido, mood swings, anxiety
    8. Behavioral: lowered work performance, food cravings, alcohol and drug overindulgence, confusion, sleeplessness, lack of coordination, suicide, lethargy, child abuse, assaultive behavior
    9. Other: allergies, hypoglycemia, joint pain, backache, palpitations, water retention
- Management is focused on eliminating uncomfortable symptoms and is highly individualized:

P

1. Dietary measures, such as limiting sugar, red meat, alcohol, coffee, tea, chocolate, caffeine, salt, sodium, and vitamins A, B_6, and C to relieve symptoms
2. Drug therapy, which is controversial: diuretics, progesterone therapy, and bromocriptine mesylate
3. Education about PMS and its symptoms
4. Self-help groups and support groups

PRESBYOPIA

See Refractive Errors.

PRIAPISM

- Priapism is an uncontrolled and long-maintained erection without sexual desire, which causes the penis to become large, hard, and painful.
- Priapism occurs from neural, vascular, or pharmacologic causes.
- Common causes are thrombosis of the veins of the corpus cavernosum, leukemia, sickle cell anemia, diabetes, and malignancies.
- Priapism is also associated with intake of psychotropic medications, antidepressants, and antihypertensives.
- Priapism is considered a urologic emergency because penile circulation may be compromised, and the client may not be able to void with an erect penis.
- Conservative treatment measures include
    1. Prostatic massage
    2. Sedation
    3. Bed rest
    4. Warm enemas to cause venous dilation and increase outflow of trapped blood
    5. Meperidine (Demerol) for its hypotensive effect
- Urinary catheterization is required if the client is unable to void.

- Aspiration of the corpora cavernosa with a large-bore needle or surgical intervention may be required.
- Priapism should be resolved within the first 24 to 30 hours to prevent penile ischemia, gangrene, fibrosis, and impotence.

PROGRESSIVE SYSTEMIC SCLEROSIS

See Sclerosis, Progressive Systemic.

PROLAPSE, MITRAL VALVE

- Mitral valve prolapse occurs as a result of mitral valve leaflet enlargement, prolapsing into the left atrium during systole.
- Mitral valve prolapse is usually benign but may progress to a stage of pronounced mitral regurgitation.
- The cause is associated with endocarditis, myocarditis, and acute or chronic rheumatic heart disease.
- A familial occurrence is well established.
- Signs and symptoms include
    1. Atypical chest pain
    2. Dizziness and syncope
    3. Palpitations
    4. Atrial or ventricular dysrhythmias
    5. Non-ejection systolic click
- Valve replacement surgery is indicated only when pronounced mitral regurgitation follows.

PROLAPSE, UTERINE

- Uterine prolapse is more serious than uterine displacement.

- Three stages are described, according to the degree of descent of the uterus:
    1. *Grade I:* The uterus bulges into the vagina, but the cervix does not protrude through the entrance to the vagina.
    2. *Grade II:* The uterus bulges further into the vagina, and the cervix protrudes through the entrance to the vagina.
    3. *Grade III:* The body of the uterus and cervix protrudes through the vaginal entrance; the vagina is turned inside out.
- Uterine prolapse is caused by congenital defects, persistent high intra-abdominal pressure related to heavy physical labor or exertion, or any cause that weakens pelvic support.
- Physical findings include
    1. Client's report of "something in the vagina"
    2. Dyspareunia
    3. Backache
    4. Feeling of heaviness or pressure in the pelvis
    5. Bowel or bladder problems, such as incontinence
    6. Protrusion of the cervix during pelvic examination
- Interventions are based on the degree of prolapse:
    1. Insertion of a pessary
    2. Surgical vaginal hysterectomy

PROSTATIC CANCER

See Cancer, Prostatic.

PROSTATIC HYPERPLASIA, BENIGN

OVERVIEW

- Glandular units in the prostate undergo tissue hyperplasia, resulting in benign prostatic hypertrophy (BPH).

- The enlarged prostate extends upward into the bladder and inward, narrowing the prostatic urethral channel.
- The prostate obstructs urine flow by encroaching on the bladder opening, resulting in a hyperirritable bladder and producing urgency and frequency, bladder wall hypertrophy, and hydronephrosis and hydroureter.
- Urinary retention or incomplete bladder emptying results in urinary tract infections.

Considerations for Elderly Clients

1. The development of BPH is almost a universal condition in older men.

Transcultural Considerations

1. Worldwide, BPH is most common in Caucasians.
2. The reported incidences of BPH in African-American and Caucasian men in the United States are similar.
3. The incidence of BPH in Asian countries, such as China and Japan, is lower than that in the Caucasian and African-American populations.

COLLABORATIVE MANAGEMENT
Assessment

P

- The nurse records the client's
  1. Age
  2. Urinary pattern and symptoms (prostatism):
     a. Frequency
     b. Nocturia
     c. Hesitancy
     d. Intermittency
     e. Diminished force and caliber of stream
     f. Sensation of incomplete bladder emptying
     g. Postvoid dribbling (overflow incontinence)
     h. Hematuria
- The nurse assesses for
  1. Distended bladder
  2. Client readiness for digital prostatic examination (BPH causes an elastic, nontender prostate enlargement; cancer causes the prostate to become stone-hard and nodular)
  3. Laboratory findings, including possible urinary tract infection

Interventions

Nonsurgical Management

- Finasteride (Proscar) may be used to shrink the prostate gland and improve urine flow. Finasteride lowers dihydrotestosterone, a major cause of prostate growth; the major side effects are impotence and decreased libido, although they are uncommon.
- Prostatic fluid may be released by prostatic massage, frequent intercourse, and masturbation.
- The nurse teaches the client to
    1. Avoid drinking large amounts of fluid in a short period
    2. Avoid alcohol and diuretics
    3. Void as soon as the urge is felt
    4. Avoid medications that increase urinary retention, such as anticholinergics, antihistamines, and decongestants

Surgical Management

- Surgery is performed for acute urinary retention, chronic urinary tract infections secondary to residual urine in the bladder, hematuria, hydronephrosis, and bladder neck obstruction symptoms, such as urinary frquency and nocturia.
- The usual surgical interventions to treat BPH include
    1. *Transurethral resection of the prostate (TURP),* which involves the insertion of a resectoscope though the urethra and resection of the enlarged portion of the prostate (the safest procedure)
    2. *Suprapubic,* or *transvesical, prostatectomy,* which involves a low abdominal incision to expose the bladder; the prostate gland is enucleated through the bladder cavity, and repair to the bladder is done, if required
    3. *Retropubic,* or *extravesical, prostatectomy,* which is accomplished by an abdominal incision above the symphysis pubis; a small incision is made into the prostate gland, and the gland is enucleated
    4. *Perineal prostatectomy,* which is used primarily to remove prostate glands filled with calculi, to treat prostatic abscesses, to repair complications, or to treat poor surgical risks; the surgeon makes a U-shaped incision between the ischial tuberosities, the scrotum, and the rectum; the prostatic capsule is opened and enucleated

- The nurse provides preoperative care:
  1. Informs the client to expect an indwelling bladder catheter and possibly continuous bladder irrigation
  2. Tells the client to expect hematuria and blood clots
  3. Provides information about sexual functioning and continence
- The nurse provides postoperative care:
  1. Informs the client that he may feel the urge to void because of the large diameter of the three-way Foley catheter and the pressure of the balloon on the internal sphincter
  2. Instructs the client to try not to void around the catheter, which will cause the bladder to spasm
  3. Maintains continuous bladder irrigation with normal saline solutions, as ordered
  4. Monitors the color of the output and adjusts the rate of the irrigation accordingly to keep the urine clear
  5. Hand irrigates the catheter, as ordered, to remove obstructive blood clots
  6. Monitors for frank bleeding, hyponatremia, and anemia
  7. Assesses the suprapubic catheter (in suprapubic prostatectomy), the catheter site, and the drainage system, if necessary
  8. After removal of the catheter, instructs the client to increase fluid intake
  9. Observes voided urine for clots, color, and consistency
  10. Administers antispasmodics and analgesics, as ordered
  11. Monitors the dressing and drains (in open surgical procedures)
  12. Avoids rectal procedures (in perineal prostatectomy)

P

Considerations for Elderly Clients

1. If the postoperative client becomes restless and confused, restraints should be avoided; familiar personal objects can be given to the client for distraction.
2. The elderly client susceptible to congestive heart failure may not be able to tolerate large amounts of fluid.

Continuing Care

- The nurse provides postoperative discharge instructions:
  1. Recognize that temporary loss of control of urination is normal and will improve.
  2. Contract and relax the urinary sphincter frequently to reestablish urinary control.
  3. Increase water intake to keep urine flowing freely.
  4. Avoid strenuous activities to prevent injury.
  5. Notify the physician of persistent hematuria.
  6. Consume alcohol, soft drinks, and spicy foods in moderation to prevent irritation to remaining prostatic tissue and overstimulation of the bladder.
  7. Keep the area around the suprapubic catheter clean; report decreased drainage or redness at the catheter insertion site (in suprapubic prostatectomy).

Prostatic hypertrophy, benign

See Prostatic Hyperplasia, Benign.

Prostatitis

- Prostatitis is an inflammatory condition of the prostate.
- The most common cause is abacterial prostatitis, which can occur after a viral illness or result from a sudden decrease in sexual activity.
- Bacterial prostatitis is usually associated with urethritis or an infection of the lower urinary tract.
- Common causative organisms include *Escherichia coli, Enterobacter, Proteus,* and group D streptococci.
- Bacterial prostatitis is manifested by
  1. Fever and chills
  2. Dysuria

3. Urethral discharge
4. Boggy, tender prostate
5. Decreased sexual function
6. Urinary tract infections
7. White blood cells in the prostatic secretions

- *Chronic prostatitis* is manifested by
    1. Backache
    2. Perineal pain
    3. Mild dysuria
    4. Urinary frequency
    5. Hematuria (possible)
    6. An irregularly enlarged, firm, and lightly tender prostate
- Complications include epididymitis and cystitis.
- Treatment includes antimicrobials, such as carbenicillin indanyl sodium (Geocillin) or fluroquinolones (ciprofloxacin), and comfort measures such as sitz baths, stool softeners, and analgesia.
- Health teaching includes measures that will drain the prostate, including intercourse, masturbation, and prostatic massage.
- The nurse teaches the client with chronic prostatitis the importance of increasing fluid intake and of long-term antibiotic therapy, such as trimethoprim (Protprin).

PSEUDOCYSTS, PANCREATIC

- Pancreatic pseudocysts develop as a complication of acute or chronic pancreatitis.
- Two percent to 20% of clients with pancreatitis experience pseudocysts, with a 10% mortality.
- These "false cysts" do not have an epithelial lining and are encapsulated sac-like structures that form on or surround the pancreas.
- The pancreatic wall is inflamed, vascular, and fibrotic, containing large amounts of straw-colored or dark brown viscous fluid (enzyme exudate from the pancreas).
- The pseudocyst may be palpated as an epigastric mass in 50% of cases.
- The primary symptom is epigastric pain radiating to the back.

553

- Complications include hemorrhage; infection; obstruction of the gut, biliary tract, or splenic vein; abscess or fistula formation; and pancreatic ascites.
- A pseudocyst may spontaneously resolve or may rupture and cause hemorrhage.
- Surgical intervention with internal drainage is accomplished by creating an ostomy between the pseudocyst and the stomach, jejunum, or duodenum; external drainage is provided by insertion of a sump drainage tube to remove pancreatic exudate and secretions.
- Pancreatic fistulas are common postoperative complications, with skin breakdown.

PSORIASIS

OVERVIEW

- Psoriasis is a scaling skin disorder with underlying dermal inflammation characterized by exacerbations and remissions.
- Abnormal proliferation of epidermal cells in the outer skin areas results in cell shedding every 4 to 5 days.

COLLABORATIVE MANAGEMENT

Assessment

- The nurse records the client's
    1. Precipitating factors, including skin trauma, upper respiratory tract infections, operation, past and current medications, and stress
    2. Family history of psoriasis
    3. Age at onset
    4. Description of progression and patterns of recurrences
    5. Gradual or sudden onset of episode
    6. Description of lesion location
    7. Associated symptoms such as fever and pruritus
    8. Previous treatment modalities
- *Psoriasis vulgaris* is the most common type and is characterized by

1. Thick erythematous papules or plaques surmounted by silvery-white scales
2. Sharply defined borders between lesions and normal skin distributed symmetrically, with the scalp, elbows, trunk, knees, sacrum, and extensor surfaces of the limbs commonly involved
3. Associated nail involvement
- *Exfoliative psoriasis* (erythrodermic psoriasis) is characterized by generalized erythema and scaling without obvious lesions.

Interventions

- The nurse
  1. Applies topical steroids, as ordered, to skin lesions, followed by warm, moist dressings to increase absorption
  2. Applies tar preparations, as ordered, which contain crude coal tar and derivations and are available in solution, ointment, lotion, gel, and shampoo
- Ultraviolet light therapy decreases epidermal growth rate.
- Systemic treatment with a cytotoxic agent is given for severe, debilitating psoriasis.
- The nurse

P

  1. Identifies precipitating factors
  2. Explains the rationale of the treatment plan and the importance of compliance
  3. Teaches the proper application and side effects of the therapeutic agents
  4. Emphasizes the control of symptoms by the identification of precipitators and complying with treatment
  5. Emphasizes the importance of follow-up visits with the physician(s)

PSS

See Sclerosis, Progressive Systemic.

PTOSIS

- Ptosis is the drooping of, or the inability to use, the upper eyelid.
- Causes of ptosis include
    1. Congenital, resulting from muscle dysfunction
    2. Mechanical, caused by abnormal weight of the eyelids from edema
    3. Inflammation, tumors, or injury to the third cranial nerve
- Treatment is palliative; surgery may be indicated if visual acuity or appearance is adversely affected.
- Nursing management after surgery consists of
    1. Assessing the eye for drainage and infection
    2. Applying cool compresses, ophthalmic antibiotic, or an antibiotic-steroid combination ointment
    3. Teaching the client
        a. The procedure to instill the ointment
        b. To keep the eye as clean as possible
        c. To avoid rubbing the eye

PUD

See Ulcers, Peptic.

PULMONARY CONTUSIONS

See Contusions, Pulmonary.

PULMONARY DISEASE, OCCUPATIONAL

- There are several occupational pulmonary diseases.

- *Pneumoconiosis* refers to chronic respiratory diseases related to the inhalation of dust.
- *Acute occupational diseases* include
    1. *Byssinosis,* a pulmonary disease of textile workers caused by excess inhalation of certain vegetable fibers and characterized by chest tightness, coughing, wheezing, and dyspnea; it is especially prominent on the first day back to work following an absence
    2. *Toxic pneumonitis,* caused by excess exposure to irritant gases such as ammonia, sulfur dioxide, chlorine, ozone, and nitrogen dioxide, which cause inflammation or edema of the respiratory system
- *Chronic occupational diseases* include
    1. *Silicosis,* a chronic fibrosing disease of the lungs caused by excess inhalation of free crystalline silica dust over a long period
        a. Hazardous exposure includes mines and quarries, foundries, tunneling, sandblasting, pottery making, stone masonry, and the manufacture of glass, tile, and bricks.
        b. The disease is characterized by the formation of selective nodules in the pulmonary parenchyma accompanied by massive fibrosis.
        c. Clients experience dyspnea on exertion, malaise, anorexia, weight loss, and marked reduction in lung volumes.
    2. *Asbestosis,* a diffuse interstitial fibrosis with diffuse pleural thickening and diaphragmatic calcification caused by exposure to asbestos
        a. At risk are asbestos miners, millers, and building trade and shipyard workers, including loggers, insulation workers, pipe fitters, steam fitters, sheet metal workers, and welders.
        b. Restrictive ventilatory defects result, and frequent repsiratory infections are common.
    3. *Talcosis,* a fibrosis occurring after years of exposure to high concentrations of talc dust in the production of paints, ceramics, asphalt, roofing materials, cosmetics, and rubber goods
    4. *Pneumoconiosis and chronic bronchitis,* which is caused by coal workers' chronic excess exposure to coal dust
    5. *Berylliosis,* which is caused by exposure to beryllium in an operation in which metals are heated to fumes or machined to dust; there is higher likelihood of progression of advanced irreversible diseases

P

- Preventive measures include wearing special masks and ensuring adequate ventilation.
- Interventions are based on the fact that restrictive pulmonary disease is present (deficits in chest wall compliance, vital capacity, and total lung volume).
- Oxygen therapy is indicated for hypoxemic clients.
- Respiratory therapy to promote sputum clearance is essential.

PULMONARY EMBOLISM

See Embolism, Pulmonary.

PULMONARY EMPYEMA

See Empyema, Pulmonary.

PULMONARY SARCOIDOSIS

See Sarcoidosis, Pulmonary.

PULMONARY TUBERCULOSIS

See Tuberculosis, Pulmonary.

PUMP FAILURE

See Heart Failure.

Purpura, Autoimmune Thrombocytopenic

See Thrombocytopenic Purpura, Autoimmune.

Pyelonephritis

OVERVIEW

- Pyelonephritis is a bacterial infection of the renal pelvis; it refers to the active presence of microorganisms or the effects remaining from previous infections within the kidney.
- Microorganisms enter the renal pelvis and activate the inflammatory response, which results in mobilization of white blood cells and local edema.
- The infection is generally classified as acute or chronic.
- Complications include renal abscess, perinephric abscess, emphysematous pyelonephritis, and septicemia.
- Pregnancy, diabetes mellitus, and chronic renal calculi increase the risk for acute pyelonephritis.
- Stones, obstruction, and neurogenic impairment involving the voiding mechanism often lead to chronic pyelonephritis.

COLLABORATIVE MANAGEMENT

Assessment

- The nurse records the client's
  1. History of pyelonephritis
  2. History of urinary tract infections, especially if associated with pregnancy
  3. History of diabetes mellitus, stone disease, or other structural or functional abnormalities of the genitourinary tract
- The nurse assesses the client for
  1. Flank or abdominal discomfort
  2. Hematuria, cloudy urine
  3. General malaise

559

4. Chills and fever
5. Asymmetry, edema, or erythema of the costovertebral angle
6. Anxiety, embarrassment, or guilt
7. Presence of white blood cells and bacteria in the urine

Planning and Implementation

✦ NDx: Pain

- The nurse
  1. Administers analgesics and anesthetics, as ordered
  2. Encourages the client to eat a balanced diet and to drink 2 to 3 liters of fluids per day
- Preoperatively, the nurse
  1. Administers antibiotics, as ordered
  2. Teaches the client about the nature and purpose of the surgery, the expected outcome, and his or her role postoperatively
- Surgical procedures include
  1. Pyelolithotomy, removal of a stone from the renal pelvis
  2. Nephrectomy, removal of a kidney
  3. Ureteral diversion or reimplantation of the ureter to restore the bladder drainage mechanism
- Postoperatively, the nurse provides routine postoperative care.

✦ NDx: Potential for Renal Failure

- The nurse
  1. Ensures that antibiotic therapy is administered as ordered
  2. Assesses for signs of impending renal failure, such as decreased urinary output

Continuing Care

- The nurse instructs the client about
  1. Medication administration:
     a. Purpose
     b. Timing
     c. Frequency
     d. Duration
     e. Possible side effects
  2. Nutrition and fluid intake
  3. Balance between rest and activity
  4. Limitations after surgery

RA

See Arthritis, Rheumatoid.

Raynaud's Disease

See Raynaud's Phenomenon and Raynaud's Disease.

Raynaud's Phenomenon and Raynaud's Disease

- Raynaud's phenomenon and disease are caused by vasospasm of the arterioles and arteries of the upper and lower extremities.
- Cutaneous vessels are constricted, causing blanching of the extremities, followed by cyanosis.
- When the vasospasm is relieved, the tissue becomes reddened or hyperemic.
- *Raynaud's phenomenon* usually occurs unilaterally in people older than 30 years of either sex.
- *Raynaud's disease* occurs bilaterally in persons between the ages of 17 and 50 years and is more common in females.
- Clinical manifestations include
    1. Color changes in the extremity or digits, ranging from blanched to reddened to cyanotic
    2. Numbness of the extremity or digits
    3. Coldness of the extremity or digits
    4. Pain
    5. Swelling
    6. Ulcerations
    7. Aggravation of symptoms by cold or stress

R

8. Gangrene of digits in severe cases
- Interventions include
  1. Drug therapy to prevent vasoconstriction
  2. Lumbar sympathectomy to relieve symptoms in the feet
  3. Sympathetic ganglionectomy to relieve symptoms in the upper extremities
- Health teaching emphasizes methods to minimize vaso-constriction:
  1. Decreasing exposure to cold
  2. Decreasing stress
  3. Wearing warm clothes, socks, and gloves
  4. Keeping the home at a comfortable, warm temperature

RECTOCELE

- A rectocele is a protrusion of the rectum through a weakened vaginal wall.
- A rectocele may develop as a result of the pressure of a baby's head during a difficult delivery, a traumatic forceps delivery, or a congenital defect of the pelvic support tissues.
- Assessment findings include
  1. Constipation
  2. Hemorrhoids
  3. Fecal impaction
  4. Feelings of vaginal or rectal fullness
  5. Bulge of the posterior vaginal wall during pelvic examination
- Management is focused on promoting bowel elimination:
  1. High-fiber diet
  2. Stool softeners
  3. Laxatives
- The surgical intervention is a posterior colporrhaphy or posterior repair.
- Care is similar to other rectal surgeries.
- If both a cystocele and a rectocele are repaired, the client has an anterior and posterior repair.

REFRACTIVE ERRORS

- Refractive errors result from problems in the ability of the eye to focus images on the retina.
- Types of refractive errors include
    1. *Myopia* (nearsightedness), a defect in which distant objects appear blurred
    2. *Hyperopia* (farsightedness), a defect in which close objects appear blurred
    3. *Presbyopia,* the inability of the lens to alter its shape to focus the eye for close work
    4. *Astigmatism,* a refractive defect that prevents focusing of sharp, distinct images
    5. *Aphakia,* the absence of the crystalline lens
- Treatment of refractive errors includes
    1. Eyeglasses
    2. Contact lenses (complications include corneal edema, corneal abrasions, and giant papillary cell conjunctivitis)
    3. Surgery:
        a. *Radial keratotomy* to treat mild to moderate myopia; complications include overcorrection or undercorrection of the refractive error, corneal scars, and failure to achieve adequate correction.
        b. *Epikeratophakia* is the surgical grafting of donor corneal tissue onto the client's own cornea to alter its refractive ability.

REGIONAL ENTERITIS

See Crohn's Disease.

RENAL ABSCESSES

See Abscesses, Renal.

RENAL ARTERY STENOSIS

See Stenosis, Renal Artery.

RENAL CELL CARCINOMA

See Cancer, Renal.

RENAL FAILURE, ACUTE

OVERVIEW
- Acute renal failure (ARF) is the rapid deterioration of renal function associated with an accumulation of nitrogenous wastes in the body (azotemia).
- There are three types of acute renal failure:
  1. *Prerenal azotemia:*
     a. This can be reversed by establishing normal intravascular volume, blood pressure, and cardiac output.
     b. Prolonged hypoperfusion can lead to tubular necrosis and ARF.
  2. *Intrarenal acute renal failure:*
     a. Synonyms include acute tubular necrosis (ATN) and lower nephron nephrosis.
     b. Causes include infections, drugs, infiltrating tumors, inflammation of the glomeruli, and a major obstruction to blood flow.

3. *Postrenal azotemia:* Failure results from an obstruction of formed urine anywhere in the genitourinary tract.

- There are four phases of ARF:
    1. The *onset phase,* beginning with the precipitating event and continuing until oliguria is observed, lasts hours to several days. Clinical manifestations are rising blood urea nitrogen (BUN) and creatinine levels.
    2. During the *oliguric phase* urine output is 100 to 400 mL; this usually lasts 8 to 15 days but can last several weeks, especially in older clients.
    3. The *diuretic phase* begins when the BUN level starts to fall and lasts until it reaches normal levels. Normal renal tubular function is reestablished. Diuresis can result in an output of up to 10 L/day.
    4. During the *convalescence phase* the client returns to normal activities but functions at a lower energy level.

COLLABORATIVE MANAGEMENT

Assessment

- The nurse records the client's
    1. Exposure to nephrotoxins
    2. Recent surgery or trauma
    3. Transfusions
    4. Known renal disease
    5. History of diabetes mellitus, systemic lupus erythematosus, and chronic malignant hypertension
    6. History of acute illnesses, including influenza, colds, gastroenteritis, and sore throat or pharyngitis
    7. History of intravascular volume depletion
    8. History of urinary obstructive disease
- The nurse assesses for
    1. Cardiovascular manifestations:
        a. Chest pain
        b. Tachycardia
        c. Hypotension
        d. Decreased cardiac output
        e. Decreased central venous pressure
        f. Peripheral edema
        g. Cardiac irritability
    2. Respiratory symptoms:
        a. Shortness of breath

R

        b. Pulmonary edema
        c. Friction rub
    3. Neurologic manifestations:
        a. Lethargy
        b. Somnolence
        c. Tremors
        d. Headache
        e. Mental confusion
        f. Muscle cramps
        g. Generalized weakness
        h. Seizures
        i. Flaccid paralysis
        j. Coma
    4. Gastrointestinal (GI) manifestations:
        a. Nausea
        b. Vomiting
        c. GI bleeding
        d. Constipation
        e. Diarrhea
        f. Flank pain
    5. Genitourinary manifestations:
        a. Decreased urinary output
        b. Hematuria
        c. Changes in urine stream
        d. Difficulty starting urination
        e. Dysuria
        f. Urgency
        g. Incontinence
    6. Integumentary manifestations:
        a. Ecchymoses
        b. Yellow pallor

Interventions

- Nursing diagnoses, goals, and interventions for the client with chronic renal failure also apply to the client with ARF (see Renal Failure, Chronic).
- The client with ARF receives multiple medications, as does the client with chronic renal failure (see Renal Failure, Chronic).
- Fluid challenges and diuretics are frequently used to promote renal perfusion.
- A low-dose dopamine infusion may be used to promote renal perfusion.
- Hypercatabolism results in the breakdown of muscle for protein, which leads to increased azotemia; clients require increased calories. Total parenteral nutrition

(TPN) with intralipid infusion may be required to reduce catabolism.

- Indications for hemodialysis or peritoneal dialysis in
patients with ARF are symptoms of uremia, persistent
hyperkalemia, uncompensated metabolic acidosis, fluid
volume excess, uremic pericarditis, and uremic encephalopathy. (See Renal Failure, Chronic, for a discussion of dialysis.)
- Continuous arteriovenous *hemofiltration* (CAVH), and
continuous arteriovenous hemodialysis and filtration
(CAVHD), alternatives to dialysis, may be used.
- CAVH is used to treat massive fluid overload states
when hemodynamic stability is not present.
- CAVHD uses a dialysate delivery system to remove
nitrogenous or other waste products, in clients with
limited cardiac output or significant hypotension.

Continuing Care

- The needs of the client vary depending on the status of
the disease on discharge. Refer to "Continuing Care"
under Renal Failure, Chronic.
- Follow-up care may include medical visits, laboratory
tests, consultation with a dietitian, temporary dialysis,
home nursing care, and social work assistance.

R

RENAL FAILURE, CHRONIC

OVERVIEW

- Chronic renal failure (CRF) is a condition in which
the kidney ceases to remove metabolic wastes and excessive water from the blood.
- The progression toward CRF occurs in three stages:
  1. *Stage I,* or *diminished renal reserve:*
     a. There is a reduction in renal functioning with-
     out accumulation of metabolic wastes.
     b. The unaffected kidney may compensate.
  2. *Stage II,* or *renal insufficiency:*
     a. Metabolic wastes begin to accumulate in the
     blood because the unaffected nephrons no
     longer compensate.

b. The degree of insufficiency is determined by the decreasing glomerular filtration rate and is classified as mild, moderate, or severe.

3. *Stage III,* or *end-stage renal disease* (ESRD):
   a. ESRD occurs when excessive amounts of metabolic wastes accumulate in the blood.
   b. The kidneys are unable to maintain homeostasis and require dialysis.

- Pathologic alterations include disruptions in the glomerular filtration rate (GFR), abnormalities of urine production and water excretion, electrolyte imbalance, and metabolic anomalies.
- Metabolic alterations include disturbances in blood urea nitrogen (BUN) and creatinine excretion.
- *Urea* is the primary product of protein metabolism and is normally excreted by the kidney; BUN varies with dietary intake of protein.
- *Creatinine* is derived from creatine and phosphocreatine; the normal rate of excretion depends on muscle mass, physical activity, and diet.
- *Azotemia* is the increased accumulation of nitrogenous waste in the blood; it is a classic indicator of renal failure.
- Variations in sodium excretion occur, depending on the stage of CRF.
- *Hyponatremia,* or sodium depletion, in early CRF is due to obligatory loss.
- Sodium retention occurs when the kidney's ability to excrete sodium decreases as urine production decreases.
- *Hyperkalemia* results from an increase in potassium load, including ingestion of potassium in medications, failure to restrict potassium in the diet, blood transfusions, and excess bleeding.
- Other pathologic occurrences include numerous metabolic disturbances, such as changes in pH (metabolic acidosis), calcium (hypercalcemia) and phosphorus (hyperphosphatemia) imbalances, and vitamin D insufficiency.
- Renal *osteodystrophy* caused by hypocalcemia and phosphorus retention results in skeletal demineralization manifested by bone pain, pseudofractures, sclerosis of the spine, skull demineralization, osteomalacia, reabsorption of bone, and loss of tooth lamina.
- Cardiovascular alterations include anemia, hypertension, congestive heart failure, and pericarditis.

COLLABORATIVE MANAGEMENT

Assessment

- The nurse records the client's
    1. Age and sex
    2. Height and weight
    3. Current and past medical conditions
    4. Medications, prescription and nonprescription
    5. Family history of renal disease
    6. Dietary and nutritional habits
    7. Change in food tastes
    8. History of gastrointestinal (GI) problems, such as nausea, vomiting, anorexia, diarrhea, or constipation
    9. Current energy level
    10. Recent injuries and abnormal bruising or bleeding
    11. Weakness
    12. Shortness of breath
    13. Detailed urinary elimination
- The nurse assesses for
    1. Cardiovascular abnormalities:
        a. Hypertension
        b. Cardiomyopathy
        c. Uremic pericarditis
        d. Peripheral edema
        e. Congestive heart failure
        f. Pericardial friction rub or effusion
    2. Respiratory manifestations:
        a. Breath that smells like urine (uremic fetor or halitosis)
        b. Deep sighing or yawning
        c. Tachypnea
        d. Pulmonary edema or pleural effusion
        e. Kussmaul's respirations
        f. Uremic lung or hilar pneumonitis
    3. Neurologic manifestations:
        a. Lethargy or daytime drowsiness
        b. Insomnia
        c. Shortened attention span
        d. Paresthesia
        e. Slurred speech
        f. Muscle twitching, tremors, jerky movements
        g. Seizures
        h. Coma

R

4. GI disruptions:
   a. Anorexia
   b. Nausea
   c. Vomiting
   d. Unpleasant or metallic taste
   e. Constipation
   f. Diarrhea
   g. Uremic gastritis (possible GI bleeding)
5. Genitourinary findings:
   a. Change in urinary frequency
   b. Hematuria
   c. Change in urine appearance
   d. Proteinuria
6. Integumentary or dermatologic manifestations:
   a. Pale, yellow skin
   b. Uremic frost (urea crystals on the face and eyebrows) (rare)
   c. Severe itching (pruritus)
   d. Dry skin
   e. Purpura
   f. Ecchymoses
7. Hematologic findings:
   a. Anemia
   b. Abnormal bleeding
8. Immunologic considerations: susceptibility to infections

Planning and Implementation

✦ **NDx:** Altered Nutrition: Less than Body Requirements

- Dietary principles are based on the regulation of protein intake; limitation of fluid intake; restriction of potassium, sodium, and phosphorus intake; administration of vitamin and mineral supplements; and providing adequate calories.
- The nurse
  1. Limits the client's protein intake:
     a. Chronic uremia: 0.55 to 0.60 g/kg of body weight per day
     b. Hemodialysis: 1.0 to 1.2 g/kg of body weight per day
     c. Peritoneal dialysis: 1.2 to 1.4 g/kg of body weight per day
  2. Closely monitors the client's fluid intake:
     a. Chronic uremia: 1500 to 3000 mL/day

b. Hemodialysis: 700 mL/day plus amount of urinary output
c. Peritoneal dialysis: fluid restrictions based on fluid weight gain and blood pressure

3. Monitors and restricts sodium intake:
   a. Nondialyzed client with uremia: 1 to 3 g/day
   b. Hemodialysis: 2 to 4 g/day
   c. Peritoneal dialysis: restrictions based on the fluid weight gain and blood pressure
4. Monitors potassium intake and serum potassium levels with allowance of 60 to 70 mEq/day
5. Monitors phosphorus levels in clients with renal failure to avoid osteodystrophy
6. Administers vitamin and mineral supplements, as ordered
7. Collaborates with the dietitian or nutritionist
8. Assists the client in adapting the diet to food preferences, ethnic background, and the budget

✦ NDx: Fluid Volume Excess

- The nurse
  1. Administers diuretics, as ordered (diuretics are not given to clients with ESRD)
  2. Weighs the client daily on the same scale and at the same time
  3. Measures and records intake and output
  4. Maintains fluid restriction, as ordered

✦ NDx: Decreased Cardiac Output

- The nurse
  1. Administers calcium channel blockers, angiotensin-converting enzyme (ACE) inhibitors, alpha- and beta-adrenergic blockers, and vasodilators
  2. Teaches the family to measure the client's blood pressure and weight daily and to bring these records when visiting the physician, nurse, or dietitian
  3. Monitors the client for decreased cardiac output, heart failure, congestive heart failure, and dysrhythmias

✦ NDx: Risk for Infection

- The nurse
  1. Notifies the physician of signs and symptoms of the effects of medications or drug toxicity

R

571

2. Administers cardiotonic drugs such as digoxin or digitoxin and monitors the client for signs of toxicity, including nausea, vomiting, anorexia, visual disturbances, cardiac irregularities, and bradycardia
3. Administers agents to control phosphorus excess, such as calcium acetate, calcium carbonate, and aluminum hydroxide
4. Monitors the client for hypercalcemia and hypophosphatemia
5. Instructs the client to avoid compounds containing magnesium
6. Administers opioid analgesics cautiously because the effects may last longer and uremic clients are sensitive to the respiratory depressant effects

✦ NDx: Risk for Injury

- The nurse
  1. Monitors the client closely for drug-related complications
  2. Teaches the client to avoid certain medications that can increase renal damage
  3. Teaches clients to avoid medications that contain magnesium

✦ NDx: Fatigue

- The nurse
  1. Administers vitamin and mineral supplements, as ordered
  2. Administers recombinant erythropoietin to treat anemia, as ordered

✦ NDx: Anxiety

- The nurse
  1. Observes the client's behavior for signs of anxiety
  2. Evaluates the client's support system
  3. Explains all procedures, tests, and treatments
  4. Provides instruction on ESRD appropriate to the client's needs and ability to understand
  5. Encourages the client to discuss current problems, fears, or concerns and to ask questions
  6. Facilitates discussion with family members concerning the client's prognosis and potential impacts on the client's lifestyle

✦ NDx: Potential for Pulmonary Edema

- The nurse
  1. Assesses for early signs of pulmonary edema, such as restlessness, dyspnea, and crackles
  2. Manages the client aggressively to alleviate pulmonary edema
- *Hemodialysis* is used to remove the body's excessive fluid and waste products and to restore chemical and electrolyte balance.
- Hemodialysis is based on the principle of diffusion, in which the client's blood is circulated through a semipermeable membrane that acts as an artificial kidney.
- Client selection for hemodialysis includes
  1. Fatal, irreversible renal disease
  2. Absence of illness that would complicate hemodialysis
  3. Expectation of rehabilitation
  4. Client's acceptance of the regimen
- Dialysis settings include acute care facility, free-standing centers, and the home.
- Total dialysis time is usually 12 hours per week, generally divided into three 4-hour treatments.
- Vascular access route is needed to perform hemodialysis.
- Long-term vascular access for hemodialysis is accomplished by
  1. Arteriovenous (AV) fistula
  2. AV graft
- Complications of vascular access include
  1. Thrombosis or stenosis
  2. Infection
  3. Ischemia
  4. High-output heart failure
  5. Aneurysm formation
- Temporary vascular access for hemodialysis is accomplished by an AV shunt or specially designed catheter inserted into the subclavian, internal jugular, or temporal vein.
- Nurses are specially trained to perform hemodialysis.
- After hemodialysis, the nurse
  1. Closely monitors for side effects:
     a. Hypotension

R

          b. Headache
          c. Nausea
          d. Malaise
          e. Vomiting
          f. Dizziness
          g. Muscle cramps
    2. Obtains the client's weight and vital signs
    3. Avoids invasive procedures for 4 to 6 hours because of heparinization of the dialysate
    4. Monitors for signs of bleeding
    5. Monitors laboratory results
- Complications of hemodialysis include
    1. Dialysis disequilibrium
    2. Infectious disease
    3. Hepatitis
    4. Human immunodeficiency virus infection

🅔 Considerations for Elderly Clients

    1. ESRD occurs more frequently in people over 65 years of age.
    2. Clients over 65 receiving dialysis are more at risk for dialysis-induced hypotension.

- *Peritoneal dialysis* (PD), an alternative and slower dialysis method, is accomplished by the surgical insertion of a silicone rubber catheter (Tenckhoff's catheter) into the abdominal cavity to instill dialysis solution into the abdominal cavity.
- Candidates for PD include
    1. Clients who are hemodynamically unstable
    2. Clients who are unable to tolerate anticoagulation
    3. Clients who lack vascular access
    4. Elderly or pediatric clients
- The PD process occurs by means of a transfer of fluid and solutes from the bloodstream through the peritoneum.
- There are three types of PD:
    1. Intermittent
    2. Continuous ambulatory (CAPD)
    3. Continuous cycle
    4. Multiple bag-continuous
    5. Automated
- Complications of PD include
    1. Peritonitis

        2. Pain
        3. Insufficient flow of the dialysate
        4. Leakage of the dialysate
        5. Exit site and tunnel infection
- The nurse
        1. Implements and monitors PD therapy and instills, dwells, and drains the solution, as ordered
        2. Maintains PD flow data and monitors for negative or positive fluid balances
        3. Obtains baseline and daily weights
        4. Monitors laboratory results to measure the effectiveness of the treatment
        5. Maintains accurate intake and output record
        6. Takes vital signs regularly
        7. Performs an ongoing assessment for signs of respiratory distress or pain
- *Renal transplantation* is appropriate for select clients.
- Candidates for a kidney transplant are free from medical problems that could increase risk:
        1. Advanced incorrectible cardiac disease
        2. Active infection
        3. Intravenous drug abuse
        4. Malignancies
        5. Severe obesity
        6. Active vasculitis
        7. Severe psychologic problems
        8. Long-standing pulmonary disease
- Treatment of some diseases must be completed before transplantation occurs:
        1. Gastrointestinal system disorders, peptic ulcer, diverticulitis
        2. Ureteral or bladder abnormalities
        3. Metabolic diseases, such as diabetes mellitus, gout, or hyperparathyroidism
- Donor kidneys are obtained from a living related donor or a cadaver.
- After a suitable donor kidney is found, the client undergoes a *nephrectomy,* removal of the diseased kidney, with reimplantation of the donor organ.
- Postoperative care of the renal transplant recipient is similar to that for other abdominal surgeries.
- The nurse
        1. Monitors for the return of renal function by assessing hourly urine output

2. Obtains daily urinalysis, glucose level, acetate, and culture
3. Monitors the client for oliguria:
    a. Administers diuretic and osmotic agents to increase urinary output
    b. Weighs the client daily
    c. Observes for fluid overload, which could lead to hypertension, congestive heart failure, and pulmonary edema
4. Monitors the client for diuresis:
    a. Observes for electrolyte imbalance, such as hypokalemia and hyponatremia
    b. Observes for hypovolemia, which may lead to hypotension episodes
5. Monitors the client for complications:
    a. Rejection:
        (1) Hyperacute rejection occurs immediately after transplantation surgery.
        (2) Acute rejection occurs 1 week to 2 years after surgery and is treated with increased dosages of immunosuppressive drugs. It is manifested by oliguria or anuria, fever, enlarged tender kidney, fluid retention, increased blood pressure, chronic fatigue, and changes in urinalysis and blood chemistry.
        (3) Chronic rejection signs and symptoms include gradually increasing BUN and serum creatinine levels, fluid retention, and changes in serum electrolyte.
    b. Vascular complications:
        (1) Stenosis of the renal artery
        (2) Vascular leakage or thrombosis
    c. Wound complications, such as hematomas and abscesses
    d. Genitourinary tract complications:
        (1) Ureteral leakage, fistula, or obstruction
        (2) Formation of calculi
        (3) Bladder neck contracture
        (4) Scrotal swelling
        (5) Graft rupture
6. Administers medications, as ordered:
    a. Immunosuppressives
    b. Corticosteroids
    c. Antilymphocyte preparations
    d. Monoclonal antibodies
    e. Cyclosporine

Continuing Care

- The nurse provides in-depth health teaching about diet and pathophysiology of renal disease and drug therapy.
- The nurse
  1. Provides information and emotional support to assist the client with decisions about treatment course, personal lifestyle, support systems, and coping
  2. Teaches the client who selects in-home hemodialysis the principles and care of the vascular system and makes referrals for the installation of the needed equipment at home
  3. Provides extensive teaching in the procedures of PD and assists the client to obtain the needed equipment and supplies
  4. Provides renal transplant patients with detailed instructions about the prescribed immunosuppressive drug therapy
  5. Assists the client and family to adjust to the diagnosis and treatment regimen
  6. Refers the client to a home health nurse and to local and state support groups and agencies

RENAL TRAUMA

See Trauma, Renal.

R

RENAL TUBERCULOSIS

See Tuberculosis, Renal.

RESPIRATORY ACIDOSIS

See Acidosis, Respiratory.

RESPIRATORY ALKALOSIS

See Alkalosis, Respiratory.

RESPIRATORY FAILURE, ACUTE

OVERVIEW

- Acute respiratory failure can be classified three ways:
    1. *Ventilatory failure,* or hypoventilation, occurs when the client is unable to eliminate CO_2 from the alveoli and hypoxemia occurs as a result. It is usually the result of a mechanical abnormality of the lungs or chest wall, a defect in the respiratory control center of the brain, or an impairment in the function of the respiratory muscles. The most common cause is chronic airflow limitation.
    2. *Oxygenation failure* occurs when oxygen is able to reach the alveoli, but it is unable to be absorbed or utilized properly. Causes include impaired diffusion at the alveolar level, right-to-left shunting of blood in the pulmonary vessels, ventilation-perfusion mismatching, breathing air with too low a concentration of oxygen, or abnormal hemoglobin that fails to absorb the oxygen.
    3. A *combination* of both ventilatory and oxygenation failure.

COLLABORATIVE MANAGEMENT
Assessment

- The nurse assesses the client for
    1. Dyspnea, the hallmark of respiratory failure
    2. Orthopnea
    3. Change in respiratory rate and quality
    4. Decreased oxygen saturation on pulse oximetry

Interventions

- The nurse
    1. Administers oxygen therapy, as ordered
    2. Monitors mechanical ventilation, if needed
    3. Assists the client in finding a position of comfort for easier breathing
    4. Assists the client with relaxation and diversion techniques to decrease the anxiety typically associated with dyspnea
    5. Administers pulmonary medications systemically or by inhaler for bronchodilation, as ordered
    6. Encourages deep breathing and other breathing exercises

Retinal Holes, Tears, and Detachments

OVERVIEW

- A *retinal hole* is a break in the integrity of the peripheral sensory retina and is frequently associated with trauma and aging.
- A *retinal tear* is a more jagged and irregularly shaped break in the retina that occurs as a result of traction on the retina.
- *Retinal detachment* is the separation of the sensory retina from the pigmented epithelium.
- Rhegmatogenous detachments occur after the development of a hole or tear in the retina creates an opening for the vitreous to filter into the subretinal space.
- Traction detachments are created when the retina is pulled away from the epithelium by bands of fibrous tissue in the vitreous humor.
- Exudative detachments are caused by fluid accumulation in the subretinal space as a result of an inflammatory process.

COLLABORATIVE MANAGEMENT

- Indirect ophthalmoscopic examination reveals gray bulges or folds in the retina that quiver with movement; a hole or tear may be seen.

R

579

- Repair of retinal holes or tears is done by surgery.
- Treatment is directed toward sealing the break by creating an inflammatory response that will bind the retina and choroid together around the break:
  1. *Cryotherapy*
  2. *Photocoagulation*
  3. *Diathermy*
- For repair of *retinal detachments,* the treatment is directed toward placing the retina in contact with the underlying structures.
- The *scleral buckling* procedure is most often performed.
- During the scleral buckling procedure, the ophthalmologist repairs wrinkles or folds in the retina so that the retina can assume its normal smooth position.
- The nurse provides preoperative care:
  1. Provides routine preoperative care
  2. Maintains activity restrictions
  3. Maintains the eyepatch over the affected eye to reduce eye movement
  4. Administers topical medications, as ordered, to inhibit accommodation and constriction
- The nurse provides postoperative care:
  1. Provides routine postoperative care
  2. Reports any drainage to the physician immediately
  3. Does not remove the initial eyepatch and shield without a specific order
  4. Positions the client, as ordered, to allow gas that may have been used to promote reattachment to float against the retina:
     a. The client lies on the abdomen with the head turned so that the unaffected eye is down.
     b. The client sits on the side of the bed with the head on a bedside stand.
  5. Withholds food and fluids until the client is fully awake and nausea has passed; administers antiemetics, as ordered
  6. Administers analgesics, as ordered, such as meperidine (Demerol), acetaminophen (Tylenol), or oxycodone (Endocet◆)
  7. Instructs the client to avoid activities that will increase intraocular pressure, such as sneezing, straining at stool, and bending over from the waist
  8. Administers antibiotic-steroid drops, as ordered, which are given to prevent infection

9. Administers cycloplegic agents, as ordered, which dilate the pupil and rest the muscles used for accommodation
10. Enforces activity restrictions, including avoidance of reading, writing, and performing close work, such as needlepoint

Rheumatoid Arthritis

See Arthritis, Rheumatoid.

Rhinitis

- Rhinitis is an inflammation of the nasal mucosa, and is the most common disorder affecting the nose and sinuses of adults.
- *Acute rhinitis* is caused by allergens, bacteria, or virus; the offending substance causes release of vasoactive mediators, which induce vasodilation and increased capillary permeability, with resultant edema and swelling of the nasal mucosa.
- Symptoms of acute rhinitis include headache, nasal irritation, sneezing, nasal congestion, rhinorrhea, and itchy, watery eyes.
- *Allergic rhinitis* (hay fever) is initiated by sensitivity reactions to allergens and occurs as acute seasonal episodes.
- *Chronic rhinitis* presents intermittently or continuously on exposure to allergens such as dust, animal dander, wool, and foods.
- *Rhinitis medicamentosa* occurs after excessive use of nosedrops or sprays as a rebound effect, causing nasal congestion.
- *Acute viral rhinitis* (the common cold) is caused by one of more than 30 viruses and spreads via droplet nuclei from sneezing and coughing.
- The common cold is usually self-limiting; complications include otitis media, sinusitis, and bronchitis.

R

- Complications occur more often in the elderly or in immunosuppressed individuals.
- Measures to relieve symptoms include
    1. Antihistamines and decongestants
    2. Antipyretics for fever
    3. Proper rest
    4. Adequate fluid intake
- The client at risk should avoid contact with people who are susceptible to infections.
- Thorough hand washing is important to avoid spread of the infection.
- Antibiotic therapy is given for secondary bacterial infections.
- Allergy testing and desensitization used in clients with allergic rhinitis.

RIB FRACTURES

See Fractures, Rib.

ROTATOR CUFF INJURIES

- The function of the rotator cuff is to stabilize the head of the humerus in the glenoid cavity during shoulder abduction.
- It undergoes degenerative changes as one gets older.
- Older adults tend to have small tears related to aging, repetitive motions, or falls.
- Younger adults usually sustain tears of the cuff by trauma, including falls, throwing a ball, or heavy lifting.
- Clinical manifestations include shoulder pain and inability to initiate or maintain abduction of the arm at the shoulder.
- Treatment involves nonsteroidal anti-inflammatory drugs, physical therapy, sling support, and ice and heat applications.
- Surgery may be required to treat injuries that do not respond to conservative treatment.

SARCOIDOSIS, PULMONARY

- Pulmonary sarcoidosis is a chronic interstitial or fibrotic lung disease associated with an intense cellular immune response in the alveolar structures.
- The hallmark of sarcoidosis is noncaseating granuloma of the alveolar structures composed of lymphocytes, macrophages, epithelioid cells, and giant cells.
- Interstitial fibrosis results in a loss of lung compliance and functional ability to exchange gases.
- Cor pulmonale (right-sided congestive heart failure) develops due to the heart's inability to pump against the noncompliant, fibrotic lung.
- The disease affects African Americans ten times more frequently than Caucasians and develops between the ages of 20 and 40 years.
- Indications for treatment vary.
- If the client is asymptomatic, with no abnormalities in pulmonary function tests, there is no treatment.
- For reduced pulmonary function, steroids are administered.

SCABIES

- Scabies is a contagious skin disease characterized by epidermal curved or linear ridges and follicular papules associated with severe pruritus.
- Hypersensitivity reactions result in excoriated erythematous papules, pustules, and crusted lesions on the elbows, nipples, lower abdomen, buttocks, thighs, and axillary folds.
- Scabies are transmitted by close and prolonged contact with an infested companion or bedding.
- Scabies mites are carried by pets and occur endemically among schoolchildren, institutional elderly clients, and clients of lower socioeconomic status.
- Treatment consists of chemical disinfection with scabicides such as lindane (Kwell, Kwellada◆) or topical sulfur preparations.
- Clothes and personal items are laundered in hot water.

SCLERODERMA, SYSTEMIC

See Sclerosis, Progressive Systemic.

SCLEROSIS, AMYOTROPHIC LATERAL

See Amyotrophic Lateral Sclerosis.

SCLEROSIS, MULTIPLE

OVERVIEW

- Multiple sclerosis (MS) is a progressive degenerative disease that affects the myelin sheath and conduction pathway of the central nervous system.
- MS is one of the leading causes of disability in persons 20 to 40 years of age.
- The four types are
    1. *Relapsing-remitting,* with exacerbations followed by remission that returns the client to baseline
    2. *Relapsing-progressive,* which is characterized by the absence of remission and does not return the client to baseline
    3. *Chronic-progressive,* which is similar to relapsing-progressive, but its initial presentation is more insidious with spinal cord and cerebellar symptoms
    4. *Benign,* or *stable,* which presents with a few episodes of mild attacks; there is minimal or no disability

 Transcultural Considerations

1. People living in colder climates of the Northeast, Great Lakes, and Pacific Northwest are at higher risk for the disease.

2. Caucasians of higher socioeconomic status have a greater prevalence of MS than other ethnic groups.
3. Women are affected slightly more often than men.

COLLABORATIVE MANAGEMENT

Assessment

- The nurse assesses for
  1. Progression of symptoms (often the client reports noticing symptoms several years previously but they disappeared and medical attention was not sought)
  2. Factors that aggravate symptoms
     a. Stress
     b. Fatigue
     c. Overexertion
     d. Temperature extremes
     e. Hot shower or bath
  3. Personality or behavior changes (the nurse verifies this information with family or friends of the client)
  4. Changes in neurologic status
     a. Vision: decreased acuity, blurred vision, diplopia, scotoma (changes in peripheral vision), nystagmus
     b. Motor: fatigue, stiffness of legs, flexor spasms, increased deep-tendon reflexes, clonus, positive Babinski's reflex, absent abdominal reflexes
     c. Cerebellar: ataxic gait, intention tremor, dysmetria, tinnitus, vertigo
     d. Cranial nerve: hearing loss, facial weakness, swallowing difficulties
     e. Speech pattern: dysarthria; slow, scanning speech
     f. Sensation: hypalgesia, paresthesia, facial pain
     g. Changes in mental status (late in the disease process): memory loss, decreased ability to perform calculations, inattention, impaired judgment
  5. Changes in bowel and bladder function
  6. Changes in sexuality: impotence, difficulty sustaining an erection
  7. Apathy, emotional lability, and depression
  8. Body image disturbance

S

585

Interventions

- As a result of weakness and fatigue, the client requires more time to complete activities of daily living (ADL).
- The nurse teaches, in collaboration with physical and occupational therapy,
  1. Exercise program to strengthen and stretch muscles
  2. Ambulation as tolerated, with assistive devices as appropriate, such as a cane, walker, or electric (Amigo) cart
  3. How to use assistive-adaptive devices to help the client remain independent in ADL
  4. Importance of avoiding rigorous activities that lead to an increase in body temperature, which may lead to fatigue, decreased motor ability, and visual acuity
- The nurse gives medications as ordered:
  1. Steroids: adrenocorticotropic hormone, corticosteroids
  2. Adjunctive therapy to treat muscle spasticity, paresthesia
  3. Immunosuppressive therapy: cyclophosphamide (Cytoxan), interferon beta-1a (Avonex)
- The nurse
  1. Applies an eye patch to relieve diplopia and switches the eye patch every few hours
  2. Teaches scanning techniques to compensate for peripheral vision deficits
  3. Provides a hazard-free and standardized environment
  4. Tests the temperature of the water before bathing (teaches the client to do this at home before placing hands in hot water)
  5. Teaches the client to avoid overexposure to heat or cold
- Clients using complementary therapies, such as nutritional supplements and bee stings, report improvement in their condition, but these modalities have not been scientifically tested.

Continuing Care

- The nurse
  1. Encourages the client to remain independent in all activities for as long as possible
  2. Refers the client for vocational counseling, if necessary

    3. Encourages the client to ventilate feelings of frustration, anger, or both
- The nurse
    1. Ensures that the client can correctly use all adaptive-assistive devices ordered for home use
    2. Provides drug information, as needed
    3. Teaches an exercise program in collaboration with physical and occupational therapy
        a. ADL and the use of adaptive equipment
        b. Strengthening and stretching exercises
        c. Positioning techniques
    4. Reviews the established bowel and bladder, skin care, and nutrition program
    5. Refers the client to a support group
    6. Encourages the client to engage in regular social activities, obtain adequate rest, and avoid stress
    7. Refers to local and national support groups, as needed

$\underline{S}$CLEROSIS, PROGRESSIVE SYSTEMIC

OVERVIEW

- Progressive systemic sclerosis (PSS), also referred to as *systemic scleroderma,* is a chronic connective tissue disease characterized by inflammation, fibrosis, and sclerosis and is similar to lupus erythematosus.

COLLABORATIVE MANAGEMENT
Assessment

- PSS is manifested by arthralgia; stiffness; painless, symmetric, pitting edema of the hands and fingers, which may progress to include the entire upper and/or lower extremities and face; and taut and shiny skin that is free from wrinkles.
- In PSS, inflammation is replaced by tightening, hardening, and thickening of skin tissue; the skin loses its elasticity, and range of motion is markedly decreased.

- Joint contractures may develop, and the client is unable to perform activities of daily living (ADL).
- Major organ involvement is manifested in
  1. *Gastrointestinal tract:* hiatal hernia, esophageal reflux, dysphagia, reflux of gastric contents that can cause esophagitis, partial bowel obstruction, and malabsorption
  2. *Cardiovascular system:* Raynaud's phenomenon, digit necrosis, vasculitis, myocardial fibrosis, dysrhythmias, and chest pain

Interventions

- Treatment of PSS is directed toward forcing the disease into remission and slowing its progress and includes
  1. Drugs such as steroids and immunosuppressants in large doses
  2. Local skin measures, such as using mild soap, lotion, and gentle cleaning
  3. Bed cradle and footboard
  4. Constant room temperature
  5. Small, frequent meals, minimizing foods that stimulate gastric secretion (e.g., spicy foods, caffeine, alcohol) and having the client sit up for 1 to 2 hours after meals (if there is esophageal involvement)
- Refer to Arthritis, Rheumatoid, for care of joint pain.

Continuing Care

- Health teaching and discharge planning are similar to those for the client with lupus (see Lupus Erythematosus).

SCOLIOSIS

- Scoliosis is a C- or S-shaped lateral curvature of the vertebral spine.
- Scoliosis is generally diagnosed and treated in adolescence.
- Deviations of more than 50 degrees can compromise cardiopulmonary function.

- Treatment for the adult involves a surgical fusion and the insertion of instrumentation.
  1. The *Harrington* rod
  2. *Dwyer* cable isntrumentation
  3. The *Luque* rod system
  4. The *Cotrel-Dubousset* (C-D) system
- Nursing care is similar to that for a client undergoing a laminectomy or spinal fusion.

SDAT

See Alzheimer's Disease.

SEIZURE DISORDERS

OVERVIEW

- Epilepsy is a chronic disorder characterized by recurrent seizure activity.
- A seizure is an abnormal, sudden, excessive discharge of electrical activity within the brain.
- Three major types of epilepsy include
  1. *Generalized*
     a. *Tonic-clonic* (formerly called a grand mal seizure), characterized by stiffening or rigidity of the muscles, followed by rhythmic jerking of the extremities. Immediate unconsciousness occurs, and the client may be incontinent of urine or stool and/or frothing of the mouth may occur.
     b. *Absence* (formerly called petit mal seizure), consisting of a brief (often seconds) period of loss of consciousness (as though the client is daydreaming).
     c. *Myoclonic,* a brief, generalized jerking or stiffening of the extremities, which may occur singly or in groups.

     d. *Atonic* (formerly called "drop attacks"), characterized by sudden loss of muscle tone, which in most cases causes the client to fall.
  2. *Partial* (focal) seizure
     a. *Complex* (often called a psychomotor seizure or a temporal lobe seizure), which causes the client to lose consciousness or black out for a few seconds. Characteristic behavior, known as automatism may occur, such as lip smacking, patting, and picking at clothes.
     b. *Simple,* which consists of a déjà vu phenomenon, perception of an offensive smell, or sudden onset of pain.
  3. *Unclassified,* or idiopathic seizure, which occurs for no known reason

- *Primary* seizures are usually inherited and are often age-related.
- *Secondary* seizures often result from underlying brain pathology, such as a head injury, vascular disease, brain tumors, aneurysm, opportunistic infections from acquired immunodeficiency syndrome (AIDS), or meningitis. They may also occur in the presence of metabolic and electrolyte disorders, drug withdrawal, acute alcohol intoxication, water intoxication, or kidney and liver failure.

COLLABORATIVE MANAGEMENT

Assessment

- The nurse records the following concerning the seizures
  1. How often they occur
  2. The type of movement or activity and if more than one type occurs
  3. Sequence of progression
  4. How long they last
  5. Presence and description of aura or precipitating events
  6. Postictal status
  7. Length of time before the client returns to preseizure status
  8. If the client is incontinent during the seizure
  9. When the last seizure took place
- The nurse records the client's

1. Current medications, including dosage, frequency of administration, and the time at which the medication was last taken
2. Compliance with the medication schedule and reason(s) for noncompliance, if appropriate
- The nurse assesses for
  1. Any changes in normal neurologic function
  2. Self-concept disturbances
  3. Impaired social interactions or denial of the problem, which may be caused by the client's fear that a seizure may occur at work or in social situations.
  4. Electroencephalographic changes
- During a seizure, the nurse assesses for
  1. Type and progression of seizure activity
  2. Factors that may have precipitated the event
  3. All physical manifestations, including eye fluttering, changes in pupil size, head and eye deviation automatism, changes in level of consciousness, apnea, and cyanosis
  4. Postictal status

Interventions

Nonsurgical Management

- Drug therapy is the major component of management; the physician introduces one anticonvulsant at a time to achieve seizure control.
- The nurse administers drug therapy, as ordered
  1. Carbamazepine (Tegretol, Mazepine◆) is contraindicated if glaucoma, cardiac, renal, or hepatic disease is present.
  2. Clonazepam (Klonopin, Rivotril◆) is contraindicated if glaucoma is present; the complete blood count (CBC) should be followed.
  3. Diazepam (Valium, Apo-Diazepam◆) is given to stop the motor activity associated with status epilepticus; if the intravenous route is selected, the nurse monitors the client closely for respiratory distress.
  4. Ethosuximide (Zarontin) is contraindicated in renal or liver disease; the nurse monitors CBC and liver function tests.
  5. Phenobarbital (Barbita, Luminal◆) potentiates phenothiazines; the nurse monitors for drowsiness, depression, and cognitive impairment.

S

6. Phenytoin (Dilantin) and fosphenytoin (Cerebyx) are used to control seizures. The nurse monitors CBC and calcium levels. If phenytoin is administered intravenously, the nurse flushes the catheter with saline before and after administering and gives the drug slowly.
7. Primidone (Myidone, Sertan◆) is potentiated by isoniazid; drug interactions are the same as for phenobarbital.
8. Divalproex (Depakote) and Valproic acid (Depakene) are used for all types of seizures; the nurse monitors CBC, PT/PTT, and AST, as well as bruising and other indications of bleeding.
9. Gabapentin (Neurontin), lamotrigine (Lamictal), and Topiramate are given for partial seizures.

- The nurse follows agency policy for the implementation of seizure precautions
  1. Keeps oxygen and suctioning equipment available at the bedside
  2. Maintains a saline lock that may be indicated for clients at risk for tonic-clonic seizures
  3. Recognizes that padded tongue blades do *not* belong at the bedside and nothing should be inserted into the client's mouth after a seizure begins
  4. Takes action appropriate for the type of seizure (e.g., observes the partial seizure or turns the client with a tonic-clonic seizure on his or her side)
  5. Applies protective head gear for clients with atonic seizures, as appropriate
  6. Keeps the bed in the low position and side rails up at all times
  7. Carefully observes the seizure and documents the time when the seizure began, the part or parts of the body affected, the progression of the seizure, eye deviation, nystagmus, changes in pupil size, the client's condition throughout the seizure, and postictal status

- *Status epilepticus* is a seizure that lasts longer than 4 minutes or occurs in rapid succession. It is a neurologic *emergency* and must be treated promptly, or brain damage and possibly death from anoxia, cardiac dysrhythmias, or lactic acidosis may occur.
- The nurse
  1. Establishes an airway (intubation may be necessary)

2. Monitors the client's respiratory status carefully
3. Administers oxygen
4. Establishes an IV line and starts 0.9% saline infusion
5. Has medications available that are used to treat status epilepticus
6. Monitors vital signs frequently

Surgical Management

- Several procedures may be performed when traditional methods fail to maintain seizure control:
    1. *Vagal nerve stimulation,* being studied in the United States, which involves placing a vagal nerve stimulating device below the left clavicle to control partial seizures
    2. *Corpuscallostomy,* which involves severing the corpus callosum to prevent neuronal discharges from passing through the two hemispheres of the brain; used to treat tonic-clonic or atonic seizures
    3. Other procedures, including anterior temporal lobe resection for complex partial seizures of temporal origin; cortical resection; and hemispherectomy, in which part or all of a cerebral hemisphere is removed
- For nursing care for this procedure, see "Surgical Management" under Tumors, Brain.
- The nurse
    1. Helps the family identify coping strategies used successfully in the past
    2. Provides a complete education program on epilepsy

Continuing Care

- Most clients are treated on an outpatient basis, and little home care preparation is needed.
- The nurse provides drug information
    1. Taking all medications in the correct dosage, at the right time, and by the right route and being sure not to stop the medications
    2. What to do if a dose is missed or if complications or side effects occur
- The nurse explains
    1. Precautions to take when ill, under stress, fatigued, or when workload or social activities increase

2. Diet and effects of alcohol (alcohol should be avoided)
3. Driving restrictions, if any
4. Importance of follow-up visits with the physician(s)
5. Need to wear a Medic-Alert bracelet or necklace
6. State law, which prohibits discrimination against people who have epilepsy
7. Refers the client to the Epilepsy Foundation of America, National Epilepsy League, or National Association to Control Epilepsy; and local support groups

SENILE DEMENTIA, ALZHEIMER'S TYPE

See Alzheimer's Disease.

SHOCK

OVERVIEW

- Shock is a pathologic condition rather than a disease process.
- Shock is characterized by generalized abnormal cellular metabolism, which occurs as a direct result of inadequate delivery of oxygen to body tissues or inadequate usage of oxygen by body tissue.
- The classification of shock includes four types:
    1. *Hypovolemic* shock
        a. There is a loss of circulating fluid volume from the central vascular space to the extent that mean arterial pressure (MAP) decreases and the body's total need for tissue oxygenation is not adequately met.
        b. The causes include hemorrhage and dehydration, or shifting of fluid from the central vascular space to the interstitial space.

2. *Cardiogenic* shock
    a. Occurs when the heart muscle is unhealthy and contractility is impaired.
    b. The result is inadequate cardiac output.
        (1) *Direct pump failure* can result from myocardial infarction (MI), cardiac arrest, serious dysrhythmias, valvular pathologic changes, and myocardial degeneration associated with inadequate myocardial circulation, systemic infection, and exposure to chemical toxins.
        (2) *Indirect pump failure* can result from cardiac tamponade, electrolyte imbalances (especially hyperkalemia and hypocalcemia), administration of drugs that decrease the rate and vigor of cardiac contractility, and injuries to the cardioregulatory areas of the brain.
3. *Distributive* shock
    a. There is a loss of sympathetic tone, vasodilation, pooling of blood in the venous and capillary beds, and increased vascular permeability, which all contribute to decreased MAP.
    b. The origin of this set of reactions is neural (neurogenic shock) or chemical (anaphylaxis).
    c. Conditions that cause loss of sympathetic tone include severe pain, prolonged exposure to heat, and neurologic damage.
    d. Chemical-induced shock has three common origins:
        (1) Anaphylaxis
        (2) Sepsis
        (3) Capillary leak syndrome
4. *Obstructive* shock
    a. Results from conditions that affect the ability of the heart muscle to pump effectively
    b. Causes include
        (1) Cardiac tamponade
        (2) Pulmonary embolism
        (3) Pulmonary hypertension
        (4) Arterial stenosis
        (5) Constrictive pericarditis

COLLABORATIVE MANAGEMENT

Assessment

- The nurse records the client's
    1. Risk factors for shock

2. Age
3. History of recent illness, trauma, and/or procedures, and/or chronic conditions that may lead to shock
4. Current medications
5. Allergies
6. Intake and output for the previous 24 hours

- The nurse assesses for general clinical manifestations of shock
  1. Cardiovascular changes:
     a. Decreased cardiac output
     b. Increased pulse rate
     c. Thready pulse
     d. Decreased blood pressure (it is important to consider the client's baseline blood pressure when shock is suspected)
     e. Narrowed pulse pressure
     f. Postural hypotension
     g. Low central venous pressure (CVP)
     h. Flat neck and hand veins in dependent positions
     i. Slow capillary refill in the nail beds
     j. Diminished peripheral pulses; as shock progresses, possible absence of superficial peripheral pulses
  2. Respiratory changes:
     a. Increased respiratory rate
     b. Shallow respirations
     c. Decreased arterial carbon dioxide partial pressure and oxygen tension
     d. Cyanosis, especially around the lips and nail beds
  3. Neuromuscular changes:
     a. Anxiety and restlessness
     b. Decreased level of consciousness
     c. Generalized muscle weakness
     d. Diminished or absent deep-tendon reflexes
     e. Sluggish pupillary response to light
  4. Renal changes:
     a. Decreased urinary output
     b. Increased specific gravity
     c. Sugar and acetone present in the urine
  5. Integumentary changes:
     a. Color changes: first evident in mucous membranes and in the skin around the mouth; as shock progresses, color changes noted in the extremities

        b. Cool to cold
        c. Moist and clammy
        d. Pale to mottled to cyanotic
        e. Mouth dry, paste-like coating present
    6. Gastrointestinal changes:
        a. Decreased motility
        b. Diminished or absent bowel sounds
        c. Nausea and vomiting
        d. Constipation
        e. Increased thirst
- If septic shock is suspected, the nurse assesses for the following in addition to the general clinical manifestations
    1. Normal skin color with pink mucous membrane and warmth
    2. Disseminated intravascular coagulation (DIC)
    3. Adult respiratory distress syndrome (ARDS)
    4. Change in behavior or verbal response
    5. Positive results of blood and urine cultures

Interventions

- The nurse provides emergency care for the client in hypovolemic shock:
    1. Ensures a patent airway
    2. Assesses the client for evidence of injury or apparent bleeding
    3. Covers any wound with a clean cloth or dressing and applies pressure to a wound if bleeding appears to be originating from an artery
    4. Inserts an intravenous (IV) line and infuses Ringer's lactate or normal saline, blood or blood products, as ordered
    5. Applies military antishock trousers (MAST), if indicated
    6. Administers oxygen, as ordered
    7. Elevates the client's feet, keeping the head flat or elevated 30 degrees
    8. Administers medications, as ordered, to increase venous return and improve myocardial contractility or perfusion
    9. Monitors vital signs and neurologic signs
    10. Monitors CVP, pulmonary artery pressure, and pulmonary wedge pressure
    11. Prepares the client for surgery, if necessary, to treat the underlying cause

- The nurse provides care for the client in sepsis-induced distributive shock:
    1. Ensures a patent airway
    2. Starts and maintains an IV line
    3. Administers oxygen, as ordered
    4. Obtains blood, urine, wound, and sputum specimens for cultures, as indicated
    5. Examines the client for overt bleeding, especially at the gums or injection or IV sites
    6. Elevates the client's feet, keeping the head flat
    7. Takes frequent vital signs
    8. Administers medications, as ordered:
        a. Antibiotics
        b. Anticoagulants
        c. Clotting factors
    9. Maintains a safe environment, including strict adherence to aseptic technique during invasive procedures and dressing changes

---

SIADH

See Syndrome of Inappropriate Antidiuretic Hormone.

SICKLE CELL ANEMIA

See Anemia, Sickle Cell.

SILICOSIS

See Pulmonary Disease, Occupational.

SIMPLE VAGINITIS

See Vaginitis.

SINUS CANCER

See Cancer, Nasal and Sinus.

SJÖGREN'S SYNDROME

- Sjögren's syndrome is a disorder in which inflammatory cells and immune complexes obstruct secretory ducts and glands.
- The disorder is manifested by dry eyes (sicca syndrome), dry mouth (xerostomia), dry vagina, swelling of the parotid and lacrimal areas, fever, fatigue, and associated connective tissue disease.
- Treatment includes steroids; meticulous mouth, eye, and perineal care; and use of artificial tears and saliva.

SKIN CANCER

See Cancer, Skin.

SKIN INFECTIONS

See Infections, Skin.

Skin Infections, Fungal

See Infections, Skin.

Skin Infections, Viral

See Infections, Skin.

SLE

See Lupus Erythematosus.

Spastic Bowel

See Irritable Bowel Syndrome.

Spastic Colon

See Irritable Bowel Syndrome.

Spinal Cord Injury

See Trauma, Spinal Cord.

600

SPINAL CORD TUMORS

See Tumors, Spinal Cord.

SPRAINS

- A sprain is the excessive stretching of a ligament, typically caused by twisting motions from a fall or sports activity.
- Sprains are classified by their severity:
    1. *First-degree* sprain (*mild* sprain) involves tearing of a few fibers of the ligament; joint function is not impaired.
    2. *Second-degree* sprain (*moderate* sprain) involves many torn fibers of the ligament: the joint is stable.
    3. *Third-degree* sprain (*severe* sprain) involves tearing of fibers to the point that the joint is unstable.
- Pain and swelling characterize ligament injuries.
- The therapy for mild sprains is minimal. Ice and a compression bandage are used to reduce swelling and provide joint support.
- Clients with second-degree sprains usually require casting for 4 to 6 weeks until the tear heals.
- Clients with third-degree sprains typically require surgery to repair the ligament tear, followed by a period of casting. Artificial ligament implants may be used, especially for knee ligament injuries.
- Complete healing of knee ligaments can take 6 to 9 months or longer.

SQUAMOUS CELL CARCINOMA

See Cancer, Skin.

STENOSIS, AORTIC

OVERVIEW

- In a client with aortic stenosis, the aortic valve orifice narrows, obstructing the left ventricular outflow during systole.
- Increased resistance to ejection or afterload results in left ventricular hypertrophy.
- As stenosis progresses, cardiac output becomes fixed.
- The left atrium has incomplete emptying, and the pulmonary system becomes congested; right-sided heart failure may develop.
- Congenital valvular disease or malformation is the main cause.

🕮 Considerations for Elderly Clients

1. Atherosclerosis and degenerative calcification of the aortic valve are the predominant causative factors in people older than 70 years.
2. Aortic stenosis has become the most common valvular disorder in countries with an aging population; 80% of clients with aortic stenosis are men.

COLLABORATIVE MANAGEMENT

- Signs and symptoms include
  1. Dyspnea on exertion
  2. Angina
  3. Syncope on exertion
  4. Fatigue
  5. Debilitation
  6. Peripheral cyanosis
  7. Diamond-shaped systolic crescendo-decrescendo murmur
- Aortic valve surgery is the treatment of choice.
- Balloon valvuloplasty may be performed to repair the valve; a balloon catheter is inserted through the femoral artery and advanced to the aortic valve where the balloon is inflated, enlarging the orifice of the valve.
- In aortic valve replacement surgery, the valve is excised during cardiopulmonary bypass surgery, then re-

placed with a prosthetic (synthetic) or biologic (tissue) valve.
- The postoperative client requires lifetime anticoagulation therapy to prevent thrombus formation on the valve.
- For preoperative and postoperative care, see Surgical Management under Coronary Artery Disease.

STENOSIS, MITRAL

OVERVIEW

- Mitral stenosis is the thickening of the mitral valve by fibrosis and calcification.
- Valve leaflets fuse together, becoming stiff; the chordae tendineae contract and shorten; the valvular orifice narrows, preventing normal blood flow from the left atrium to the left ventricle; and as a result, the left atrial pressure rises, the left ventricle dilates, pulmonary artery pressures increase, and the right ventricle hypertrophies.
- Pulmonary congestion and right-sided heart failure occur.
- Rheumatic fever is most often the cause of mitral stenosis.
- Nonrheumatic causes include atrial myxoma, calcium accumulation, and thrombus formation.

S

COLLABORATIVE MANAGEMENT

- Signs and symptoms include
  1. Orthopnea
  2. Dyspnea on exertion
  3. Paroxysmal nocturnal dyspnea
  4. Hemoptysis
  5. Hepatomegaly
  6. Neck vein distention
  7. Pitting edema
  8. Atrial fibrillation
  9. Rumbling, apical diastolic murmur
- *Mitral commissurotomy,* the procedure of choice for pure mitral stenosis, is performed during cardiopulmonary bypass surgery by incising the fused commissures, widening the orifice.

- *Balloon valvuloplasty* is performed for older clients, high-risk surgical clients, and those who refuse operative treatment.
- The surgeon passes a balloon from the femoral vein through the atrial septum to the mitral valve.
- The balloon is inflated, enlarging the mitral orifice.
- After the procedure, the nurse
    1. Monitors the client closely for bleeding from the catheter insertion site
    2. Monitors heart sounds and cardiac output
    3. Observes for indications of systemic emboli
- The nurse
    1. Provides health teaching information regarding
        a. Medications
        b. Oral hygiene
        c. Plan of work, activity, and rest to conserve energy
        d. Importance of taking an antibiotic before any procedures (e.g., dental work, surgery)
    2. Refers the client to community resources, such as the American Heart Association
- *Mitral valve replacement* is indicated if the leaflets are calcified and immobile; the valve is excised during cardiopulmonary bypass surgery, and a new valve is sutured into place.
- The postoperative client requires lifetime anticoagulant therapy to prevent thrombus formation on the valve.
- For preoperative and postoperative care, see care of the client undergoing a coronary artery bypass grafting procedure under Coronary Artery Disease.

STENOSIS, RENAL ARTERY

- Renal artery stenosis involves pathologic processes affecting the renal arteries, resulting in severe narrowing of the lumen and reducing blood flow to the renal parenchyma.
- Uncorrected stenosis leads to ischemia and atrophy of renal tissue.
- Renal artery stenosis is suspected when a sudden onset of hypertension occurs.

- Atherosclerotic changes in the renal artery are associated with corresponding disease of the aorta and other major vessels.
- Fibromuscular changes of the vessel wall occur throughout the length of the renal artery between the aortic junction and branching into the renal segmental arteries.
- The location of the defect, the overall condition of the client, and the size of the atrophied kidney influence the decision for therapeutic intervention.
- Treatment includes
    1. Antihypertensive drugs
    2. Percutaneous transluminal balloon angioplasty
    3. Renal artery bypass surgery

STONES, URINARY

See Urolithiasis.

STRAINS

- A strain, sometimes referred to as a "muscle pull," is an excessive stretching of a muscle and/or tendon when it is weak or unstable.
- Strains may be caused by falls, lifting heavy items, and exercise.
- Strains are classified according to their severity:
    1. *First-degree* strain (*mild* strain) causes mild inflammation manifested by swelling, ecchymosis (minimal bleeding), and tenderness.
    2. *Second-degree* strain (*moderate* strain) involves tearing of the muscle or tendon, possibly resulting in impaired muscle function.
    3. *Third-degree* strain (*severe* strain) involves a ruptured muscle or tendon and causes severe pain and disability.

- Management usually involves cold and heat applications, activity limitations, progressive exercise, anti-inflammatory drugs, and analgesics.
- Clients with third-degree strains may require surgery to repair the muscle or tendon.

STRICTURE, URETHRAL

See Hydronephrosis, Hydroureter, and Urethral Stricture.

STROKE

See Cerebral Vascular Accident.

SUBCLAVIAN STEAL SYNDROME

- Subclavian steal syndrome occurs in the upper extremities from a subclavian artery occlusion and results in altered blood flow and ischemia in the arm.
- The disorder occurs at any age but is more common with risk factors for atherosclerosis.
- Clinical manifestations include
    1. Paresthesias
    2. Lightheadedness
    3. Dizziness
    4. Pain and discomfort when the arms are elevated
    5. Difference in blood pressure between arms
    6. Subclavian bruit on the occluded side
    7. Subclavian pulse decreased on the occluded side
    8. Discoloration of the affected arm

- Surgical intervention involves one of three procedures: endarterectomy of the subclavian artery, carotid-subclavian bypass, or dilation of the subclavian artery.
- Nursing interventions include
    1. Frequent brachial and radial pulse checks
    2. Observation for ischemic changes of the extremity
    3. Observation for edema and redness

SUBLUXATION

See Dislocation and Subluxation.

SYNDROME OF INAPPROPRIATE ANTIDIURETIC HORMONE

OVERVIEW

- Syndrome of inappropriate antidiuretic hormone (SIADH) occurs when ADH (vasopressin) is secreted in the presence of low plasma osmolality because feedback mechanisms that regulate ADH do not function properly.
- Water is retained, which results in dilutional hyponatremia and expansion of extracellular fluid volume.
- SIADH is associated with
    1. Oat cell carcinoma of the lung
    2. Carcinoma of the pancreas, duodenum, and genitourinary tract
    3. Ewing's sarcoma
    4. Hodgkin's and non-Hodgkin's lymphoma
    5. Viral and bacterial pneumothorax, lung abscess, active tuberculosis, pneumothorax, chronic obstructive pulmonary disease

6. Central nervous system disorders, such as trauma, cerebral vascular accident, infections, tumors, porphyria, and lupus erythematosus
7. Drugs such as exogenous ADH, chlorpropamide, vincristine, cyclophosphamide, carbamazepine, general anesthetic agents, and tricyclic antidepressants

COLLABORATIVE MANAGEMENT
Assessment
- The nurse records the client's
  1. Medical history
  2. Weight, especially a history of weight gain
- The nurse assesses for
  1. Gastrointestinal disturbances, such as loss of appetite, nausea, and vomiting
  2. Water retention
  3. Lethargy, headache, hostility, uncooperativeness, and disorientation
  4. Seizure activity
  5. Decreased or sluggish deep-tendon reflexes
  6. Vital sign changes (tachycardia, hypothermia)
  7. Irritability, anxiety
  8. Hyponatremia, decreased serum osmolality

Interventions
- The nurse
  1. Restricts fluid intake, as ordered (may be as low as 500 to 600 mL/day)
  2. Weighs the client daily
  3. Carefully measures intake and output
  4. Provides frequent mouth care
  5. Suggests hard candy to relieve dryness of the mouth
- The nurse administers diuretics as ordered, particularly if congestive heart failure results from fluid overload
- The nurse
  1. Monitors neurologic status
  2. Promotes a safe environment

Continuing Care
- The nurse teaches the client

1. To restrict fluids if SIADH is not completely resolved
2. To use the same scale for daily weights
3. To avoid over-the-counter medications such as aspirin or nonsteroidal anti-inflammatory drugs, which may contribute to hyponatremia

SYPHILIS

OVERVIEW

- Syphilis is a classic sexually transmitted disease.
- The primary population affected is young adults in their early 20s; the number of cases is declining.
- The causative organism is *Treponema pallidum,* a spirochete with a slender, spiral shape.
- In *primary* syphilis, the chancre is the first lesion developing at the site of inoculation or entry of the organism.
- During the highly infectious stage, the chancre begins as a small papule; within 3 to 7 days, it breaks down into its characteristic appearance—a painless, indurated, smooth, weeping lesion.
- Without treatment, the chancre disappears within 6 weeks; however, the organism disseminates throughout the bloodstream.
- *Secondary* syphilis, which develops from 6 weeks to 6 months after the onset of primary syphilis, becomes a systemic disease because spirochetes circulate throughout the bloodstream.
- Symptoms of secondary syphilis include malaise, low-grade fever, headache, muscular aches and pains, and sore throat.
- A generalized rash usually evolves from papules, to squamous papules, to pustules.
- *Latent* syphilis is a later stage of the disease.
- *Early latent* syphilis occurs during the first year after infection, and infectious lesions can recur.
- *Late latent* syphilis is a disease of more than 1 year's duration after infection; it is noninfectious except to the fetus of a pregnant woman.

S

- *Late* syphilis develops after a highly variable period—from 4 to 20 years in untreated cases.
- Manifestations of late syphilis include benign lesions of the skin, mucous membranes, and bones; aortitis and aneurysms; and neurosyphilis.

COLLABORATIVE MANAGEMENT

- Assessment includes
  1. Sexual history
     a. Type and frequency of sexual activity
     b. Number of contacts
     c. Past history of sexually transmitted diseases
     d. Potential sites of infection
     e. Sexual preferences
  2. Chief complaint
  3. Inspection of the external genitalia for a chancre lesion and other physical findings, such as enlarged lymph nodes
  4. Positive results from Venereal Disease Research Laboratory (VDRL) and fluorescent treponemal antibody absorption tests
- Management includes antibiotic therapy with penicillin.
- Client education includes
  1. Treatment and side effects
  2. Complications of untreated syphilis
  3. Follow-up care
  4. Treatment for sexual partners
  5. Disease reported to the health department
  6. Contagiousness of the disease

SYSTEMIC LUPUS ERYTHEMATOSUS

See Lupus Erythematosus.

Talcosis

See Pulmonary Disease, Occupational.

TB

See Tuberculosis, Pulmonary.

Tension Pneumothorax

See Pneumothorax, Tension.

Testicular Cancer

See Cancer, Testicular.

T

Tetanus

- Tetanus, also known as lockjaw, is caused by *Clostridium tetani* and is easily prevented through immunization.
- Tetanus is characterized by muscle rigidity, opisthotonos, cramps, muscle spasms, stiffness, and headache.
- Treatment includes prompt (within 72 hours) intramuscular antitoxin human tetanus immune globulin, or hyperimmune equine or bovine serum.

- Antibiotics may be needed for superimposed infections.
- Sedation, antianxiety agents, and muscle relaxants to decrease muscle spasms and increase the client's comfort are provided.
- Propranolol (Inderal) or other anti-dysrhythmic agent may be given to treat cardiac irregularities, and the client may need aggressive respiratory support.

THECA-LUTEIN CYSTS

See Cysts, Ovarian.

THORACIC OUTLET SYNDROME

- Thoracic outlet syndrome is a compression of the subclavian artery at the thoracic outlet by anatomic structures, such as a rib or muscle.
- Damage of the arterial wall produces thrombosis or embolization to distal arteries of the arm.
- The common sites of compression of the thoracic outlet are the interscalene triangle; between the coracoid process of the scapula and the pectoralis minor tendon; and, most common, the costoclavicular space.
- Clinical manifestations include
    1. Neck, shoulder, and arm pain
    2. Numbness of the extremity
    3. Moderate edema of the extremity
    4. Increasing pain and numbness when the arm is held over the head or out to the side.
- Conservative treatment includes
    1. Physical therapy
    2. Exercise
    3. Avoidance of aggravating positions
- Surgical treatment involves resection of the anatomic structures compressing the artery.

THROMBOANGIITIS OBLITERANS

See Buerger's Disease.

THROMBOCYTOPENIC PURPURA, AUTOIMMUNE

OVERVIEW

- Autoimmune thrombocytopenic purpura was known as idiopathic thrombocytopenic purpura (ITP) before the underlying cause was identified.
- The total number of circulating platelets is greatly diminished, although bone marrow platelet production is normal.
- An antibody (antiplatelet antibody) is made and coats the surface of the platelets, making the platelets more susceptible to attraction and destruction by phagocytic leukocytes.
- The spleen is the primary site of platelet destruction.
- When the rate of platelet destruction exceeds the rate of platelet production, the number of circulating platelets decreases, and blood clotting slows.

COLLABORATIVE MANAGEMENT
Assessment

- The nurse assesses for
    1. Ecchymoses (bruises) on the arms, legs, upper chest, and back
    2. Petechial rash
    3. Mucosal bleeding
    4. Anemia
    5. Neurologic dysfunction (as a result of an intracranial bleed)

Interventions

* The nurse
    1. Administers immunosuppressant drugs, such as corticosteroids and azathioprine (Imuran), as ordered, to inhibit immune system synthesis of autoantibodies directed against platelets
    2. Administers low-dose chemotherapy with agents such as cyclophosphamide (Cytoxan), as ordered
    3. Administers platelet transfusions for acute, life-threatening bleeding (less than 20,000 mm^3)
    4. Maintains a safe environment
* A splenectomy is performed for clients not responding to drug therapy.

THYROID CANCER

See Cancer, Thyroid.

THYROIDITIS

OVERVIEW

* Thyroiditis is the inflammation of the thyroid gland.
* There are three types of thyroiditis.
    1. *Acute suppurative thyroiditis,* caused by bacterial invasion of the thyroid gland and manifested by neck tenderness, pain, fever, malaise, and dysphagia
    2. *Subacute granulomatous thyroiditis,* which results from a viral infection of the thyroid gland and is manifested by fever, chills, dysphagia, and muscle and joint pain; on palpation, the gland feels hard
    3. *Chronic thyroiditis* (Hashimoto's disease), believed to be an autoimmune disease, which is manifested by dysphagia, painless enlargement of the thyroid gland, low serum thyroid levels, and increased thyroid-stimulating hormone secretion, which causes

a euthyroid state for some time, followed by the development of hypothyroidism

COLLABORATIVE MANAGEMENT

- Acute suppurative thyroiditis is treated symptomatically and with antibiotics.
- Subacute granulomatous thyroiditis is treated with rest, fluids, and acetylsalicylic acid (aspirin); severe cases may be treated with corticosteroids.
- Chronic thyroiditis is usually treated with thyroid hormone; a subtotal thyroidectomy may be necessary. See Surgical Management under Hyperthyroidism.

TONSILLITIS

- Tonsillitis is an inflammation and infection of the tonsils and lymphatic tissue of the oropharynx.
- Tonsillitis is a contagious airborne or food-borne infection.
- The acute form lasts 7 to 10 days and is caused by a bacterial organism, usually *Streptococcus,* and viruses.
- Acute symptoms begin with the sudden onset of a mild to severe sore throat, fever, muscle aches, chills, dysphagia, ear pain, headache, anorexia, and malaise.
- The tonsils are swollen and red with pus and covered with white or yellow exudate.
- The uvula may be edematous and inflamed, and the cervical lymph nodes are tender and enlarged.
- Treatment includes
    1. Systemic antibiotics for 7 to 10 days
    2. Warm saline gargles
    3. Analgesics
    4. Antipyretics
    5. Antiseptic anesthetic lozenges
    6. Tonsillectomy and adenoidectomy
- Tonsillectomy and adenoidectomy are indicated for
    1. Recurrent acute infections or chronic infections unresponsive to antibiotic therapy
    2. Peritonsillar abscess
    3. Hypertrophy of tonsils and adenoids, causing airway obstruction

4. Diphtheria carriage
- The chronic form of tonsillitis results from unresolved acute infections or recurrent infections.

Toxic shock syndrome

- The pathophysiology of toxic shock syndrome (TSS) is not fully understood.
- Certain strains of *Staphylococcus aureus* produce a toxin associated with TSS.
- Menstrual-related TSS theories focus on tampon use and conclude that toxins readily cross the vaginal mucosa.
- Highly absorbent tampons rub the vaginal walls and cause ulceration, which allows transport of the toxins; prolonged or continued tampon use can cause chronic vaginal ulcerations through which *S. aureus* is absorbed; and plastic tampon inserters can cause ulceration.
- Diaphragms, cervical caps, and vaginal contraceptives have also been implicated.
- Physical findings include
  1. Fever (temperature greater than 102° F)
  2. Diffuse rash
  3. Hypotension
  4. Influenza-type symptoms, including sore throat, vomiting, diarrhea, and generalized rash
- Primary treatment includes
  1. Fluid replacement due to dehydration
  2. Antibiotics (e.g., oxacillin, nafcillin, and cephalosporin)
  3. Administration of platelets, if needed
  4. Corticosteroids for skin changes
- Client education is focused on prevention, including instructions on proper tampon, vaginal sponge, and diaphragm use.

TRACHEOBRONCHIAL TRAUMA

See Trauma, Tracheobronchial.

TRACHOMA

- Trachoma is a chronic, bilateral scarring form of conjunctivitis caused by *Chlamydia trachomatis.*
- Trachoma is the leading cause of blindness in the world. Manifestations include tearing, photophobia, edema of the eyelids, conjunctival edema, profuse drainage, eyelid scars, and turns inward, leading to corneal abrasion.
- Treatment includes oral tetracycline (Achromycin, Apo-Tefra◆) or erythromycin (E-Mycin, E.E.S., Apo-Erythro◆) which may also be used as a topical ointment.
- The client is taught to
    1. Use warm water to clean the face and eye
    2. Not share washcloths for bathing and to launder them separately in hot water
    3. Wash the hands before and after touching the eyes
    4. Complete the prescribed course of treatment.

TRANSPLANTATION, LIVER

- Liver transplantation is done to treat diseases including
    1. Primary or secondary cirrhosis and chronic active hepatitis with cirrhosis
    2. Hepatic metabolic diseases, such as protoporphyria and Wilson's disease

617

  3. Budd-Chiari syndrome (hepatic vein syndrome)

  4. Primary sclerosing cholangitis

- Extensive physiologic and psychologic assessment of the client is required.
- After a donor organ is retrieved, the liver transplant surgical procedure requires 6 to 18 hours to complete.
- Liver transplantation involves five anastomoses between recipient and donor organs, including the suprahepatic inferior vena cava, infrahepatic vena cava, portal vein, hepatic artery, and biliary tract.
- Immunosuppression therapy with cyclosporin A, azathioprine (Imuran), prednisone (Deltasone), and/or FK506, is given to prevent organ rejection, which may be acute or chronic.
- Clinical manifestations of acute rejection include

  1. Tachycardia

  2. Fever

  3. Right upper quadrant or flank pain

  4. Decreased bile pigment and volume

  5. Increasing jaundice

  6. Elevated serum bilirubin, aminotransaminases, prothrombin time, and alkaline phosphatase

- Treatment of rejection includes the administration of additional steroids and antibodies to lymphocytes, such as OKT3.
- Immunosuppression increases the client's susceptibility and risk for opportunistic infections.
- Other complications include hemorrhage, hepatic artery thrombosis, fluid and electrolyte imbalances, atelectasis, acute renal failure, chronic graft rejection, and psychologic maladjustment.
- The nurse monitors for signs of complications

  1. Fever

  2. Increased abdominal pain, distention, and rigidity

  3. Change in neurologic status

  4. Coagulopathy

TRAUMA, ABDOMINAL

OVERVIEW

- Abdominal injuries account for 25% of deaths from trauma.

- Two broad categories are
    1. *Blunt trauma,* 50% resulting from automobile accidents and the balance caused by assaults and falls, commonly affecting multiple abdominal organs
    2. *Penetrating trauma,* most often caused by gunshot wounds and stab wounds; the liver and small bowel are most commonly involved in stab wounds, and the small bowel in gunshot wounds
- The major cause of death is hemorrhage.

● Transcultural Considerations

In the United States, injury from violence and abuse is highest for young, African-American men between 19 and 24 years of age who are separated or divorced; those who earn less then $10,000 per year; and residents of large cities.

COLLABORATIVE MANAGEMENT
Assessment

- Mental status and skin perfusion are *priority* nursing assessments for hypovolemic shock.
- The nurse assesses for abdominal trauma by
    1. Asking the client about the presence, location, and quality of pain
    2. Inspecting the abdomen, back, flanks, genitalia, and rectum for contusions, abrasions, lacerations, ecchymosis, penetrating injuries, and symmetry; ecchymosis around the umbilicus is known as *Cullen's sign* and may indicate retroperitoneal bleeding into the abdominal wall; ecchymosis in either flank is known as *Turner's sign*
    3. Auscultating the abdomen for absent or diminished bowel sounds and bruits
    4. Percussing for abnormal sounds such as resonance over the liver or dullness over the stomach or intestines *(Ballance's sign)*
    5. Lightly palpating the abdomen to identify areas of tenderness, guarding, rigidity, and spasm
    6. Noting blood in peritoneal lavage

Interventions
Nonsurgical Management
- The nurse
    1. Places large-bore intravenous catheters, as ordered

619

2. Infuses intravenous fluids at a rapid rate, as ordered
3. Obtains blood samples for analysis
4. Inserts an indwelling Foley catheter
5. Inserts a nasogastric tube to prevent vomiting
- The client who does not have overt signs of bleeding may be admitted to the hospital for observation.
- The nurse
  1. Assesses for abdominal or referred pain and nausea
  2. Monitors mental status, vital signs, bowel signs, urinary output, and changes in clinical findings every 15 to 30 minutes, then hourly
  3. Reports any change immediately to the physician

Surgical Management

- For clients with severe abdominal trauma, an exploratory laparotomy with repair of abdominal injuries is performed.
- Most clients with gunshot and stab wounds require an exploratory laparotomy to assess for internal damage.
- A colostomy, either temporary or permanent, may be required. (See the Surgical Management discussion under Cancer, Colorectal.)

Trauma, Bladder

OVERVIEW

- Bladder trauma occurs as a result of blunt or penetrating injury to the lower abdomen.
- The most common cause is a fractured pelvis in which bone fragments puncture the bladder.

COLLABORATIVE MANAGEMENT

- The nurse assesses the client for
  1. Anuria
  2. Hematuria
  3. Bloody urinary meatus
  4. Results of a cystogram and of a voiding cystourethrogram
- Clients with bladder trauma other than a simple contusion require surgical intervention, including closure repair of the anterior or posterior bladder wall and peritoneal membrane.

- Clients with anterior bladder wall injury require a Penrose drain and a Foley catheter.
- Clients with posterior bladder wall injury require a Penrose drain and a Foley or suprapubic catheter.

TRAUMA, ESOPHAGEAL

OVERVIEW

- Trauma to the esophagus can occur from blunt injuries or chemical burns from caustic agents as a complication of surgery or endoscopy or from the stress of protracted severe vomiting; the incidence is low in adults.

COLLABORATIVE MANAGEMENT

Assessment

- Most clients are initially evaluated and treated in the emergency room.
- The nurse assesses the client for
    1. Pain
    2. Dysphagia
    3. Vomiting
    4. Bleeding
    5. Results of x-ray and endoscopy

Interventions

- The nurse
    1. Maintains the client on a nothing-by-mouth (NPO) status to prevent further leakage of esophageal secretions
    2. Maintains the nasogastric or gastrostomy tube drainage to rest the client's esophagus
    3. Administers total parenteral nutrition (TPN), as ordered, during esophageal rest (usually for at least 10 days)
    4. Administers broad-spectrum antibiotics, corticosteroids, and analgesics, as ordered
- If nonsurgical management is not effective in healing traumatized esophageal tissue, surgery may be needed to remove the tissue; a resection or replacement of the damaged esophageal segment with small bowel tissue may be required. (See Surgical Management under Tumors, Esophageal.)

T

TRAUMA, FACIAL

OVERVIEW

- Facial trauma is defined by the specific bones that are involved, i.e., mandibular, maxillary, zygomatic, orbital, or nasal fracture and by the side of the face involved.
- Because the face is very vascular, facial trauma causes a significant amount of bleeding.

COLLABORATIVE MANAGEMENT

Assessment

- The *first* priority in the management of facial trauma is assessment for a patent airway.
- The nurse also assesses the client for
    1. Edema of soft tissues
    2. Asymmetry
    3. Pain
    4. Leakage of cerebrospinal fluid through the ears or nose (may indicate temporal or basilar skull fracture)
    5. Vision and extraocular movements
    6. Neurologic status
    7. Results of skull and facial x-rays and computed tomography (CT) scan

Interventions

- The nurse's *first* intervention is to establish and maintain a patent airway.
- The nurse
    1. Anticipates the need for emergent intubation or a tracheotomy
    2. Treats the client for shock
    3. Works with the trauma team to provide appropriate treatment
    4. Establishes intravenous access, if not already started
    5. Assists in stabilization of fractures, if present
    6. Administers antibiotics, as ordered
    7. For mandibular fixation with plates, teaches the client oral care with a water-irrigating device, soft diet restrictions, and the method for cutting wires if emesis occurs

8. Collaborates with the dietitian, as needed, to ensure adequate nutrition

TRAUMA, HEAD

OVERVIEW

- Head trauma is a traumatic insult to the brain caused by an external force that may produce a diminished or altered state of consciousness and changes in cognitive abilities, physical functioning, and/or behavioral and emotional functioning.
- The damage most frequently occurs to the frontal and temporal lobes, and may be either temporary or permanent.
- An open head injury occurs when the skull is fractured or penetrated by an object, violating the integrity of brain and dura and exposing them to environmental contaminants.
- Types of cranial fractures include
    1. *Linear,* a simple, clean break
    2. *Depressed,* in which bone is pressed inward into brain tissue to at least the thickness of the skull
    3. *Open,* in which the scalp is lacerated, creating a direct opening to the brain tissue
    4. *Basilar,* which occurs at the base of the skull, usually along the paranasal sinus, and results in a cerebrospinal fluid (CSF) leak from the nose or ear, possibly resulting in damage to cranial nerves I, II, VII, and VIII and infecton
- *Closed* head injuries, which are caused by blunt trauma and lead to concussions, contusions, and lacerations of the brain.
    1. A *concussion* is characterized by a brief loss of consciousness.
    2. A *contusion* causes bruising of the brain tissue.
    3. A *laceration* causes actual tearing of the cortical surface vessels and may lead to secondary hemorrhage.
- Secondary responses include any neurologic damage that occurs after the initial injury and may result in increased morbidity and mortality, including

1. Increased intracranial pressure (ICP)
2. Edema: vasogenic or interstitial
3. Hemorrhage: epidural, subdural, or intracranial
4. Loss of cerebral autoregulation
5. Hydrocephalus
6. Herniation

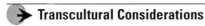 **Transcultural Considerations**

1. Head injury occurs three times more frequently in males than in females.
2. Seventy percent occur in clients between the ages of 10 and 39, with a peak incidence of 15 to 24 years of age.

Considerations for Elderly Clients

1. Clients older than 60 years of age have a higher mortality rate from head injury.

COLLABORATIVE MANAGEMENT
Assessment

- The nurse records the events surrounding the injury
  1. When, where, and how the injury occurred
  2. The client's level of consciousness immediately after the injury and upon admission to the hospital or unit and if there have been any changes or fluctuations
  3. Presence of seizure activity
- The nurse records the client's
  1. Age, sex, and race
  2. Past medical and social history
  3. Hand dominance
  4. Allergies to medications and foods, especially seafood (clients allergic to seafood are often allergic to the medium used in diagnostic testing)
  5. Alcohol and illegal drug consumption
- The nurse assesses for
  1. Impaired airway or breathing pattern
  2. Signs and symptoms of hypovolemic shock or hemorrhage, which may indicate abdominal bleeding or bleeding into soft tissue around major fractures
  3. Indications of spinal cord injury

4. Cardiac dysrhythmias from chest trauma, bruising of the heart, and/or interference with the autonomic nervous system
5. Impaired cerebral autoregulation manifested by changes in vital signs
6. Changes in neurologic status and indications of increased ICP
   a. Decreased level of consciousness (stuporous, comatose)
   b. Pupils that are large (or pinpoint) and nonreactive to light
   c. Decreased or absent motor strength in the extremities, hemiparesis or hemiplegia
   d. Inability to follow commands, confused
   e. Behavioral changes
   f. Cranial nerve dysfunction, especially I, III, V, VII, IX, and X
   g. Ataxia
   h. Aphasia
   i. Complaints of severe headache, nausea, or vomiting
   j. Seizure activity
   k. Drainage of CSF from the ear or nose ("halo" sign)
7. Indications of post-traumatic sequelae in the client who experienced a minor head injury; symptoms may persist for weeks or months
   a. Persistent headache
   b. Weakness
   c. Dizziness
8. Personality and behavior changes
9. Loss of memory
10. Problems with perception, reasoning abilities, and concept formation
11. Changes in personality and behavior, such as temper outbursts, risk-taking behavior, depression, and denial of disability
12. Loss of short-term memory and recent memory
13. Ability to learn new information, to concentrate, and to plan

Planning and Implementation

✦ **NDx:** Altered (Cerebral) Tissue Perfusion

Nonsurgical Management

- The nurse performs a neurologic assessment every 1 to 2 hours

1. Verbal response and orientation
2. Eye opening, pupil size, and reaction to light
3. Motor response
4. Vital signs, especially fever and dysrhythmias

- The nurse
  1. Elevates the head of the bed 30 to 45 degrees (unless contraindicated, e.g., spinal cord injury)
  2. Avoids activities that may increase ICP
     a. Positions the client to avoid extreme hip or neck flexion
     b. Avoids clustering nursing procedures
     c. Provides a quiet environment
- The client on a respirator may be hyperventilated to maintain an arterial carbon dioxide (PCO_2) level of 27 to 35 mmHg and an arterial oxygen level maintained at 80 to 100 mmHg.
- The client may be placed in barbiturate coma using pentobarbital (Nembutal) to decrease the metabolic demands of the brain. This requires sophisticated hemodynamic monitoring techniques, mechanical ventilation, and ICP monitoring. Complications include cardiac dysrhythmias, hypotension, and fluid and electrolyte disturbances. Some facilities use narcotic sedation rather than barbiturates.
- The nurse administers drug therapy, as ordered
  1. Glucocorticoid (dexamethasone, Medrol, methylprednisolone) to reduce edema (although the effectiveness of the intervention is being questioned)
  2. Osmotic diuretics (mannitol) given through or drawn up through a needle with a filter to eliminate microscopic crystals
  3. Loop diuretics (e.g., furosemide, Furoside◆) to treat increased ICP
  4. Codeine or fentanyl (Sublimaze) or paralytic agents (pancuronium) used if the client is mechanically ventilated to control restlessness and agitation in those at risk for increased ICP
  5. Anticonvulsants (phenytoin) to treat seizure activity
  6. Acetaminophen to reduce fever and treat headache
- The client with head trauma is at risk for hyperglycemia, diabetes insipidus, syndrome of inappropriate antidiuretic hormone, fluid overload, and/or dehydration.
- The nurse
  1. Monitors electrolytes and serum and urine osmolarity

   2. Measures intake and output every hour

   3. Measures urine specific gravity every hour

Surgical Management

- A *craniotomy* may be indicated to
  1. Evacuate a subdural or epidural hematoma
  2. Treat uncontrolled increased ICP; ischemic tissue or tips of temporal lobe removed
  3. Treat hydrocephalus
- Surgical insertion of an ICP-monitoring device is often performed. Types of devices include
  1. Intraventricular
  2. Epidural monitor
  3. Subdural bolt, catheter, or screw
  4. Fiberoptic transducer tipped pressure sensor

✦ NDx: Sensory/Perceptual Alterations

- The nurse
  1. Provides a hazard-free environment
  2. Monitors the client for nutritional deficits that may occur secondary to loss of smell and for the ability to taste, swallow, or feel food in the oral cavity
     a. Ensures that mealtime is a pleasant experience
     b. Checks the temperature of food and beverages on the tray before serving
     c. Positions the client to maximize swallowing ability
     d. Collaborates with the speech/language pathologist to develop and implement a swallowing program for the client, as needed
  3. Keeps the side rails up while the client is in bed and the seat belt on while the client is in a chair
  4. Initiates a sensory stimulation program, such as audiotapes used for no longer than 10 to 15 minutes.
  5. Orients the client to environment, time, place, and the reason for hospitalization
  6. Reassures the client that family or significant others know where he or she is and explains when the family will visit
  7. Provides simple, short explanations of procedures and activities immediately before any interventions
  8. Maintains a normal sleep-wake cycle
  9. Asks the family to bring in familiar objects, such as pictures

T

10. Monitors the client's reaction to television or radio; (the client is often unable to differentiate programs from what is happening within his or her own environment)

✦ **NDx:** Impaired Physical Mobility; Self Care Deficit

- The nurse
  1. Performs active and passive range-of-motion exercises at least once every 8 hours
  2. Positions the client carefully and uses splints and braces correctly
  3. Applies high-top athletic shoes if the client's feet are flaccid; uses them with clients who are spastic only after consultation with physical therapy
  4. Applies thigh-high antiembolism stockings to prevent pulmonary embolism
  5. Collaborates with physical and occupational therapists to plan exercise and activities of daily living (ADL) program

✦ **NDx:** Risk for Injury

- The nurse
  1. Maintains seizure precautions
  2. Keeps the bed in a low position and the side rails up
  3. Restrains the client's extremities if necessary; and, on the written order, uses hand mitts

✦ **NDx:** Impaired Gas Exchange

- The nurse
  1. Performs chest physiotherapy and encourages the client to breathe deeply
  2. Turns and repositions the client at least once every 2 hours
  3. Suctions the client as needed

✦ **NDx:** Body Image Disturbance; Altered Role Performance

- The nurse
  1. Establishes a trusting relationship with the client
  2. Allows the client to direct and participate in his or her care and decision-making regarding treatment as much as possible

3. Encourages the client to verbalize feelings, anxieties, and fears
4. Emphasizes the client's abilities while assisting the client to adapt to disabilities

✦ **NDx:** Altered Nutrition: Less than Body Requirements

- The nurse
    1. Begins nutritional support as soon as possible with hyperalimentation, tube feedings (nasal or gastrostomy), or oral feedings
    2. Weighs the client daily
    3. Monitors the client's serum albumin level and checks for signs of dehydration

Continuing Care

- The nurse
    1. Provides a detailed plan of care at the time of discharge for clients to be transferred to a rehabilitation or long-term-care facility (rehabilitation may be a lengthy process; see Rehabilitation)
    2. Refers the client to the local head injury support group
    3. Teaches the client and family measures to treat sensory dysfunctions:
        a. The home should have functioning smoke detectors (the client may have loss of sense of smell).
        b. Objects and furniture should be kept in the same place.
        c. The measures described under Sensory/Perceptual Alteration are relevant here also.
        d. The nurse helps the family and client to develop a home routine that is structured, repetitious, and consistent.

- For minor head injury, the nurse discusses symptoms of post-traumatic syndrome, informs the client this is "normal," and refers the client and family to a support group if symptoms persist.

TRAUMA, KIDNEY

See Trauma, Renal.

TRAUMA, KNEE

- *Meniscus* injuries are characterized by pain, swelling, and tenderness in the knee and sometimes by a clicking or snapping sound when moving the knee.
- A common diagnostic technique is the *McMurray test;* the examiner flexes and rotates the knee, then presses on the medial aspect while slowly extending the leg; the test result is positive if a clicking sound is palpated or heard, but a negative finding does not rule out a tear.
- Treatment of *locked* knee is manipulation followed by casting for 3 to 6 weeks.
- A *meniscectomy,* or removal of all or part of the meniscus, may be required.
- Postoperative care includes
    1. Monitoring the dressing for drainage and bleeding
    2. Circulation checks: skin temperature and color, movement, sensation, pulses, capillary refill, pain
    3. Leg exercises: quadriceps setting and straight-leg raising
    4. Knee immobilizer
    5. Elevating the leg on pillows; applying ice
- Ligament injuries result in sprains.
- Anterior cruciate ligament (ACL) injuries are characterized by a "snap"; within a few hours, the knee is swollen, stiff, and painful.
- ACL injuries are treated with exercise, bracing, and restriction of activity; surgical repair and casting may be needed.
- For a *rupture* of the *patellar tendon,* the treatment is surgical repair and casting for 6 to 8 weeks or tendon transplant. (For care of the client in a cast, see also Fracture.)

Trauma, Laryngeal

- Laryngeal trauma consists of crushing injuries, fractures, or intrinsic injuries such as prolonged endotracheal intubat ion.
- Symptoms include hoarseness, dyspnea, and aphonia; edema and bleeding also occur.
- Respiratory assessment includes monitoring for a patent airway and distress symptoms, which include tachypnea, anxiety, sternal retractions, nasal flaring, decreased oxygen saturation, and stridor.
- Management is cause specific.
- Laceration of the cricoid cartilage requires surgical repair and tracheostomy.

Trauma, Liver

- Liver trauma is the most common organ injury in penetrating abdominal trauma and the second most common organ injury after blunt abdominal trauma.
- Common injuries to the liver include simple lacerations, multiple lacerations, avulsions, and crush injuries.
- Because the liver is a vascular organ, blood loss is massive when trauma occurs.
- Signs of hemorrhagic shock from blood loss include hypotension, tachycardia, tachypnea, pallor, diaphoresis, cool, clammy skin, and confusion.
- Clinical manifestations of liver trauma include right upper quadrant pain with abdominal tenderness, distention, guarding, and rigidity and abdominal pain aggravated by deep breathing and referred to the left shoulder.
- Peritoneal lavage confirms injury.
- Exploratory laparotomy with either simple suture closure and/or packing or extensive hepatic resection may be performed depending on the extent of trauma.
- The client requires infusion of multiple blood products and massive volume to maintain hydration.

T

TRAUMA, PERIPHERAL NERVE

- Mechanisms of injury for peripheral nerve trauma include
    1. Partial or complete severance of a nerve
    2. Contusion, stretching, constriction, or compression of a nerve
    3. Ischemia
    4. Electrical, thermal, and radiation sources
- The most commonly affected nerves are the median, ulnar, and radial nerves of the arms and the peroneal, femoral, and sciatic nerves of the legs.
- Regeneration of the damaged nerve may occur.
- Nerve damage is characterized by pain, burning, and/or other abnormal sensations distal to the trauma, weakness or flaccid paralysis, and change in skin color and temperature (a warm phase and a cold phase).
- Treatment consists of immobilization of the area with a splint, cast, or traction.
- Surgery may include resection and suturing to reapproximate the severed nerve ends, nerve grafts, and nerve and tendon transplants.
- Postoperative nursing care is directed toward frequent skin care and assessment, management of pain, and instructing the client to protect the involved area from trauma.

TRAUMA, RENAL

OVERVIEW

- Renal trauma is injury to one or both kidneys.
- The injuries include
    1. *Minor* injuries: contusion, small lacerations, and disruption of the integrity of the parenchyma and the calyx
    2. *Major* injuries: lacerations to the cortex, medulla, or one of the segmental branches of the renal artery or vein; likely to follow penetrating abdominal, flank, or back wounds

3. Pedicle injuries: a laceration or disruption of the renal artery and/or vein, resulting in rapid and extensive hemorrhage

COLLABORATIVE MANAGEMENT

- The nurse records the client's
  1. History of events surrounding the trauma
  2. History of renal or urologic disease
  3. Previous surgical intervention
  4. History of diabetes or hypertension
- The nurse assesses for
  1. Abdominal and/or flank pain
  2. Presence of flank asymmetry
  3. Presence of flank bruising
  4. Penetrating injuries of the lower thorax or back
  5. Abdominal ecchymoses
  6. Abdominal distention
  7. Penetrating abdominal wounds
  8. Hemoglobin or red blood cells in the urine
  9. Decreased serum hemoglobin and hematocrit values
- The nurse
  1. Administers low-dose dobutamine, as ordered, to ensure renal perfusion
  2. Administers fluids, such as crystalloids and red blood cells, to restore circulatory blood volume; plasma volume expanders may also be given
- Depending on the extent of the injury, *nephrectomy* (the surgical removal of the kidney) may be required.
- For major vascular tearing, the kidney may be surgically removed, repaired through revascularization techniques, and then surgically reimplanted.
- The nurse
  1. Instructs the client to observe the pattern and frequency of urination and to note the color, clarity, and amount of urine produced
  2. Instructs the client to seek medical attention for feelings of bladder distention, inadequate bladder emptying, and signs of infection
  3. Describes the signs and symptoms of urinary infection, including chills, fever, lethargy, and cloudy, foul-smelling urine

T

TRAUMA, SPINAL CORD OVERVIEW

- An injury to the vertebral column and spinal cord may be caused by motor vehicle accidents, falls, sports such as diving and football, and penetrating trauma.
- As a result, a loss or decrease in motor function, sensation, reflex activity, and bowel and bladder function may occur.
- The extent of the injury can be classified as
    1. Complete when the spinal cord is transected and total motor and sensory loss occurs
    2. Incomplete, with preservation of a mixed pattern of motor, sensory, and reflex function
- Cervical spinal cord injuries may result in specific syndromes.
    1. Anterior cord is characterized by loss of motor function below the level of the injury; sensations of touch, position, and vibration remain.
    2. Posterior cord is characterized by intact motor function and changes in sensation and position sense.
    3. Brown-Seyquard is characterized by loss of motor function, proprioception, vibration, and deep touch on the same side as the injury and loss of pain and temperature on the opposite side.
    4. Central cord is characterized by loss of motor function that is more pronounced in the upper extremities than in the lower extremities.

 Transcultural Considerations

1. The typical client is an unmarried male between the ages of 15 and 30.
2. Peak incidence of injury is during the summer or warmer months.

COLLABORATIVE MANAGEMENT

Assessment

- The nurse records the client's
    1. Description of how the injury occurred and the probable mechanism of injury

2. Position immediately after the injury
3. Symptoms that occurred after the injury and what changes have occurred since then
4. Problems encountered during the extrication and transport
5. Past medical history, with particular attention to a history of arthritis of the spine, congenital deformities, osteoarthritis or osteomyelitis, cancer, previous back and spinal cord injury, and respiratory problems

- The nurse assesses for
    1. Adequate airway and breathing pattern and respiratory compromise
    2. Indication of hemorrhage or bleeding around the fracture sites or in the abdomen
    3. Decreased or absent motor strength; the ability to shrug the shoulders, flex and extend the arms, elevate the arms and legs off the bed, extend the wrist, wiggle the toes, flex and extend the feet and legs
    4. Muscle wasting, spasticity, contractures, and decreased muscle tone
    5. Decreased or absent sensation
    6. Cardiovascular dysfunction, such as bradycardia, hypotension, and cardiac dysrhythmias
    7. Change in thermoregulatory capacity, with the client's body tending to assume the temperature of the environment
    8. Indications of autonomic dysreflexia characterized by severe headache, hypertension, bradycardia, nasal stuffiness, and flushing
    9. Paralytic ileus manifested by decreased or absent bowel sounds and distended abdomen
    10. Heterotrophic ossification manifested by swelling, redness, warmth, and decreased range of motion (ROM) of the involved extremity
    11. Changes in the level of consciousness
    12. Coping strategies used in the past
    13. Body image and self-esteem disturbances

Planning and Implementation

✦ NDx: Altered (Spinal Cord) Tissue Perfusion

Nonsurgical Management

- The nurse
    1. Monitors neurologic signs and vital signs every 2 to 4 hours

2. Assesses for changes in respiratory function
3. Monitors for neurogenic shock

- The most commonly used devices for cervical injuries are cervical tongs (Gardner-Wells, Crutchfield-Vinke) and the halo fixation device to immobilize the spine.
- Traction is added, with the amount of weight to be used prescribed by the physican.
- Weights should hang free at all times; the nurse never releases the traction.
- The nurse monitors insertion sites for infection and cleans pins per hospital policy.
- The nurse administers drug therapy, as ordered
    1. Methylprednisolone (Solu-Medrol) is given in high doses within 8 hours after injury
    2. Dextran, a plasma expander, used to increase capillary blood flow with the spinal cord and to prevent or treat hypotension
    3. Atropine sulfate, used to treat bradycardia
    4. Dantrolene (Dantrium) or baclofen (Lioresal), used to treat spasticity
- Bed rest and immobilization with a brace or corset is used to treat lumbar or sacral injuries.

Surgical Management

- *Decompressive laminectomy* is performed to relieve compression from a hematoma, to remove bone fragments, or to remove a penetrating object such as a bullet.
- *Spinal fusion* or insertion of metal or steel rods to stabilize the vertebral column may be indicated.
- The nurse provides routine preoperative care.
- The nurse provides postoperative care
    1. Provides routine postoperative care
    2. Records vital signs and neurologic checks every hour and then every 4 to 6 hours, depending on the client's condition
    3. Helps the client logroll from side to side
    4. Checks the surgical site for drainage and signs of infection

    ✦ **NDx:** Ineffective Airway Clearance; Ineffective Breathing Pattern; Impaired Gas Exchange

- The nurse
    1. Performs a respiratory assessment at the beginning of each shift
    2. Turns the client at least every 2 hours

3. Encourages the client to cough and deep breathe every 1 to 2 hours
4. Teaches the client to use an incentive spirometer every 2 hours while awake
5. Performs tracheal suctioning if needed

✦ NDx: Impaired Physical Mobility; Self Care Deficit

- The nurse
  1. Repositions the client every 2 hours while the client is in bed and every 30 minutes while in a chair
  2. Inspects the skin and teaches the client to inspect the skin every shift for signs of pressure sores or reddened areas
  3. Performs ROM exercises to all extremities at least once every 8 hours
  4. Collaborates with physical and occupational therapy to determine positioning and exercise programs; determines the need for splints and a plan to prevent foot drop
  5. Assesses for signs of deep venous thrombosis, measures the calf and thigh each day
  6. Applies thigh-high antiembolism stockings
  7. Observes for orthostatic hypotension when raising the head of the bed, dangling the client on the side of the bed, and transferring the client to a chair
  8. Collaborates with physical and occupational therapy to identify techniques and assistive devices to enable the client to become as independent as possible in activities of daily living (ADL)

✦ NDx: Altered Urinary Elimination; Constipation

- The nurse establishes an individualized bowel program
  1. Schedules a consistent time for evacuation
  2. Encourages fluids unless contraindicated
  3. Provides a high-fiber diet
  4. Assesses the need for a suppository or stool softener
  5. Places the client on a bedside commode or bedpan at the time determined to be the client's normal time to have a bowel movement; allows for privacy
  6. Teaches the client to use the Valsalva maneuver or to massage the abdomen from right to left to stimulate bowel evacuation

- The nurse establishes an individualized bladder program
    1. Begins an intermittent catheterization program as soon as possible
    2. Catheterizes the client every 4 hours and more frequently if the urinary output is greater than 500 mL
    3. Recognizes that over time, intervals between catheterization are increased and adjusted to the client's fluid intake and sleep times
    4. Encourages fluids unless contraindicated to 2000 to 2500 mL; restricts fluids after 7 PM
    5. Teaches the client with upper motor injury that he or she may be able to stimulate voiding by stroking the inner thigh, performing the Valsalva maneuver, or tightening the abdominal muscles
    6. Catheterizes for residual urine after the client voids to ascertain the effectiveness of the aforementioned maneuvers

---

✦ **NDx:** Impaired Adjustment

- The nurse
    1. Invites the client to ask questions and answers honestly and openly
    2. Refers questions about prognosis and potential for complete recovery to the physician because the timing and extent of recovery vary greatly
    3. Explores coping strategies with the client
    4. Redirects socially unacceptable behavior
    5. Refers the client to clergy, psychiatric liaison nurse, psychologist, social worker, or financial counselor

Continuing Care

- The nurse
    1. Identifies and suggests corrections for hazards in the home
    2. Ensures that the client can correctly use all assistive-adaptive devices ordered for home use
    3. Ensures that assistive-adaptive equipment is installed in the home before discharge
    4. Prepares the client for the reaction of people outside the hospital
    5. Refers the client to local, state, and national support groups

6. Provides the telephone number for the spinal cord injury hotline
- The nurse teaches the client and family in collaboration with other health team members
    1. Training in ADL
    2. Structured exercise program
    3. Correct use of adaptive-assistive equipment
    4. Transfer skills
    5. Diet
    6. Bowel and bladder program
    7. Drug information as needed
    8. Skin care

Trauma, TRACHEOBRONCHIAL

- Most tears of the tracheobronchial tree are the result of severe blunt trauma, primarily involving the mainstem bronchi.
- Injuries to the cervical trachea occur at the junction of the trachea and cricoid cartilage.
- Clients with laceration of the trachea develop massive air leaks, which produce pneumomediastinum (air in the mediastinum) and extensive subcutaneous emphysema.
- Upper airway obstruction may occur, producing severe respiratory distress and inspiratory stridor.

- Most cervical tears are managed by cricothyroidotomy or tracheostomy below the level of the injury.
- The nurse
    1. Assesses for hypoxemia
    2. Administers oxygen, as ordered
    3. Maintains mechanical ventilation, if required
    4. Assesses for subcutaneous emphysema
    5. Auscultates the lungs to assess for further complications
    6. Provides care to the tracheostomy, if needed
    7. Monitors for hypotension and shock

TSS

See Toxic Shock Syndrome.

TUBERCULOSIS, PULMONARY

OVERVIEW

- Pulmonary tuberculosis (TB) is a highly communicable disease typically caused by *Mycobacterium tuberculosis.*
- The tubercule bacillus is transmitted via aerosolization (airborne route) to a susceptible site in the lung's bronchi or alveoli and freely multiplies.
- Granulomatous inflammation is surrounded by collagen, fibroblasts, and lymphocytes; areas of caseation localize and undergo reabsorption, hyaline degeneration, and fibrosis.
- Calcification and liquefaction occur.
- The initial infection is seen most often in the middle or lower lobes, with the upper lobes being the most common sites of reinfection.

➤ Transcultural Considerations

1. The incidence of TB is higher in African-Americans, Asians, Pacific Islanders, Native Americans, Alaskan Natives, and Hispanics.
2. Foreign-born people from Asia, Africa, the Caribbean, and Latin America are also at high risk for TB.
3. Clients with human immunodeficiency virus (HIV) infection are at high risk to convert from TB infection to active TB.
4. The elderly, homeless, and lower socioeconomic groups are at-risk populations, as well as those living in crowded conditions, such as prison inmates.

COLLABORATIVE MANAGEMENT

Assessment

- The nurse records the client's
    1. Past exposure to TB
    2. Country of origin
    3. Travel to foreign countries
    4. Prior TB tests
    5. History of bacille Calmette-Guérin vaccine
- The nurse assesses for
    1. Progressive fatigue
    2. Lethargy
    3. Anorexia, nausea
    4. Weight loss
    5. Irregular menses
    6. Low-grade fever
    7. Night sweats
    8. Cough with mucoid, blood-streaked, mucopurulent sputum
    9. Chest tightness
    10. Dull, aching chest pain
    11. Dullness with chest percussion
    12. Bronchial breath sounds and/or rales
    13. Increased transmission of spoken or whispered sounds
    14. Localized wheezing
    15. Positive result on a tuberculin (Mantoux) test
- Management of the client with TB includes
    1. Drug therapy, including isoniazid (INH) and rifampin throughout the course of treatment, with pyrazinamide added for the first two months; most clients undergo this therapy for 6 months
    2. Airborne precautions in a well ventilated room
    3. Client teaching
    4. Rest
    5. Careful monitoring of sputum cultures
    6. Diet rich in iron, protein, and vitamin C
    7. Emotional support
    8. The nurse wears a N95 or HEPA respirator when caring for the client

Continuing Care

- The nurse teaches the client and family
    1. Adherence to the prescribed drug regimen for 6 to 12 months, as ordered

2. Side effects of medications and ways to minimize them to ensure compliance
3. Need to resume usual activities gradually
4. Maintenance of proper nutrition
5. Identification of people who have been exposed to the client to determine infection with TB
6. Importance of follow-up visits with the physician(s)
7. To take chemotherapeutic drugs at bedtime to minimize the effects of nausea
8. To increase the intake of foods rich in iron, protein, and vitamin C
9. Importance of covering the mouth and nose when coughing or sneezing and proper disposal of tissues
10. To wear a mask when in crowds until the medication is effective, usually in 2 to 3 weeks

TUBERCULOSIS, RENAL

- Renal tuberculosis, or granulomatous nephritis, occurs when the kidney is invaded by *Mycobacterium tuberculosis,* usually by the blood-borne route.
- Normal renal parenchyma is replaced by scar tissue or a granuloma.
- Symptoms include
    1. Urinary frequency
    2. Dysuria
    3. Hypertension
    4. Hematuria
    5. Proteinuria
    6. Renal colic
- Treatment includes
    1. Chemotherapy
    2. Surgical excision of diseased tissue

Tumors, Benign Bone

OVERVIEW

- Benign bone tumors are often asymptomatic and may be discovered on routine radiographic examination or as the cause of pathologic fractures.
- Types of benign tumors include
    1. Chondrogenic (from cartilage)
        a. Osteochondroma is the most common and generally involves the femur and tibia; it usually begins in childhood but may not be diagnosed until adulthood. Males are affected more often than females.
        b. Chondroma, or endochondroma, primarily affects the hands, feet, ribs, sternum, spine, and long bones and frequently causes pathologic fractures after trivial injury. These tumors affect women and men equally of any age.
    2. Osteogenic (from bone)
        a. Osteoid osteoma most frequently involves the femur and tibia and causes unremitting bone pain; it occurs most often in male children and in young adults.
        b. Osteoblastoma, often called the giant osteoid osteoma, affects the vertebrae and long bones; it affects male adolescents and young adults of both sexes.
        c. Giant cell tumors, unlike most other benign tumors, affect women older than 20 years of age. These tumors are aggressive and can metastasize to the lung, even though the tumors are benign.

COLLABORATIVE MANAGEMENT

Assessment

- The nurse assesses for
    1. Severity, nature, and location of pain
    2. Local swelling around the involved area
    3. Muscle spasms or atrophy
    4. Anxiety and fear about diagnosis and surgery

Interventions

- The nurse
    1. Maintains a hazard-free environment
    2. Increases dietary protein, vitamins C and D, calcium, and iron to promote healing
    3. Administers analgesics and nonsteroidal anti-inflammatory drugs (NSAIDs), such as ibuprofen (Motrin), as ordered
    4. Applies heat or cold
    5. Teaches imagery and relaxation techniques
- Curettage, a surgical procedure, is performed to excise the tumor tissue; bone grafting may be needed.

TUMORS, BRAIN

OVERVIEW

- Brain tumors arise anywhere within the brain structure and are named according to the cell or tissue from which they originate.
- *Primary* tumors originate within the central nervous system (CNS) and occur as a rapid proliferation or abnormal growth of cells normally found within the CNS.
- *Secondary* tumors occur as a result of metastasis from other areas of the body, such as the lungs, breast, kidney, or gastrointestinal tract.
- Complications of brain tumors include cerebral edema, increased ICP, and pituitary dysfunction.
- Malignant tumors include
    1. *Gliomas,* which arise from the neuroglial cells and infiltrate and invade surrounding brain tissue; the peak incidence is between 60 and 80 years of age
    2. *Astrocytoma,* grades 2 to 4, which are found anywhere within the cerebral hemispheres
    3. *Oligodendrogliomas,* which are generally located within the temporal lobes of the brain and are slow growing
    4. *Glioblastomas,* which are highly malignant, rapidly growing, invasive astrocytomas
    5. *Ependymomas,* which arise from the lining of the ventricles and are difficult to treat because of their location

- Benign tumors include
    1. *Grade I astrocytoma* (may undergo changes and become malignant)
    2. *Meningiomas,* which are highly vascular and arise from the meninges; although complete removal is possible, they tend to recur
    3. *Pituitary tumors,* which result in a wide variety of symptoms caused by their effect on the pituitary gland
    4. *Acoustic neuromas,* which arise from the sheath of Schwann cells in the peripheral portion of cranial nerve VIII; they compress brain tissue and tend to surround adjacent cranial nerves (V, VII, IX, and X)
- The remainder of adult tumors are of miscellaneous origin.
- Brain tumors in adults are most common in clients between 40 and 60 years of age.

🕭 Considerations for Elderly Clients

1. Meningiomas are seen more frequently in middle-aged and elderly women.
2. Gliomas are seen slightly more often in men than in women.

COLLABORATIVE MANAGEMENT
Assessment
- The nurse assesses for changes in neurologic status:
    1. Headaches—usually more severe upon awakening in the morning
    2. Nausea and vomiting
    3. Visual symptoms
    4. Seizures
    5. Changes in mentation or personality
    6. Papilledema (swelling of the optic disk)

Interventions
Nonsurgical Management
- The nurse
    1. Performs a neurologic assessment every 4 hours or more often if clinically indicated
    2. Elevates the head of bed 30 to 45 degrees
    3. Administers analgesic for headache, as ordered

4. Administers dexamethasone (Decadron) to control cerebral edema, as ordered
5. Administers phenytoin (Dilantin) to prevent seizures, as ordered
6. Administers ranitidine (Zantac) or Axid to prevent stress ulcers, as ordered
7. Administers prochlorperazine (Compazine) or other antiemetics for nausea, as ordered

- Radiation therapy is used alone or in combination with surgery and chemotherapy.
- The radiation dose is based on tumor type and location as well as on the client's response to or toleration of the treatment.
- Radiation often causes the skin to be reddened and irritated.
- Chemotherapy may be given alone or in combination with surgery and radiation therapy.
- The medications are usually injected intrathecally; a reservoir is inserted into the ventricles to give intraventricular medications.
- Radiosurgical procedures are alternatives to traditional surgery, including the gamma knife. The gamma knife, primarily used for inaccesible tumors, employs a single high dose of ionized radiation to destroy intracranial lesions, while preserving healthy tissue.

Surgical Management

- A craniotomy may be performed, depending on the tumor type, size, and location.
- The nurse provides preoperative care
    1. Provides routine preoperative care
    2. Informs the client that all or part of his or her hair will be shaved
    3. Provides information about the intensive care unit (ICU) if the client will go there after surgery
- The nurse or assistive nursing personnel provides postoperative care
    1. Monitors vital signs every 30 to 60 minutes until they are stable
    2. Monitors neurologic signs every 30 to 60 minutes until they are stable
    3. Accurately records intake and output every hour; checks urine specific gravity every hour or with every voiding
    4. Implements cardiac monitoring while in the ICU
    5. Does not position the client on the operative site

6. Monitors serum electrolytes, CBC, and osmolarity
7. Applies thigh-high antiembolism stockings
8. Helps the client turn, cough, and deep breathe every 2 hours
9. Elevates the head of the bed 30 to 45 degrees
10. Checks the head dressing for drainage every 1 to 2 hours
11. Measures output from the surgical (Hemovac) drain every 8 hours
12. Applies cool compresses to the client's eyes to decrease periorbital edema
13. Observes for and reports complications of cranial surgery (craniotomy)
    a. Clinical manifestations of ICP include
       (1) Change in level of consciousness, restlessness, or irritability
       (2) Pupils large or pinpoint and nonreactive to light
       (3) Decreased or absent motor movement
       (4) Decerebrate or decorticate posturing
       (5) Seizure activity
       (6) Bradycardia and hypertension with widened pulse pressure
    b. The clinical manifestations of epidural or subdural hematoma include the same complications as for increased ICP plus
       (1) Severe headache
       (2) Bleeding into the posterior fossa, which may cause cardiac and respiratory arrest
    c. Hydrocephalus, the clinical manifestations of which are the same as for increased ICP, plus
       (1) Blurred vision
       (2) Urinary incontinence
    d. Wound infection
       (1) The incision is reddened and puffy.
       (2) The incision may separate.
       (3) The incision is sensitive to touch and feels warm.
       (4) The client may be febrile.
       (5) Treatment is based on the severity of the symptoms.
           — Cleanse with alcohol and apply antiseptic ointment.
           — Administer systemic antibiotics, as ordered.
    e. Atelectasis, pneumonia

  f. Neurogenic pulmonary edema

  g. Meningitis

  h. Fluid and electrolyte imbalance, including diabetes insipidus and syndrome of inappropriate antidiuretic hormone (SIADH)

   (1) Hypernatremia and increased urinary output are indicative of diabetes insipidus

   (2) Hyponatremia and decreased urinary output are indicative of SIADH

Continuing Care

- The nurse or case manager

1. Identifies and suggests corrections of hazards in the home prior to discharge
2. Ensures that the client can correctly use all assistive-adaptive devices ordered for home use
3. Provides a detailed plan of care at the time of discharge for clients to be transferred to a rehabilitation or long-term-care facility (rehabilitation may be a lengthy process) (see Rehabilitation)
4. Provides drug information as needed
5. Teaches seizure precautions
6. Obtains a dietary consult to ensure adequate caloric intake for the client receiving radiation or chemotherapy
7. Emphasizes the importance of follow-up visits with the physician(s) and other therapists
8. Refers the client and family to the American Brain Tumor Association or the National Brain Tumor Association; also refers to the American Cancer Society as a community resource

TUMORS, EPITHELIAL OVARIAN

- Epithelial ovarian tumors are serous or mucinous cystadenomas that occur in women between the ages of 30 and 50.
- Serous cystadenomas usually occur bilaterally and have greater potential for malignancy than do mucinous cystadenomas.

- Both tumors can be irregular and smooth, but mucinous adenomas grow to large sizes (up to 45 kg, or 100 pounds).
- Management includes surgical unilateral salpingo-oophorectomy; small cystadenomas may be removed by cystectomy.

Tumors, Esophageal

OVERVIEW

- *Benign* tumors of the esophagus, usually in the form of leiomyomas, are uncommon and usually asymptomatic.
- *Malignant* (cancerous) tumors may develop at any point along the esophagus; they evolve as part of a slow process that begins with benign tissue changes, and they produce widespread disabling effects that are almost always fatal.
- The two types of malignant tumors are
    1. *Squamous epidermoid tumors,* which account for most esophageal cancers and usually develop in the middle third of the esophagus
    2. *Adenocarcinomas,* which develop in the lower third of the esophagus; they are believed to evolve from Barrett's epithelium, possibly created by the presence of chronic reflux
- Esophageal tumors exhibit rapid local growth and metastatic spread via the lymph nodes.

Transcultural Considerations

1. The incidence of esophageal cancer is increasing, particularly in the African-American population.
2. Esophageal cancer mortality rates for African Americans are second only to cancer of the lung.
3. In some provinces in China, residents who have esophageal cancer have a 30% to 40% probability of dying.
4. In North America, esophageal cancer affects men more than women, especially between the ages of 50 and 80.

COLLABORATIVE MANAGEMENT
Assessment

- The nurse records the client's
  1. Alcohol consumption
  2. Tobacco use
  3. History of esophageal disease or problems
  4. Severe weight loss related to anorexia, dysphagia, or discomfort
- The nurse assesses for
  1. General physical appearance
  2. Persistent and progressive dysphagia
  3. Odynophagia (painful swallowing), reported as a steady, dull, substernal pain, which may radiate
  4. Regurgitation or vomiting
  5. Foul breath
  6. Chronic hiccups
  7. Hoarseness from laryngeal spread
  8. Results of barium swallow and endoscopy, which shows the tumor

Planning and Implementation

✦ **NDx:** Altered Nutrition: Less than Body Requirements

Nonsurgical Management

- Radiation therapy reduces the tumor's size and offers consistent short-term relief of symptoms.
- Esophageal dilation achieves temporary symptomatic relief of symptoms and is used to reduce tumor obstruction and treat strictures that may occur following radiation therapy.
- A prosthesis may be inserted to bypass disabling dysphagia and maintain an open esophagus, which preserves the client's ability to take oral nutrition.
- Chemotherapy combinations, which usually include cisplatin (Platinol), have been used more frequently as part of the primary treatment for esophageal cancer.
- The nurse
  1. Administers antacids and analgesia to provide relief of heartburn
  2. Provides soft or semiliquid foods enriched with skim milk powder or commercial protein supplements to maintain adequate nutritional intake in collaboration with the dietitian

3. Provides small, frequent meals, which are better tolerated
4. Provides care for feeding tubes or parenteral nutrition systems that may be required for severe dysphagia
5. Teaches the client to remain upright for several hours after meals and to completely avoid lying flat

Surgical Management

- Radical surgery is the only definitive treatment for esophageal cancer and is the preferred intervention in healthy clients; surgeries are extensive and have a high mortality rate.
- *Subtotal or total esophagogastrectomy* is usually required because tumors are quite large and involve distant lymph nodes.
- The preferred surgical intervention, *esophagogastrostomy,* involves removing the diseased protion of the esophagus and anastomosing the cervical portion of the stomach, which is then brought up into the thorax through the esophageal hiatus, involving both laparotomy and thoracotomy incisions.
- Tumors in the upper esophagus may require *radical neck dissection laryngectomy* because of spread to the larynx.
- Tumors that spread to the stomach may require *colon interposition,* which requires removal of a section of right or left colon and bringing it up into the thorax to substitute for the esophagus.
- Preoperative care includes provision of nutritional support from 5 days to 2 to 3 weeks prior to surgery by oral supplements, tube feedings, or parenteral nutrition.
- The nurse provides preoperative care
   1. Monitors the client's weight, intake and output, and fluid and electrolyte balance
   2. Performs meticulous oral care
   3. Provides routine preoperative care and teaching
   4. Teaches the client about the incisions, wound drainage tubes, chest tubes, nasogastric (NG) tubes, and intravenous (IV) lines
   5. Encourages the client and family to talk about personal feelings and fears
- The nurse provides postoperative care
   1. Assesses the client's respiratory status
   2. Provides chest physiotherapy, as ordered

T

3. Maintains the client in a semi-Fowler's position to support ventilation and prevent reflux
4. Administers antibiotics, as ordered
5. Administers supplemental oxygen, as ordered
6. Ensures patency of the chest tube water-seal drainage system
7. Provides support of the multiple surgical incisions during turning and activity
8. Assesses for fever, fluid accumulation, general signs of inflammation, and symptoms of early shock, which could be indicative of anastomosis leakage
9. Avoids manipulation and irrigation of the surgically placed NG tube
10. Provides meticulous mouth care while the NG tube is in place
11. Maintains nothing-by-mouth (NPO) status until gastrointestinal motility is established (usually 3 to 5 days)
12. Adminsiters IV fluids and parenteral nutrition, as ordered
13. Administers 3 to 5 mL of water every 15 to 30 minutes and assesses the client's level of tolerance
14. Slowly progresses the client's diet to pureyed and semisolid foods
15. Emphasizes the importance of eating small meals and maintaining an upright position during eating

Continuing Care

- The nurse provides written postoperative instructions
  1. Respiratory care instructions to ambulate, splint incisions, and provide chest physiotherapy and to report symptoms of respiratory infection to the physician immediately
  2. Inspection of the incision for redness, tenderness, swelling, and drainage
- The nurse reinforces dietary instructions
  1. Increase dietary intake to include high-calorie, high-protein meals that contain soft and easily swallowed foods; meals should be small and frequent.
  2. Care for tube feedings and parenteral nutrition, which may be necessary; requires intensive teaching for the client and family caring for the client at home.

3. Maintain an upright position after eating and elevate the head of the bed.

- The nurse refers the client and family to appropriate community or home health care organizations, including the American Cancer Society and area hospice services.

Tumors, Malignant Bone

See Cancer, Bone.

Tumors, Spinal Cord

OVERVIEW

- Spinal cord tumors occur most frequently in the thoracic area, followed by an almost equal distribution in the lumbar and cervical regions.
- Signs and symptoms depend on the location of the tumor and on the speed of growth.
- Primary spinal cord tumors arise from the epidural vessels, spinal meninges, or glial cells of the cord.
- Secondary tumors develop as metastases from the lungs, breasts, kidney, and gastrointestinal tract.

COLLABORATIVE MANAGMENT

- The nurse assesses the client for
  1. Pain
  2. Motor deficits
     a. Weakness or paralysis
     b. Clumsiness
     c. Spasticity
     d. Hyperactive reflexes
  3. Sensory loss
     a. Slowly progressive numbness, tingling, or temperature loss
     b. Decreased appreciation of touch

      c. Inability to sense vibration and loss of position sense

    4. Loss of bowel and bladder control

- Treatment of a spinal cord tumor:
  1. Surgical removal
  2. Radiation therapy
- Postoperatively, the nurse
  1. Monitors neurologic signs and vital signs
  2. Administers pain medication, as ordered
  3. Turns and positions the client frequently
  4. Provides range-of-motion exercises every 8 hours
  5. Prevents complications of immobility
  6. Implements a bowel and bladder program as indicated

ULCERATIVE COLITIS

See Colitis, Ulcerative.

ULCERS, CORNEAL

See Corneal Disorders.

ULCERS, PEPTIC

OVERVIEW

- Peptic ulcer disease (PUD) occurs when there is a break in the continuity of the mucosa occurring in any part of the gastrointestinal tract that comes in contact with hydrochloric acid and pepsin.
- Histamine is released, resulting in acid production, vasodilation, and increased permeability.

- Certain drugs, caffeine, smoking, alcohol, radiation, and increased stress contribute to PUD; *H. pylori* is the most common infectious agent causing PUD.
- Types of peptic ulcers include
    1. *Gastric ulcer*—a break in the gastric mucosa extending to the muscularis mucosae and found in the junction of the fundus and the pylorus; most occur on the lesser curvature of the stomach near the pylorus
    2. *Duodenal ulcer*—a chronic break in the duodenal mucosa extending through the muscularis mucosa that leaves a scar with healing; characterized by high gastric acid secretion (the most common type of peptic ucler)
    3. *Stress ulcer*—an ulcer occurring after an acute medical crisis or trauma, with bleeding due to gastric erosion as the principal manifestation and multiple lesions occurring in the proximal portion of the stomach, beginning with the area of ischemia and evolving into erosions
- Complications of ulcers include
    1. *Hemorrhage:*
        a. Ulcer bleeding varies from minimal to massive hematemesis, which usually indicates bleeding at the duodenojejunal junction.
        b. Melena is more common in duodenal uclers.
        c. Hemorrhage tends to occur more often in clients with gastric uclers and in the elderly.
    2. *Perforation,* with the gastroduodenal contents emptying through the anterior wall of the stomach or duodenum into the peritoneal cavity
    3. *Pyloric obstruction:*
        a. The obstruction occurs at the pylorus.
        b. The cause is scarring, edema, and inflammation, causing vomiting.
    4. *Intractable disease:*
        a. Pain and discomfort recur.
        b. The client no longer responds to conservative management.
        c. Symptoms interfere with activities.

COLLABORATIVE MANAGEMENT

Assessment

- The nurse records the client's
    1. Tobacco use

2. Dietary intake, including alcohol, caffeine, other irritants, and patterns of eating
3. Lifestyle, including actual and perceived stress
4. Use of over-the-counter drugs, such as corticosteroids and anti-inflammatory agents
5. Symptoms, including epigastric discomfort, abdominal tenderness, cramps, indigestion, nausea, or vomiting and their onset, duration, location, and frequency, as well as aggravating and alleviating factors

- The nurse assesses for
  1. Discomfort, pain, or heartburn (relieved after eating in client with duodenal ulcer; aggravated by food in client with gastric ulcer)
  2. A feeling of fullness or hunger
  3. Melena, especially in the elderly
  4. Vomiting
  5. Orthostatic vital signs
  6. Fluid volume deficit
  7. Dizziness
  8. Low hemoglobin and hematocrit counts
  9. Results of esophagogastroduodenoscopy (EGD), which visualizes ulcer
  10. Family and individual stressors and the client's usual patterns of coping and problem solving
  11. Impact of chronic disease on the client

Considerations for Elderly Clients

1. The elderly may not experience the typical signs and symptoms, and may delay treatment.
2. Ulcer-producing drugs for chronic illnesses are often consumed by the elderly.
3. Acute stroke may put the elderly at increased risk for GI hemorrhage.

Planning and Implementation

✦ **NDx:** Pain

- The nurse
  1. Monitors the client for worsening pain
  2. Coordinates care on an ambulatory basis if possible
  3. Administers histamine antagonists, as ordered, such as ranitidine (Zantac), famotidine (Pepcid),

and nizatidine (Axid), to block gastric acid secretions

4. Administers antisecretory agents such as omeprazole (Prilosec, Losec◆) and lansoprazole (Prevacid)
5. Administers prostaglandin analogues, such as misoprostol (Cytotec), as ordered, to inhibit acid secretion and contribute to the mucosal barrier
6. Administers antacids (e.g., Maalox, Mylanta), as ordered, as buffering agents to decrease pain (given 2 hours after meals)
7. Administers mucosal barrier fortifiers, such as sucralfate (Carafate), as ordered, to provide a protective coat preventing digestive action
8. Teaches the client to avoid caffeine-containing coffee, tea, and cola and other foods that cause discomfort
9. Teaches the client to avoid alcohol and tobacco
10. Provides a bland diet with nonirritating foods during the acute phase
11. Instructs the client to avoid intense physical activity
12. Instructs the client to alter stressful work routines and to employ coping and relaxation techniques

✦ **NDx:** Potential for Hemorrhage, Perforation, and Obstruction

Nonsurgical Management

- A nasogastric (NG) tube is inserted to ascertain the presence of blood, to assess the rate of bleeding, to prevent gastric dilation, and to provide lavage.
- Blood loss of more than 1L/24 hours may cause signs and symptoms of shock:
  1. Hypotension
  2. Chills, diaphoresis
  3. Palpitations
- The nurse
  1. Documents the amount, consistency, color (bright-red or dark), and frequency of bleeding
  2. Irrigates the NG tube to maintain patency and prevent obstruction with clotted blood
  3. Maintains the client on bed rest
  4. Administers medications, such as ranitidine and antacids, as ordered

- Therapy for massive bleeding is directed toward treating shock, preventing dehydration and electrolyte imbalance, stopping bleeding, and providing rest.
- Vasopressin is administered intra-arterially by means of an infusion pump to control acute hemorrhage.
- Other treatment measures include esophagogastroduodenoscopy to identify bleeding sites, saline lavage, injection therapy, laser photocoagulation, heater probe therapy, and electrocoagulation through an endoscope.
- Treatment of perforation includes the immediate replacement of fluid, blood, and electrolytes.
- The nurse
    1. Maintains nasogastric suction to drain gastric secretions
    2. Keeps the client on nothing-by-mouth (NPO) status and monitors intake and output carefully
    3. Checks the client's vital signs at least hourly
    4. Monitors the client for septic shock
- Treatment of pyloric obstruction is directed toward restoring fluid and electrolyte balance, decompressing the dilated stomach, and, if necessary, surgical interventions.

Surgical Management

- In patients with *perforation,* surgery entails closure of the perforation after the escaped gastric contents have been evacuated.
- A *vagotomy* is done to eliminate stimulation of gastric cells and to decrease the responsiveness of parietal cells. There are three types of vagotomy procedures:
    1. *Truncal,* in which each branch of the vagus nerve may be completely cut
    2. *Selective,* in which the vagus is partially cut to preserve the hepatic and celiac branches
    3. *Superselective,* in which the nerve is partially cut so as to denervate only the parietal cell mass, thus preserving innervation of both the antrum and the pyloric sphincter
- Vagotomy and *pyloroplasty* involve cutting the right and left vagus nerves and widening the exit of the pylorus, to prevent stasis and the resultant feeling of fullness, belching, and weight loss and to enhance gastric emptying.
- Simple *gastroenterostomy* permits neutralization of gastric acid by regurgitation into the stomach of alka-

line duodenal contents; drainage of gastric contents diverts acid away from the ulcerated area to promote healing.

- *Antrectomy,* removal of the antrum of the stomach, reduces the acid-secreting portions of the stomach.
- *Subtotal gastrectomy* includes
  1. *Billroth I,* in which part of the distal portion of the stomach is removed, including the antrum, and anastomosed to the duodenum (gastroduodenostomy)
  2. *Billroth II,* which is an anastomosis of the stomach and proximal jejunum (gastrojejunostomy)
- The nurse provides routine preoperative care.
- The nurse provides postoperative care:
  1. Provides routine postoperative care
  2. Monitors the patency of the NG tube and the type of drainage
  3. Never repositions or irrigates the NG tube
  4. Assesses for fluid and electrolyte imbalances
  5. Assesses for the development of *acute gastric dilation,* in the immediate postoperative period, which is manifested by
     a. Epigastric pain
     b. Tachycardia
     c. Hypotension
     d. Feelings of fullness or hiccups
  6. Assesses for the development of the *dumping syndrome,* which occurs after gastric resection in which the pylorus is bypassed and is a postprandial problem associated with the rapid entry of food into the bowel, manifested by
     a. Vertigo
     b. Tachycardia
     c. Syncope
     d. Sweating
     e. Pallor
     f. Palpitation
     g. Epigastric fullness
     h. Abdominal distention
     i. Diarrhea
     j. Abdominal cramping
     k. Nausea with occasional vomiting
     l. Borborygmi (intestinal rumbling noise caused by gas movement)
  7. Assists in management of the dumping syndrome by

    a. Decreasing the amount of food taken by the client at one time

    b. Providing a high-protein, high-fat, low-carbohydrate diet

    c. Administering pectin in a dry powder form

    d. Placing the client in a recumbent or semirecumbent position during eating

    e. Positioning the client in a flat position after meals

    f. Administering sedatives and antispasmodics, as ordered, to delay gastric emptying

8. Assesses for the occurrence of *alkaline reflux gastritis,* which is the reflux of duodenal contents with bile acids, resulting in injury to the gastric mucosal barrier and manifested by

    a. Persistent pain

    b. Nausea and vomiting accentuated after meals

    c. Epigastric burning, partially relieved by vomiting

9. Assesses for *delayed gastric emptying,* often present after gastric surgery and usually resolving within 1 week, and which usually results from

    a. Mechanical causes, such as edema at the anastomosis or adhesions obstructing the distal loop

    b. Metabolic causes, such as hypokalemia, hypoproteinemia, or hyponatremia

10. Assesses for development of a *gastrojejunocolic fistula,* which arises from perforation of a recurrent ulceration at the gastrojejunal anastomosis site, by monitoring for

    a. Fecal vomiting

    b. Diarrhea

    c. Weight loss

    d. Anorexia

    e. Belching of fecal-smelling gas

11. Assesses for development of *afferent loop syndrome,* which occurs when the duodenal loop is partially obstructed after a Billroth II resection, by monitoring for

    a. Painful contractions

    b. Vomiting

12. Administers vitamin B_{12}, folic acid, and iron preparations to prevent *problems of nutrition,* which develop from removal of the stomach including deficiencies of vitamin B_{12}, folic acid, and iron; impaired calcium metabolism; and reduced absorption of calcium and vitamin D

Continuing Care

- The nurse
    1. Assists the client in identifying gastric irritants and lifestyle stressors to develop strategies to make lifestyle changes
    2. Teaches the client the symptoms that should be brought to the attention of the health care provider:
        a. Abdominal pain
        b. Nausea and vomiting
        c. Black, tarry stools
        d. Weakness and dizziness
- The nurse teaches the client relaxation techniques to help with coping in order to decrease ulcer recurrence.
- The nurse, in collaboration with the dietitian, instructs the client to modify the diet, including avoiding gastric irritants and having smaller, more frequent meals.

UPPER AIRWAY OBSTRUCTION

See Obstruction, Upper Airway.

URETHRAL STRICTURE

See Hydronephrosis, Hydroureter, and Urethral Stricture.

URETHRITIS

- Urethritis is inflammation of the urethra.
- Urethritis in the *male* client presents as
    1. Burning on urination
    2. Difficult urination

      3. Discharge from the urethral meatus
- Urethritis in the *female* client presents as
      1. Bacterial cystitis (mimics)
      2. Painful urination
      3. Difficulty with urination
      4. Lower abdomen discomfort
      5. Pyuria
- The most common cause in males is gonorrhea.
- In postmenopausal women, it is probably caused by tissue changes related to low estrogen and is treated with estrogen vaginal cream.
- Nonspecific urethritis may be caused by *Ureaplasma, Chlamydia,* or *Trichomonas vaginalis.*

URINARY INCONTINENCE

See Incontinence, Urinary.

UROLITHIASIS

OVERVIEW

- Urolithiasis is the presence of calculi (stones) in the urinary tract; the exact mechanism of formation is not known.
- A supersaturation of urinary filtrate with a particular element is believed to be the primary factor contributing to calculi formation.
- Other factors include the acidity or alkalinity of the urine, urinary stasis, and other substances, such as pyrophosphate, magnesium, and citrate.
- Calculi may be formed from calcium, phosphate, oxalate, uric acid, struvite, and cystine crystals, with most stones containing calcium as one component.
- *Nephrolithiasis* refers to calculi formed in the renal parenchyma; formation of calculi in the ureter is referred to as *ureterolithiasis.*

Transcultural Considerations

1. An increased incidence in the United States is seen in the Southeast.
2. Urolithiasis is more common in men than in women and tends to occur in young adulthood or early middle adulthood.

COLLABORATIVE MANAGEMENT

Assessment

- The nurse records the client's
    1. History of renal stones
    2. Family history of renal stones
    3. Diet history
    4. Previous interventions to eliminate stones
- The nurse assesses for
    1. Presence, location, severity, and duration of pain
    2. Nausea and vomiting
    3. Hematuria, oliguria, or anuria
    4. Flank pain
    5. Ureteral spasm or colic
    6. Increased turbidity and odor of urine
    7. Bladder distention
    8. Diaphoresis
    9. Pale, ashen skin
    10. Presence of red blood cells, white blood cells, and bacteria in the urine

Planning and Implementation

+ **NDx:** Pain

U

Nonsurgical Management

- The nurse administers drug therapy, as ordered:
    1. Opioid agents, such as morphine sulfate
    2. Spasmolytic agents, such as oxybutynin chloride (Ditropan) and propantheline bromide (Pro-Banthine, Propanthel◆)
- The nurse
    1. Assesses the client's response to interventions
    2. Assists the client to find a comfortable position and to use relaxation techniques
- Extracorporeal shock wave lithotripsy (ESWL) is the application of ultrasound or dry shock wave energies

to fragment the calculus. The client receives conscious sedation as the lithotriptor and fluoroscope locate and break up the calculus.

Surgical Management

- Stone removal procedures include
    1. *Cystoscopy, retrograde ureteroscopy:* use of an endoscope through the urethra to visualize stones and to extract stones with a basket or use of a laser to fragment stones; stents may be used to dilate the ureter
    2. *Percutaneous antegrade nephrostoureterolithotomy:* use of an endoscope to visualize the stone with a special attachment to extract the calculus (through a small flank incision)
    3. *Laparoscopic ureterolithotomy:* use of a laparoscope through the ureter to remove the calculus
    4. *Pyelolithotomy:* direct visualization of the renal pelvis through a large flank incision and removal of the stone
    5. *Nephrolithotomy:* direct visualization of the kidney through a large flank incision and removal of the stone
    6. *Pyeloureterolithotomy:* direct visualization of the ureter through a large flank or lower abdominal incision and removal of the stone
- The nurse provides preoperative care:
    1. Provides routine preoperative care
    2. Provides individualized instructions dependent on the procedure to be performed
- The nurse provides postoperative care:
    1. Provides routine postoperative care
    2. Monitors the amount of bleeding from the incisions
    3. Monitors the client for hematuria
    4. Records and monitors urinary output
    5. Strains the client's urine, as ordered

✦ **NDx:** Risk for Infection

- The nurse
    1. Administers broad-spectrum antibiotics, such as aminoglycosides and cephalosporins, as ordered
    2. Ensures adequate caloric intake representing a balance of all food groups
    3. Encourages intake of 2 to 3 liters of fluid per day

✦ **NDx:** Risk for Injury

- The nurse
  1. Administers drugs, as ordered, to prevent hypercalciuria, such as thiazide diuretics, orthophosphate, and sodium cellulose phosphate
  2. Administers drugs, as ordered, to prevent hyperoxaluria, such as allopurinol (Zyloprim) or vitamin B_6 (pyrodoxine)
  3. Administers drugs, as ordered, for hyperuricuria, such as allopurinol
  4. Administers antibiotics, as ordered, such as aminoglycosides and cephalosporins
  5. Provides diet modifications dependent on stone type, in consultation with the dietitian
  6. Limits calcium intake for calcium stones
  7. Limits dark green foods, such as spinach because oxalate increases as calcium decreases
  8. Reduces purine intake, such as boned fish and organ meats, for clients with uric acid stones
  9. Encourages ambulation to promote calculi passage
  10. Provides and encourages a liberal fluid intake
  11. Strains urine in filter paper to collect passed stone fragments

Continuing Care

- The nurse instructs the client on
  1. Importance of finishing all medications
  2. Importance of balancing regular exercise with rest
  3. Diet instructions depending on stone type

- The nurse
  1. Encourages continued adequate fluid intake, including the rationale for preventing dehydration and promoting urine flow
  2. Provides postoperative care instructions, including keeping the incision dry, showering instead of bathing, and monitoring the incision for redness, swelling, and drainage
  3. Teaches the client to report symptoms of recurrent infection or formation of another stone, such as pain, fever, chills, and difficulty with urination

UROTHELIAL CANCER

See Cancer, Urothelial.

UTERINE BLEEDING, DYSFUNCTIONAL

See Bleeding, Dysfunctional Uterine.

UTERINE CANCER

See Cancer, Endometrial.

UTERINE DISPLACEMENT

See Displacement, Uterine.

UTERINE LEIOMYOMA

See Leiomyoma, Uterine.

UTERINE PROLAPSE

See Prolapse, Uterine.

UVEITIS

OVERVIEW

- *Uveitis* is a general term for inflammatory diseases of the uveal tract of the eye.
- *Anterior uveitis*
  1. Includes an inflammation of the iris, an inflammation of the ciliary body, or both
  2. Is manifested by moderate periorbital aching, tearing, blurred vision, and photophobia; small, irregularly shaped, nonreactive pupil; purplish discoloration of the cornea; and an accumulation of purulent material in the anterior chamber
- *Posterior uveitis*
  1. Includes retinitis, an inflammation of the retina, and chorioretinitis, an inflammation of both the retina and choroid
  2. Is manifested by slow, insidious onset of symptoms, including visual impairment; small, irregularly shaped, nonreactive pupil; and vitreous opacities that are seen as black dots against the background of the fundus

COLLABORATIVE MANAGEMENT

- Treatment is based on symptoms:
  1. Cycloplegic agents to put the ciliary body to rest
  2. Steroid drops to decrease inflammation
  3. Analgesics for pain
  4. Antibiotics for posterior uveitis
  5. Warm compresses
  6. Darkened room, sunglasses
- The nurse teaches the client the signs and symptoms of increased intraocular pressure.

VAGINAL CANCER

See Cancer, Vaginal.

VAGINITIS

OVERVIEW

- Vaginitis is an inflammation of the lower genital tract.
- Vaginitis develops when there is a disturbance of hormone balance and bacterial interaction in the vagina, caused by changes in normal flora, alkaline pH, insertion of foreign objects such as tampons or condoms, chemical irritants such as douches or sprays, and medications, especially antibiotics.

COLLABORATIVE MANAGEMENT

- Client history includes
  1. Onset of symptoms
  2. Characteristics and color of discharge
  3. Odor of discharge
  4. Associated symptoms such as itching and dysuria
  5. Type of contraceptive used
  6. Recent antibiotic use
  7. Sexual activity
  8. History of previous vaginal infections
  9. Hygiene practices, such as douching and tampon use
- Physical examination includes
  1. Abdominal palpation for tenderness and pain
  2. External genitalia inspection for erythema, edema, excoriation, odor, and discharge
  3. Vaginal examination to note the source of the discharge and inflammation
- Interventions include special hygiene practices:
  1. Cleaning the perineum from front to back after urination and defecation
  2. Wearing cotton underwear

3. Avoiding strong douches and feminine hygiene sprays
4. Avoiding tight-fitting pants
- Health teaching focuses on preventive measures and information on infection transmission.

VARICOSE VEINS

See Veins, Varicose.

VASCULAR DISEASE, PERIPHERAL

See Arterial Disease, Peripheral, and Venous Disease, Peripheral.

VEINS, VARICOSE

OVERVIEW

- Varicose veins are distended, protruding veins that appear darkened or tortuous.
- The vein walls weaken and dilate; venous pressure increases, and the valves become incompetent.
- Incompetent valves enhance vessel dilation, and veins become tortuous and distended.
- Varicose veins occur primarily in clients subjected to prolonged standing; they also occur in pregnant women and in clients with systemic problems, such as heart disease, obesity, and a family history of varicose veins.

COLLABORATIVE MANAGEMENT

- Clinical manifestations include

1. Pain after standing
2. Fullness in the legs
3. Distended, protruding veins

- The Trendelenberg test assists in diagnosis: As the client sits up from a supine position with legs elevated, varicose veins fill from the proximal end rather than from the normal distal end.
- Conservative treatment measures include
    1. Wearing elastic stockings
    2. Elevating the extremities as often as possible
    3. Sclerotherapy, in which the physician injects a chemical to sclerose the vein, is performed on small or a limited number of varicosities
- Surgical intervention entails *ligation* (tying) and *stripping* (removal) of the affected veins under general anesthesia.
- Postoperatively, the nurse
    1. Assesses the groin and entire leg through the elastic (Ace) bandage dressing
    2. Instructs the client to keep the legs elevated and to perform range-of-motion (ROM) exercises
    3. Discharges the client to the home, as ordered, by the first postoperative day and instructs the client to
        a. Continue wearing elastic stockings
        b. Exercise by walking
        c. Limit sitting for long intervals, and keep the legs elevated when seated
        d. Avoid standing in one place

Venous Disease, Peripheral

OVERVIEW

- Peripheral vascular disease (PVD) is a group of diseases that alter the natural flow of blood through the arteries and veins of the peripheral circulation.
- Veins must be patent and have functioning valves.
- Venous blood flow may be altered by thrombus formation and defective valves.

- A *thrombus* (blood clot) results from an endothelial injury, venous stasis, or hypercoagulability.
- *Thrombophlebitis* occurs when a thrombus is associated with inflammation in superficial veins.
- *Phlebothrombosis* is the presence of a thrombus without inflammation.
- *Deep venous thrombosis* (DVT) usually occurs in the deep veins of the lower extremities and presents a major risk for pulmonary embolism; risk factors include hip or open prostate surgeries, heart failure, and immobility.
- *Venous insufficiency* occurs from prolonged venous hypertension, which stretches the veins and damages valves, resulting in venous stasis ulcers with swelling and cellulitis.

COLLABORATIVE MANAGEMENT

Assessment

- For the client with DVT, the nurse assesses for
    1. Calf or groin tenderness and pain
    2. Leg swelling
    3. Pain in the calf on dorsiflexion of the foot (Homan's sign)
    4. Warmth and edema of the extremity
    5. Size comparison with the contralateral limb
    6. Localized pitting edema
- For the client with venous insufficiency, the nurse assesses for
    1. Discoloration along the ankles, extending up to the calf
    2. Ulcer formation:
        a. Arterial ulcers develop on the toes, between the toes, or on the upper aspect of the foot. They are painful.
        b. Diabetic ulcers develop on the plantar surface of the foot, over metatarsal heads, or on the heel and pressure areas. They may not be painful.
        c. Venous stasis ulcers occur at the ankles. Minimal pain is present.

Interventions

- For DVT, the nurse
    1. Initiates interventions to prevent pulmonary emboli and an increase in the size of the thrombus

2. Elevates the extremity
3. Applies warm, moist soaks to the affected area
4. Teaches the client the importance of maintaining bed rest
5. Administers anticoagulants, such as heparin and warfarin (Coumadin), as ordered
6. Assists the client to apply antiembolism stockings

- Thrombolytic therapy with tissue plasminogen activator (t-PA) or urokinase may be effective for dissolving the thrombus.
- For venous insufficiency, the nurse
  1. Assists the client to apply elastic or compression stockings
  2. Teaches the client to use a sequential gradient compression device, as ordered
  3. Treats open venous ulcers, as ordered, with occlusive dressings and topical agents, with or without antibiotics to chemically debride the ulcer
- Surgery is performed to treat massive occlusion that does not respond to medical treatment:
  1. Thrombectomy
  2. Inferior vena cava interruption (filter)
  3. Ligation or external clipping of the inferior vena cava

Continuing Care

- Clients recovering from venous disease are usually discharged from the hospital on a regimen of warfarin.

𝓔 Considerations for Elderly Clients

1. Warfarin is used with caution in the elderly or debilitated clients to prevent bleeding.
2. A reduced dose may be used due to decreased liver and/or kidney function.

- The nurse teaches anticoagulation instructions to the client and family:
  1. Avoid potential trauma.
  2. Observe and report signs and symptoms of bleeding:
     a. Hematuria
     b. Frank or occult blood in the stool
     c. Ecchymoses
     d. Petechiae
     e. Altered level of consciousness

f. Pain
3. Apply direct pressure to bleeding sites.
4. Seek medical assistance immediately if bleeding occurs.
5. Wear a Medic-Alert bracelet or necklace and carry a Medic-Alert card at all times.
6. Inform other health care providers, such as dentists, about the therapy.
7. Avoid other medications, unless prescribed by the same physician.
8. Avoid high-fat and vitamin K–rich foods.
9. Have routine monitoring of prothrombin time or INR levels.

- The nurse teaches the client with chronic venous status to
    1. Avoid standing still or sitting for long periods
    2. Avoid crossing the legs when sitting
    3. Avoid constrictive garments
    4. Wear support hose or antiembolism stockings, as prescribed
    5. Follow the prescribed exercise program
    6. Follow the prescribed weight reduction plan, if needed
    7. Follow written and oral foot care instructions (see Continuing Care under Arterial Disease, Peripheral)
    8. Keep follow-up appointments with the health care provider(s)

$\mathbf{V}$ITAMIN B$_{12}$ DEFICIENCY ANEMIA

See Anemia, Vitamin B$_{12}$ Deficiency.

$\mathbf{V}$ULVAR CANCER

See Cancer, Vulvar.

VULVITIS

OVERVIEW

- Vulvitis is an inflammatory condition of the vulva associated with pruritus (itching) and a burning sensation.
- The vulvar skin is sensitive to hormonal, metabolic, and allergic influences; symptoms can be caused by systemic conditions, by direct contact with an irritant, or by extension of infections from the vagina.
- The most common skin disease affecting the vulva is contact dermatitis caused by irritants, such as feminine hygiene sprays, fabric dyes, soaps and detergents, and allergens.
- Primary infections affecting the vulva include herpes genitalis and condyloma acuminatum (venereal warts).
- Secondary infections are caused by organisms responsible for vaginitis, including candidiasis.
- Common parasitic infections include pediculosis pubis (crab lice) and scabies (itch mites).
- Other causes include atrophic vaginitis, vulvar kraurosis (a postmenopausal disorder causing dryness and atrophy), vulvar leukoplakia (postmenopausal atrophy and thickening of vulvar tissue), cancer, and urinary incontinence.

COLLABORATIVE MANAGEMENT

- Physical findings include
    1. Itching
    2. Burning sensation
    3. Erythema, edema, and superficial skin ulcerations
    4. White and thickened vulvar tissue
    5. Dry and scaly skin
- Treatment depends on the cause and includes
    1. Antibiotics
    2. Removal of irritants or allergens
    3. Treatment for pediculosis and scabies
    4. Interventions to relieve itching, such as sitz baths, Burow's solution compresses, and topical steroids
- Health teaching focuses on preventive measures.

WARTS

- Warts, or verrucae, are small tumors caused by infection of the keratinocytes with papillomavirus.
- Warts occur singly or in groups.
- *Common warts* are raised, flesh-colored papules with a rough, hyperkeratotic surface, commonly occurring on the hands and fingers.
- *Flat warts* appear as elevated reddish-brown or flesh-colored papules with flat tops and minimal scale.
- *Plantar warts* are painful warts occurring on the bottom of the foot and usually covered with thick callus.
- Wart treatment is aimed at destroying keratinocytes containing the virus and includes

    1. Cryosurgery (preferred)
    2. Surgical excision
    3. Electrodesiccation and curettage
    4. Topical caustic agents

GUIDE TO
HEAD-TO-TOE PHYSICAL
ASSESSMENT OF ADULTS

Guide to Head-to-Toe Physical Assessment of Adults*

Nursing Activity	Typical Finding	Changes Associated with Aging
NEUROLOGIC SYSTEM		
1. Determine level of consciousness.	1. Alert	1. None
2. Test for orientation.	2. Oriented	2. None
SKIN		
1. Inspect skin during each part of assessment.	1. Intact, warm, dry, elastic skin	1. Excessive dryness; presence of wrinkles; presence of "age spots" and hemangiomas; inelastic, sagging skin
2. Palpate any lesions.	2. No lesions	2. Presence of ecchymotic areas as a result of increased capillary fragility

HEAD AND FACE

1. Inspect and palpate the scalp, hair, and skull.
2. Inspect face for symmetry of expression.
3. Palpate the temporal arteries.
4. Palpate temporomandibular joints (TMJs).

1. No lesions, shiny hair
2. Symmetric expression
3. Faint pulsation
4. No tenderness

1. Thinning and dullness of hair
2. None
3. None
4. Possible tenderness or crepitus

EYE

1. Inspect the external eye structures.

2. Inspect the conjunctivae, sclerae, corneas, and irides.

3. Use a penlight to test pupillary response (direct and consensual).

4. Test vision by asking the client to read (if able). (*Note:* Be sure that glasses or contact lenses are in place, if used.)

1. No structural abnormalities

2. No abnormalities; round irides

3. Pupils are equal and round and react to light and accomodation

4. No vision impairment

1. Presence of an entropion (inverted eye-lid) or extropion (everted eyelid)
2. None

3. None

4. Presence of presbyopia (farsightedness)

Table continued on following page

Appendix

679

Guide to Head-to-Toe Physical Assessment of Adults *Continued*

Nursing Activity	Typical Finding	Changes Associated with Aging
EAR		
1. Inspect the external structure.	1. No structural abnormalities	1. No major change
2. Inspect the auditory meatus for drainage.	2. No drainage; small amount of cerumen may be present	2. None
3. Test hearing by whispering to the client while turning head away. (*Note:* Be sure that hearing aid, if used, is in place.)	3. No difficulty in hearing	3. Presence of presbycusis (loss of ability to hear high-pitched sounds)
MOUTH		
1. Use a penlight to inspect mouth, teeth, and gums.	1. No lesions, extensive dental caries, or gum disease.	1. None

NECK

1. Inspect for symmetry, lesions, pulsations, and jugular venous distention (JVD).
   1. Symmetric, without lesions or JVD

2. Palpate the carotid pulse, one side at a time; check for bruits.
   2. No bruits; pulses equal

3. Palpate the cervical lymph nodes.
   3. Unable to palpate

4. Test range-of-motion (ROM).
   4. No limitations

CHEST (POSTERIOR, ANTERIOR, AND LATERAL)

1. Inspect the chest for deformity, symmetry, expansion, and lesions; note pulsations or heaves (lifts).
   1. Symmetric; without lesions; anteroposterior/lateral ratio of 1:2; no heaves
   1. Slight change in anteroposterior/lateral ratio (1:1.5)

2. Palpate any chest lesions.
   2. No lesions
   2. None

3. Locate the point of maximal impulse (PMI).
   3. PMI at the left midclavicular line (MCL), fifth intercostal space (ICS)
   3. None

4. Palpate each vertebra of the spine.
   4. No tenderness or bony spurs
   4. Thoracic kyphosis

5. Auscultate breath sounds throughout all lung fields
   5. Unlabored excursion of air; no adventitious sounds
   5. Shallow respirations

6. Auscultate apical rate and rhythm; auscultate heart sounds.
   6. Presence of S_1 and S_2 heart sounds
   6. Possible S_4 heart sound

Table continued on following page

681

Guide to Head-to-Toe Physical Assessment of Adults* Continued

Nursing Activity	Typical Finding	Changes Associated with Aging
UPPER EXTREMITIES		
1. Inspect and palpate joints for swelling, tenderness, and deformity.	1. No swelling, tenderness, or deformity	1. Tenderness of one or more joints
2. Palpate brachial and radial arteries; assess for pulse deficit.	2. Pulses equal and within normal limits	2. None
3. Test range of motion in all joints and sensation.	3. No restriction	3. Slight decrease in ROM; possible crepitus
4. Test muscle strength of arms, hands, and shoulders.	4. 5/5 movement against resistance	4. Slight decrease (4+/5 or 4/5)
5. Palpate axillary nodes.	5. Nodes not palpable	5. None
ABDOMEN		
1. Inspect for contour, symmetry, lesions, and pulsations.	1. Symmetric; without lesions or pulsations	1. None

Assessment	Normal Findings	Variations
2. Auscultate bowel sounds in all four quadrants.	2. Five to 15 sounds per minute in each quadrant	2. May be slightly decreased (hypoactive)
3. Auscultate over abdominal aorta for bruit.	3. No bruit	3. None
4. Palpate for liver enlargement.	4. Liver not below costal margin	4. None

LOWER EXTREMITIES

Assessment	Normal Findings	Variations
1. Inspect and palpate for swelling, tenderness, and deformity.	1. No swelling, tenderness, or deformity	1. Tenderness of one or more joints
2. Test ROM and sensation.	2. No limitation	2. Slight decrease, possible crepitus
3. Test muscle strength.	3. 5/5 movement against resistance fifth intercostal space (ICS)	3. Slight decrease (4+/5 or 4/5)
4. Palpate femoral, popliteal, and pedal pulses.	4. Pulses equal and within normal range	4. Pedal pulses may be weak or not palpable
5. Palpate inguinal nodes.	5. Nodes not palpable	5. None

GENITALIA

Assessment	Normal Findings	Variations
1. Inspect external genitalia for lesions or drainage.	1. No lesions or drainage	1. None

* Additional assessments may be needed, depending on the client's concerns and the medical diagnoses. For more information on physical assessment, see Ignatavicius, Workman, and Mishler: Medical-Surgical Nursing, 3rd edition.

Appendix

CONSIDERATIONS FOR ETHICAL DECISION-MAKING

Considerations for Ethical Decision-Making

Definition of ethics	Ethics is the study of what is right or what people ought to do in a specific situation. Each clinical ethical issue is unique.
Resources to be used when making an ethical decision	Ethical theories and principles
	Legal statutes
	Decision-making models
	Values of the person involved
	Professional codes
	Institutional policies and procedures
	Ethicists
	Institutional ethics committees
Four major ethical principles	
Non-maleficence	Requires that no matter what other outcomes are achieved during an ethical issue, the nurse must prevent harm
Beneficence	Holds that, in addition to doing no harm, the nurse acts in the patient's best interest and promotes good
Justice	Is concerned with how resources are divided between individuals and/or groups in society; usually concerned with resources in short supply, such as organ transplants
Autonomy	Requires that a person be involved in decisions that affect his or her life
Variables that influence ethical decision-making	Nurse's knowledge, education, moral reasoning, values and beliefs, age, maturity, self-image, and previous experience
	Amount of time available to make a decision, complexity of the decision, and perceived costs and benefits
	Health care agencies, policies and procedures; conflicting loyalties between the client, professional, and institution; diverse expectations of the client; laws of the state; public beliefs about how resources should be allocated; and current events in the media

Steps in ethical decision-making

Assessment
Investigate the facts.
Identify all persons to be involved in decision-making.
Assess the decision-making environment:
  Time available to make the decision
  Events that preceded the current situation

Analysis
Identify the major ethical issues or questions to be resolved.
Identify and consider alternatives or options.

Planning
Use the four major ethical principles as a basis for the interventions.
Non-maleficence is a minimal outcome; beneficence toward the client should be fostered; and client autonomy is to be
  promoted to the greatest extent possible.
Explore options and discuss them with the client.

Intervention
Identify any task, participant, or environmental variables that were not identified during the assessment phase.
Identify competing variables.
Identify and consult resources.
Implement a choice.

Evaluation
Evaluate the decision-making process and its outcome. Were the outcomes achieved?
If not, why?
  Did the correct persons make the decision?
  What actions will be taken to prevent similar situations from occurring?
  How do the various participants feel?

Appendix

687

Appendix 3

ELECTROCARDIOGRAPHIC COMPLEXES, SEGMENTS, AND INTERVALS

Appendix

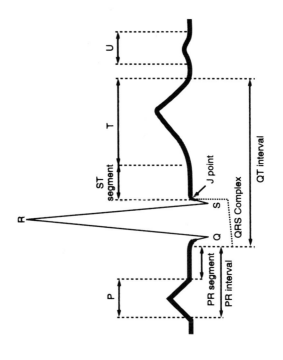

I. The first step in reading an electrocardiogram is to analyze the aspects of the heart rhythm:

P wave — Represents atrial depolarization

PR segment — Represents the time required for the impulse to travel through the atrioventricular (AV) node, where it is delayed, and through the bundle of His, bundle branches, and Purkinje fiber network, just before ventricular depolarization.

PR interval — Represents the time required for atrial depolarization as well as impulse travel through the conduction system and Purkinje fiber network, inclusive of the P wave and PR segment. It is measured from the beginning of the P wave to the end of the PR segment.

Measured from the beginning of the P wave to the end of the PR segment. Normally measures 0.12 to 0.20 second in duration.

QRS complex — Represents depolarization of both ventricles and is measured from the beginning of the Q (or R) wave to the end of the S wave.

Measured from the end of the PR interval to the J point. Normally measures from 0.04 to 0.10 second.

J point — Represents the junction where the QRS complex ends and the ST segment begins.

ST segment — Represents early ventricular repolarization.

Measured from the J point to the beginning of the T wave.

T wave — Represents ventricular repolarization.

Appendix continued on following page

U wave	Represents late ventricular repolarization. Not normally seen in all leads.
QT interval	Represents the total time required for ventricular depolarization and repolarization.
	Measured from the beginning of the QRS complex to the end of the T wave. Normally measures from 0.32 to 0.40 second.
QT interval	Represents the total time required for ventricular depolarization and repolarization and is measured from the beginning of the QRS complex to the end of the T wave.

2. Next, estimate the heart rate by counting the number of P-P or R-R intervals in 6 seconds and multiply that number by 10.

3. Finally, interpret the rhythm.

Normal Sinus Rhythm

Both atrial and ventricular rhythms are essentially regular (a slight variation in rhythm is normal). Atrial and ventricular rates are both 92/minute. There is one P wave before each QRS complex, and all the P waves are of a consistent morphology (shape). The PR interval measures 0.14 second and is constant; the QRS complex measures 0.08 second and is constant. The T waves vary in amplitude, from flat to positive, because of respirations (flat with inspiration, positive with expiration).

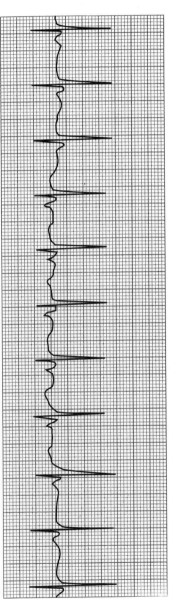

Appendix continued on following page

Appendix

693

Sinus Arrhythmia

All the P waves have the same morphology, indicating that they are all from the sinus node. The rhythm is irregular, with the shortest R-R interval (0.72 second) varying more than 0.12 second from the longest R-R interval (1.0 second).

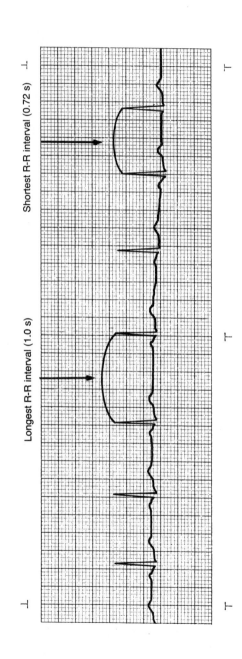

Longest R-R interval (1.0 s)　　　　Shortest R-R interval (0.72 s)

Sinus Rhythms

A, Sinus tachycardia (HR = 110/minute, PR = 0.12 second, QRS = 0.08 second). *B*, Sinus bradycardia (HR = 35/minute, PR = 0.16 second, QRS = 0.10 second). *C*, Sinus pause (underlying HR = 60/minute, PR = 0.20 second, QRS = 0.08 second, with just under a 5-second pause).

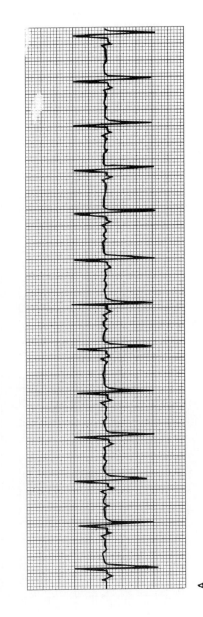

Illustration continued on following page

A

695

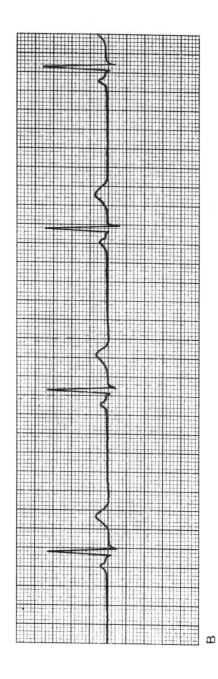

B

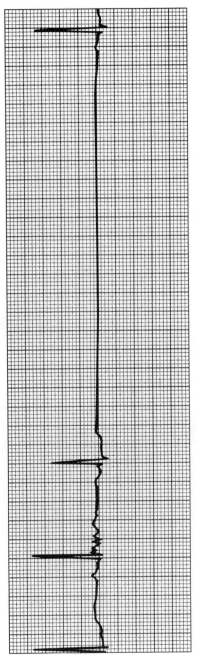

C

Normal Sinus Rhythm with a Premature Contraction

A, Normal sinus rhythm with a premature ventricular contraction (PVC). There is a complete compensatory pause following the PVC, indicated by the fact that the sinus P wave following the pause comes exactly when it was due to occur. The P wave can also be determined by the R-R intervals, measuring between two complete intervals, with the R wave following the pause coming exactly when it was due to occur. *B,* Normal sinus rhythm with a premature atrial contraction (PAC). There

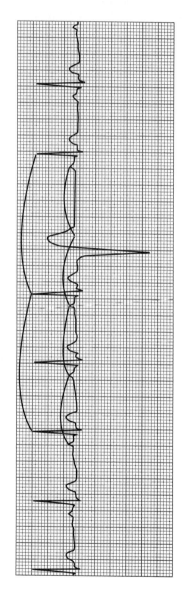

A

is an incomplete or noncompensatory pause following the PAC, indicated by the sinus P wave following the pause coming before it was originally due to occur. The QRS complex also comes before it would have been due.

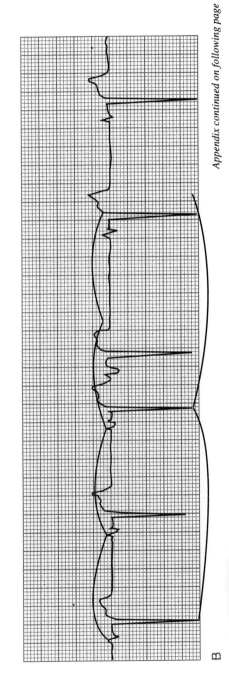

Appendix continued on following page

B

Atrial Dysrhythmias

A. Normal sinus rhythm with an 11-beat run of paroxysmal atrial tachycardia (PAT) with 1:1 conduction. *B.* Atrial tachycardia with 2:1 block. The atrial rate is 164/minute; the ventricular rate is 82/minute.

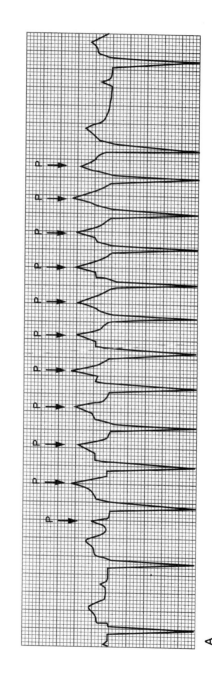

A

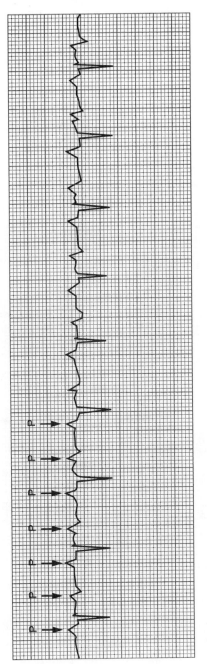

Appendix continued on following page

B

Appendix

Ventricular Dysrhythmias

A. Normal sinus rhythm with unifocal premature ventricular complexes (PVCs); note the pair of PVCs. B. Normal sinus rhythm with a three-beat run of ventricular tachycardia (three consecutive PVCs) and another unifocal PVC. C. Normal sinus rhythm with multifocal PVCs (one negative and the other positive).

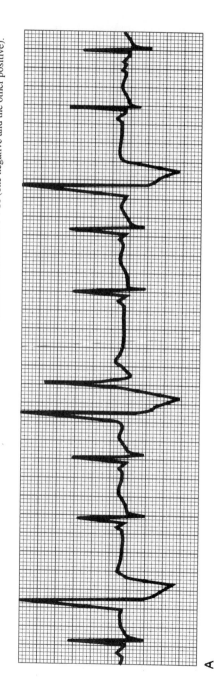

A

702

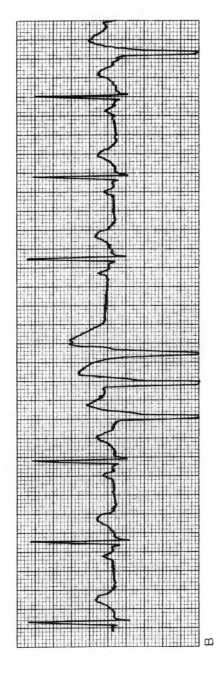

Illustration continued on following page

B

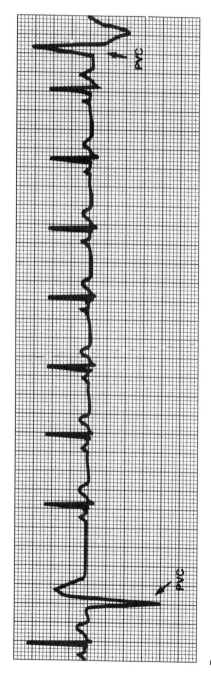

C

704

Ventricular Dysrhythmias

A, Coarse ventricular fibrillation. *B,* Ventricular asystole, initially with five P waves, then no P waves (atrial and ventricular standstill).

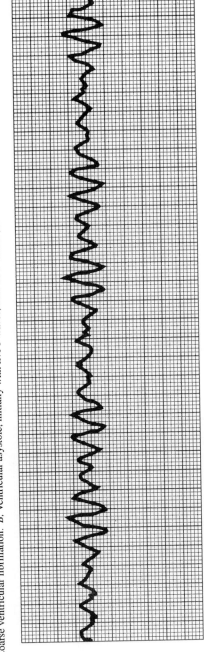

A

Illustration continued on following page

705

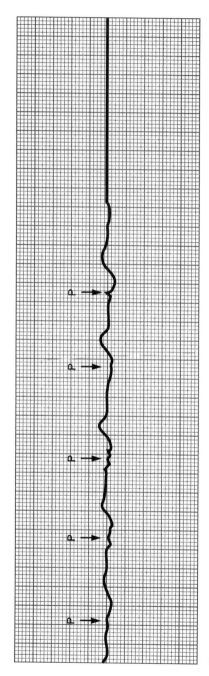

B

706

AV Blocks

A, Normal sinus rhythm with first-degree AV block (PR interval 0.28 second). B, Second-degree AV block type I (AV Wenckebach) with an irregular rhythm, grouped beating, and progressive prolongation of the PR interval until a P wave is completely blocked and not followed by a QRS complex. C, Second-degree AV block type II (Mobitz II) with 3:1 conduction and a constant PR interval.

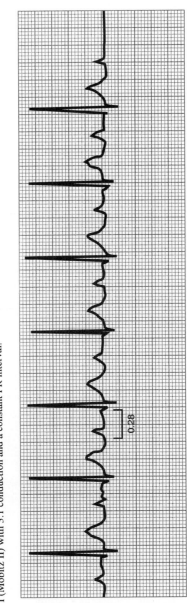

0.28

A

Illustration continued on following page

Appendix

707

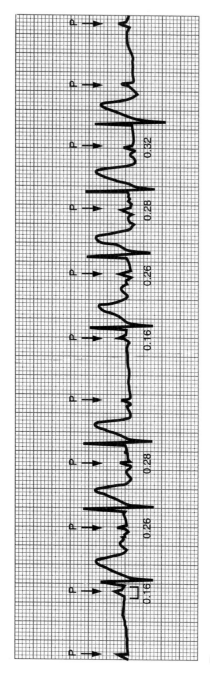

708

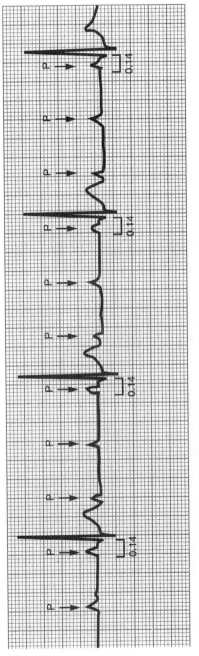

AV Blocks

A, Third-degree AV block (complete heart block) with regular atrial and ventricular rhythms, inconsistent PR intervals (AV dissociation), and a junctional escape focus (normal QRS complexes) pacing the ventricles at a rate of 38/minute. *B*, Third-degree AV block with regular atrial and ventricular rhythms, inconsistent PR intervals (AV dissociation), and a ventricular escape focus pacing the ventricles at a rate of 35/minute, with wide QRS complexes. *C*, Normal sinus rhythm with bundle branch block (wide QRS complexes measuring 0.14 second).

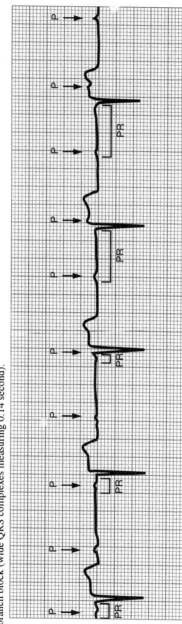

A

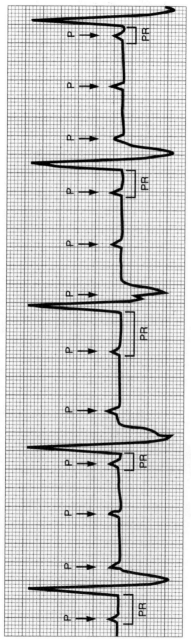

Illustration continued on following page

B

Appendix

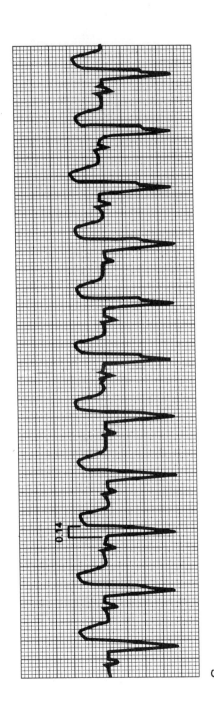

712

C

0.14

HEALTH CARE
ORGANIZATIONS AND
RESOURCES

Nursing Organizations

Academy of Medical-Surgical Nurses
East Holly Avenue
Box 56
Pitman, NJ 08071
(609) 256-2323
www.amsn.inurse.com

American Academy of Ambulatory Care Nurses
East Holly Avenue
Box 56
Pitman, NJ 08071-0056
(609) 256-2350
aaacn.inurse.com

American Academy of Nurse Practitioners
P.O. Box 12846
Austin, TX 78711
(512) 442-4262
www.aanp.org

American Association of Critical-Care Nurses
101 Columbia
Aliso Viejo, CA 92656
(800) 899-2226
www.aacn.org

American Association of Diabetes Educators
100 West Monroe, 4th Floor
Chicago, IL 60603
(312) 424-2426
www.aadenet.org

American Association of Neuroscience Nurses
224 North Des Plaines, Suite 601
Chicago, IL 60661
(312) 993-0043
www.aann.org

American Association of Nurse Anesthetists
222 South Prospect Ave.
Park Ridge, IL 60068-4001
(847) 692-7050
www.aana.com

American Association of Occupational Health Nurses
2920 Brandywine Rd., Suite 900
Atlanta, GA 30341
(800) 241-8014
www.aaohn.org

American Association of Spinal Cord Injury Nurses
75-20 Astoria Blvd.
Jackson Heights, NY 11370
(718) 803-3782
www.epva.org

American College of Nurse Practitioners
503 Capitol Ct. NE, Suite 300
Washington, DC 20002
(202) 546-4825
www.nurse.org/acnp

American Nephrology Nurses' Association
East Holly Ave., Box 56
Pitman, NJ 08071
(609) 256-2320
www.anna.inurse.com

American Nurses' Association
600 Maryland Ave SW, Suite 100 West
Washington, DC 20024-2571
(800) 274-4ANA
www.ana.org

American Society of Ophthalmic Registered Nurses
655 Beach St.
P.O. Box 193030
San Francisco, CA 94119
(415) 561-8513

American Society of Peri-Anesthesia Nurses
6900 Grove Rd.
Thorofare, NJ 08086
(609) 848-1881
www.aspan.org

American Society of Plastic and Reconstructive Surgical Nurses
East Holly Ave., Box 56
Pitman, NJ 08071-0056
(609) 256-2340
www.asprsn.inurse.com

American Thoracic Society Nursing Assembly
1740 Broadway
New York, NY 10019
(212) 315-8700
www.thoracic.org/nur

Association of Nurses in AIDS Care
11250 Roger Bacon Dr., Suite 8
Reston, VA 20190-5202
(800)260-6780
www.anacnet.org/aids/

Association of Operating Room Nurses
2170 South Parker Rd., Suite 300
Denver, CO 80231-5711
(303) 755-6300
www.aorn.org

Association for Professionals in Infection Control and Epidemiology, Inc.
1016 Sixteenth Street, NW Sixth Floor
Washington, DC 20036
(202) 296-5645
www.apic.org

Association of Women's Health, Obstetric, and Neonatal Nurses
2000 L Street NW
Washington, DC 20036
(202) 261-2400
www.awhonn.org

Dermatology Nurses Association
East Holly Ave., Box 56
Pitman, NJ 08071-0056
(609) 256-2330
www.dna.inurse.com

Emergency Nurses Association
216 Higgins Rd.
Park Ridge, IL 60068-5736
(847) 698-9400
www.ena.org

National Association of Orthopaedic Nurses
East Holly Ave., Box 56
Pitman, NJ 08071-0056
(609) 256-2310
www.naon.inurse.com

National League for Nursing
61 Broadway
New York, NY 10006
(800) 669-1656
www.nln.org

National Student Nurses' Association
555 W. 57th St.
New York, NY 10019
(212) 581-2211
www.nsna.org

Oncology Nursing Society
501 Holiday Dr.
Pittsburgh, PA 15220-2749
(412) 921-7373
www.ons.org

Sigma Theta Tau International
550 West North Street
Indianapolis, IN 46202
(317) 634-8171
http://stti-web.iupui.edu

Society of Gastroenterology Nurses and Associates, Inc.
401 North Michigan Ave.
Chicago, IL 60611-4267
www.sgna.org

Society of Urologic Nurses and Associates
East Holly Ave., Box 56
Pitman, NJ 08071-0056
(609) 256-2335
www.suna.inurse.com

WorldWide Nurse
www.wwnurse.com

Wound, Ostomy and Continence Nursing Society
1550 South Coast Highway, Suite 201
Laguna Beach, CA 92651
(888) 224-9626
www.wocn.org

Community Organizations and Other Resources

Alternative and Complementary Therapies

Alternative Medicine
http://galaxy.tradewave.com/galaxy/Medicine/therapeutics/
Alternativw-Medicine.html

Alternative Medicine (Health a-to-z)
www.healthatoz.com/categories/AM.htm

American Holistic Nurses Association
P.O. Box 2130
Flagstaff, AZ 86003-2130
(800) 278-AHNA
www.ahna.org

American Massage Therapy Association
820 Davis St., Suite 100
Evanston, IL 60201-444
(847) 864-0123
www.amtamassage.org

Complementary Therapies
www.wholenurse.com

Healing Touch International, Inc.
198 Union Blvd., Suite 202
Lakewood, CO 80228
(303) 989-7982
www.healingtouch.net

Nurses Certification Program in Interactive Imagery
P.O. Box 8177
Foster City, CA 94404
(650) 570-6157
http://members.aol.com//NCPII/NCPII.html

The Wellness Center
(704) 683-3369
www.newfrontiers.com/wellness

Cancer/Death and Dying

American Brain Tumor Association
2720 River Rd., Suite 146
Des Plaines, IL 60018
(800) 886-2282
www.abta.org

American Cancer Society
1599 Clifton Road NE
Atlanta, GA 30329
(404) 320-3333
www.cancer.org

Breast Cancer Information Clearing House
http://nysernet.org/bcic

Breast Care Helpline
(800) 462-9273

Canadian Cancer Society (National Office)
10 Alcorn Ave., Suite 200
Toronto, Ontario
Canada M4V 1E4
(416) 961-7223
www.cancer.ca

Cancer Information Hotline
(800) 4-CANCER

CDC's Tobacco Information and Prevention Source Page
www.cdc.gov/nccdphp/osh/tobacco.htm

Choice in Dying
1035 30th Street NW
Washington, DC 20007
(202) 338-9790
www.choices.org

Funeral and Memorial Societies of America
P.O. Box 10
Hinesburg, VT 05461
(802) 482-3437
www.funerals.org

Hospice Association of America
228 7th Street SE
Washington, DC 20003
(202) 546-4759
www.nahc.org

Leukemia Society of America
600 Third Ave.
New York, NY 10016
(212) 573-8484
www.leukemia.org

National Cancer Institute
Building 82
9000 Rockville Pike
Bethesda, MD 20892
(301) 496-8880
www.nih.gov/nci

NCI's CancerNet
www.nci.nih.gov

National Hospice Organization
P.O. Box 903
Falls Church, VA 22040-0903
(703) 243-5900
www.nho.org

National Ovarian Cancer Coalition
www.ovarian.org

The Quitnet
www.quitnet.org

Rory Foundation
12411 Ventura Blvd.
Studio City, CA 91604-2407
(888) RORY123
www.roryfoundation.org

Susan G. Komen Breast Cancer Foundation
www.komen.org

Cardiovascular and Hematologic Problems

American Association of Blood Banks
8101 Glenbrook Rd.
Bethesda, MD 20814-2749
www.aabb.org

American Heart Association
7272 Greenville Ave.
Dallas, TX 75231
(800) AHA USA1
www.american heart.org

American Heart Association Women's Website
7272 Greenville Ave.
Dallas, TX 75231
(888) MY HEART
www.women.americanheart.org

Heart Information Network
www.heartinfo.org

Mended Hearts, Inc.
www.mendedhearts.org

National Hemophilia Foundation
116 West 32nd Street, 11th Floor
New York, NY 10001
(212) 328-3700
www.hemophilia.org

Sickle Cell Disease Association of America, Inc.
3345 Wilshire Blvd., Suite 1106
Los Angeles, CA 90010-1880
(800) 421-8453

Diabetes Mellitus

American Diabetes Association
1660 Duke Street
Alexandria, VA 22314
www.diabetes.org

American Dietetic Association
216 West Jackson Blvd., Suite 800
Chicago, IL 60606
(312) 899-0040
www.eatright.org

CDC—Diabetes Home Pge
www.cdc.gov/nccdphp/ddt/ddthome.htm

National Institute of Diabetes and Digestive and Kidney Disease
www.niddk.nih.gov

Elderly/Gerontology

Alcohol Rehab for the Elderly
P.O. Box 267
Hopedale, IL 61747
(800) 354-7089
www.hmc.net

Alzheimer's Association
919 N. Michigan Ave., Suite 1000
Chicago, IL 60611-1676
www.alz.org

American Association of Retired Persons
601 E Street NW
Washington, DC 20049
(800) 424-3410
www.aarp.org

American Federation for Aging Research
1414 Avenue of the Americas, 18th Floor
New York, NY 10019
(212) 752-2327
www.afar.org

National Institute on Aging
www.nih.gov.nia

Eye and Ear Problems

American Foundation for the Blind
11 Penn Plaza
Suite 300
New York, NY 10001
(212) 502-7600
www.afb.org

American Speech-Language-Hearing Association
10801 Rockville Pike, Dept. AP
Rockville, MD 20852
(301) 897-5700
www.asha.org

Deafness Research Foundation
Nine East 38th Street, Seventh Floor
New York, NY 10016
(800) 535-3323
www.drf.org

Eye Bank Associations of America
1001 Connecticut Ave. NW, Suite 601
Washington, DC 20036
(202) 775-4999
www.restoresight.org

Meniere's Network of the Ear Foundation
2000 Church Street, Box 111
Nashville, TN 37236
(800) 545-4327
www.theearfound.org

Self-Help for Hard of Hearing People
7910 Woodmont Ave., Suite 1200
Bethesda, MD 20814
(301) 657-2248
www.shhh.org

Gastrointestinal Problems

American Anorexia/Bulimia Association, Inc.
members.aol.com/amanba/index.html

American Liver Foundation —Hepatitis hotline
1425 Pompton Ave.
Cedar Grove, NJ 07009
(800) 223-0179
www.liverfoundation.org

Crohn's and Colitis Foundation of America
386 Park Ave. South, 17th Floor
New York, NY 10016-8804
(800) 932-2423
www.ccfa.org

Healthy Weight
www.healthyweight.com

Immunologic Problems/Infection Control and Prevention

AIDS Treatment Data Network
www.aidsnyc.org

Allergy, Asthma, & Immunology Online
http://allergy.mcg.edu

American Academy of Allergy, Asthma, and Immunology
611 East Wells Street
Milwaukee, WI 53202
www.aaaai.org

Center for Disease Control and Prevention
1600 Clifton Rd. NE
Atlanta, GA 30333
(404) 639-3311
www.cdc.gov

HIV/AIDS Surveillance Report
Center for Disease Control and Prevention
1600 Clifton Rd. NE
Atlanta, GA 30333
(404) 639-3311
www.cdc.gov/nchstp/hiv_aids/stat

Immune Deficiency Foundation
3565 Ellicott Mills Drive, Unit B-2
Ellicott City, MD 20104
(800) 296-4433
www.primaryimmune.org

Latex Allergy Homepage
http://allergy.mcg.edu/physician/ltxhome.html

National AIDS Treatment Advocacy Project
580 Broadway, Suite 403
New York, NY 10012
(212) 219-0106
www.natap.org

The Safer Sex Page
www.safersex.org

Musculoskeletal Problems

Ankylosing Spondylitis Association
511 North La Cienega, Suite 216
Los Angeles, CA 90048
(800) 777-8189
www.spondylitis.org

Arthritis Foundation
1330 West Peachtree St.
Atlanta, GA 30309
(404) 872-7100
www.arthritis.org

Backpain Hotline
Texas Back Institute
3801 West 15th Street
Plano, TX 75075
(800) 247-2225
www.texasback.com

National Institute of Arthritis and Musculoskeletal and Skin Diseases
1 AMS Circle
Bethesda, MD 20892-3675
(301) 495-4484
www.nih.gov/niams

Osteoporosis and Related Bone Diseases—National Resource Center
1150 17th St, NW, Suite 500
Washington, DC 20036-4603
(800) 624-BONE

Neurologic Problems and Rehabilitation

American Paralysis Association
500 Morris Ave.
Springfield, NJ 07081
(800) 225-0292
www.apacure.com

Amyotrophic Lateral Sclerosis Association
21021 Ventura Blvd., Suite 321
Woodland Hills, CA 91364
(800) 782-4747
www.alsa.org

Epilepsy Foundation of America
4351 Garden City Drive, Suite 406
Landover, MD 20785
(800) 332-1000
www.efa.org

724

Epilepsy Ontario
1 Promanade Circle, Suite 338
Thornhill, Ontario
Canada L4J 4P8
(416) 229-2291
epilepsyontario.org

Huntington's Disease Society of America
140 West 22nd Street, Sixth Floor
New York, NY 10011-2420
(800) 345-4372
dsa.mgh.harvard.edu

Migraine Resource Center
www.migrainehelp.com

National Headache Foundation
5252 North Western Ave.
Chicago, IL 60625
(800) 843-2256
www.headaches.org

National Multiple Sclerosis Society
733 Third Avenue, Sixth Floor
New York, NY 10017
(800) 344-4867
www.nmss.org

National Stroke Organization
www.stroke.org

Parkinson's Disease Foundation
Columbia-Presbyterian Medical Center
650 West 168th Street
New York, NY 10032
(800) 457-6676
www.parkinsons-foundation.org

Reproductive Health Problems

All About Menopause
www.menopause.org

Atlanta Reproductive Health Center
www.ivf.com/endohtml.html

Bair PMS Home Page
www.bairpms.com

Center for Human Reproduction
www.centerforhumanreprod.com

Endometriosis Association
8585 North 76th Place
Milwaukee, WI 53223
(800) 992-3636
www.endometrios.org

Planned Parenthood Federation of America, Inc.
www.ppfa.org

The Safer Sex Page
www.safersex.org

Respiratory Problems

American Lung Association
1740 Broadway
New York, NY 10019-4374
(800) LUNG-USA
www.lungusa.org

Cystic Fibrosis Foundation
6931 Arlington Rd.
Bethesda, MD 20814
(800) 344-4823
www.cff.org

Urinary and Renal Problems

American Urogynecologic Society
www.augs.org

National Association for Continence
www.nafc.org

National Kidney Foundation
30 East 33rd Street
New York, NY 10016
(800) 622-9010
www.kidney.org

The Simon Foundation for Continence
www.simonfoundation.org

United Network for Organ Sharing
1100 Boulders Parkway, Suite 500
Richmond, VA 23225-8770
www.unos.org

Miscellaneous Resources

Agency for Health Care Policy and Research -AHCPR
www.ahcpr.gov

American Academy of Dermatology
930 N. Mecham Rd.
Schaumburg, IL 60173
(888) 462-3376
www.aad.org

American Academy of Pain Management
13947 Mono Way # A
Sonora, CA 95370
(209) 533-9744
www.aapainmanage.org

American Council on Alcoholism
5024 Campbell Blvd., Suite H
Baltimore, MD 21236
(800) 527-5344
www.aca-usa.org

American Hospital Association
www.aha.org

American Red Cross
430 17th Street
Washington, DC 20006
(202) 737-8300
www.crossnet.org

American Thyroid Association
Montefiore Medical Center
111 East 210th St.
Bronx, NY 10467
www.thyroid.org

Department of Health and Human Services (DHHS)
www.os.dhhs.org

Federal Drug Administration (FDA)
www.fda.gov

Lupus Foundation of America
Four Research Place, Suite 180
Rockville, MD 20850
(800) 558-0121
www.lupus.org/lupus

Medicare
www.medicare.gov

Medic Alert Foundation
Turlock, CA 95381
(800) 825-3785
www.medicalert.org

National Grave's Disease Foundation
www.ngdf.org

National Institutes of Health (NIH)
www.nih.gov

National Institute of Nursing Research (NINR)
www.nih.gov/ninr/

National Psoriasis Foundation
6600 SouthWest 92nd Ave., Suite 300
Portland, OR 97223
(800) 248-0886
www.psoriasis.org

World Health Organization
www.who.org

Women's Health Cosideration Resources

A Forum for Women's Health
www.womenshealth.org

All About Menopause
www.menopause.org

American Heart Association Women's Website
7272 Greenville Ave.
Dallas, TX 75231
(888) MY HEART
www.women.americanheart.org

Bair PMS Home Page
www.bairpms.com

Breast Cancer Information Clearing House
http://nysernet.org/bcic

Breast Care Helpline
(800) 462-9273

Endometriosis Association
8585 North 76th Place
Milwaukee, WI 53223
(800) 992-3636
www.endometrios.org

Healthy Weight
www.healthyweight.com

National Ovarian Cancer Coalition
www.ovarian.org

National Women's Health Hotline
www.womenshealth.com

Osteoporosis and Related Bone Diseases-National Resource Center
1150 17th St. NW, Suite 500
Washington, DC 20036-4603
(800) 624-BONE

Planned Parenthood Federation of America, Inc.
www.ppfa.org

The Safer Sex Page
www.safersex.org

The Simon Foundation for Continence
www.simonfoundation.org

Susan G. Komen Breast Cancer Foundation
www.komen.org
Women's Health Interactive
www.womens-health.com

Women to Woman America
www.wtwa.com

WWWomen!
www.wwwomen.com

SEARCH ENGINES AND ONLINE DIRECTORIES

Alta Vista
http://www.altavista.digital.com

Big Yellow
http://www.bigyellow.com

Excite
http://search.excite.com

Galaxy
http://galaxy.tradewave.com

Health A to Z
http://www.healthatoz.com

HotBot
http://www.search.hotbot.com

National Women's Health Research Center
http://www.healthywomen.org/links.html

WebCrawler
http://www.webcrawler.com

WWWomen!
http://www.wwwomen.com

Yahoo
http://www.yahoo.com

INDEX

Note: Page numbers in *italics* refer to illustrations.

Index

732

Index

Index

737

Index

C

Index

Index

Index

746

Index

Index

Index

Index

Index

Index

Index

Index

Index

765

Index

Index

Index

Index

Index

Index

Index

Index

Index

786

Index

Index